Revision Notes

for the
Final FRCR Part A

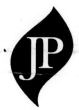

Revision Notes

for the
Final FRCR Part A

Kshitij Mankad MRCP FRCR

Neuroradiology Fellow
National Hospital for Neurology and Neurosurgery
London, UK

Edward TD Hoey MRCP FRCR

Consultant Cardiothoracic Radiologist
Heartlands Hospital
Birmingham, UK

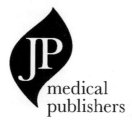

JP
medical
publishers

London • St Louis • Panama City • New Delhi

© 2010 JP Medical Ltd.
Published by JP Medical Ltd
83 Victoria Street, London, SW1H 0HW, UK
Tel: +44 (0)20 3170 8910
Fax: +44 (0)20 3008 6180
Email: info@jpmedpub.com
Web: www.jpmedpub.com

The rights of Kshitij Mankad and Edward Hoey to be identified as authors of this work have been asserted by them in accordance with the Copyright, Designs and Patents Act 1988.

All brand names and product names used in this book are trade names, service marks, trademarks or registered trademarks of their respective owners. The publisher is not associated with any product or vendor mentioned in this book.

Medical knowledge and practice change constantly. This book is designed to provide accurate, authoritative information about the subject matter in question. However readers are advised to check the most current information available on procedures included and check information from the manufacturer of each product to be administered, to verify the recommended dose, formula, method and duration of administration, adverse effects and contraindications. It is the responsibility of the practitioner to take all appropriate safety precautions. Neither the publisher nor the authors assume any liability for any injury and/or damage to persons or property arising from or related to use of material in this book.

This book is sold on the understanding that the publisher is not engaged in providing professional medical services. If such advice or services are required, the services of a competent medical professional should be sought.

ISBN: 978-1-907816-00-0

British Library Cataloguing in Publication Data
A catalogue record for this book is available from the British Library

Library of Congress Cataloging in Publication Data
A catalog record for this book is available from the Library of Congress

JP Medical Ltd is a subsidiary of Jaypee Brothers Medical Publishers (P) Ltd, New Delhi, India with offices in Ahmedabad, Bengaluru, Chennai, Hyderabad, Kochi, Kolkata, Lucknow, Mumbai and Nagpur. Visit www.jaypeebrothers.com for more details.

Publisher:	Richard Furn
Development Editor:	Alison Whitehouse
Design:	Pete Wilder, Designers Collective Ltd
Copy Editor:	Robert Whittle

Typeset, printed and bound in India.

Preface

The Final FRCR Part A examination is daunting to prepare for as it requires an in-depth knowledge of anatomy, disease, differential diagnoses and applied radiology practice.

This book has been compiled to ease the revision process by presenting the requisite core knowledge for each of the six system-based modules, namely cardiothoracic and vascular, musculoskeletal and trauma, gastrointestinal and hepatobiliary, genitourinary, gynaecology and breast, paediatrics, and central nervous system and head and neck. Each chapter has been authored by recent exam candidates and in turn edited by radiology consultants with subspecialty expertise in that field, to ensure focused and succinct coverage of high-yield exam topics.

Only the essential facts are presented, selected entirely on the basis of the scope of remembered past questions. This should speed up the revision process by reducing time spent searching through large textbooks and journals. Being revision notes, the content is designed to make the knowledge-finding process easy for the stressed candidate. Each topic is presented in a concise manner and exhaustive lists of differential diagnoses have been restricted to those that most often get tested. For ease of reading, the main reference sources have been listed in a general bibliography at the very end of the book rather than cited in the text.

Although primarily aimed at radiology trainees, this book will also be useful to physicians, surgeons, medical students and anyone with an interest in radiology.

Kshitij Mankad
Edward Hoey

Contents

Contributing Authors

Jooly Joseph
Specialty Registrar in Radiology
Leeds Teaching Hospitals NHS Trust
Leeds, UK

Amit Lakkaraju
Specialty Registrar in Radiology
Leeds Teaching Hospitals NHS Trust
Leeds, UK

Sapna Puppala
Consultant Cardiovascular and
Interventional Radiologist
Leeds Teaching Hospitals NHS Trust
Leeds, UK

Nasim Tahir
Specialty Registrar in Radiology
Leeds Teaching Hospitals NHS Trust
Leeds, UK

Prasanna Tirukonda
Specialty Registrar in Radiology
Leeds Teaching Hospitals NHS Trust
Leeds, UK

Reviewers

David Gilmour
Specialty Registrar in Ophthalmology
Leeds Teaching Hospitals NHS Trust
Leeds, UK

Sanjoy Nagaraja
Consultant Interventional Neuroradiologist
University Hospitals Coventry and
Warwickshire NHS Trust
Coventry, UK

Naveen Parasu
Assistant Professor, McMaster University
Staff Musculoskeletal Radiologist
Henderson General Hospital, Hamilton
Health Sciences
Hamilton, Ontario
Canada

Sapna Puppala
Consultant Cardiovascular and
Interventional Radiologist
Leeds Teaching Hospitals NHS Trust
Leeds, UK

Nabil el Saiety
Consultant Gastrointestinal Radiologist
University Hospital of North Staffordshire
Stoke on Trent, UK

Hemant Sonwalkar
Consultant Interventional Radiologist
Calderdale and Huddersfield Foundation
NHS Trust
Halifax, UK

Ashok Raghavan
Consultant Paediatric Radiologist
Sheffield Children's Hospital
Sheffield, UK

Chapter 1

Cardiothoracic and vascular system

- Leading cause of cancer deaths in the western world
- 60% occur in men, 40% in women (incidence increasing)
- Risk factors are smoking and exposure to asbestos, radon and nickel

WHO classification
Small cell (20% of cases)   Non-small cell: • Squamous cell (35% of cases)   • Adenocarcinoma (30% of cases)   • Large cell (10% of cases)   • Others, e.g. carcinoid (5% of cases)

Small cell lung cancer

- Arises from Kulchitsky's cells of the amine precursor uptake decarboxylase (APUD) line
- The majority arise proximally in the bronchial submucosa
- Highly malignant tumour with 30-day doubling time
- 5–10% associated with paraneoplastic syndromes
  - Syndrome of inappropriate antidiuretic hormone secretion (low sodium)
  - Cushing's syndrome (increased adrenocorticotropic hormone (ACTH) secretion)
  - Eaton–Lambert syndrome (myasthenia-like syndrome)
  - Subacute cerebellar degeneration
  - Limbic encephalopathy

Staging of small cell lung cancer

- 2009 TNM staging system stages small cell lung cancer as part of the same classification system as non-small cell carcinoma and replaces the older description system of limited and extensive stage disease

- Small cell cancer occurs almost exclusively in smokers. It is associated with rapid doubling time, early development of metastatic disease and initial sensitivity to chemotherapy and radiation
- Despite initial response to treatment, long-term survival is much worse than that of patients with non-small cell carcinoma

Non-small cell carcinoma

Squamous cell carcinoma

- Commonest histological subtype in the UK
- Slow growing tumour with a 90-day doubling time
- Strongest link with smoking
- Two thirds arise centrally, one third peripherally
- Commonest cause of a Pancoast's tumour
- May secrete parathyroid hormone-related peptide (PTHrP), causing hypercalcaemia
- Strong association with hypertrophic pulmonary osteoarthropathy (HPOA)
- Central necrosis is common, and 30% cavitate

HPOA
• Symmetrical laminated periostitis of extremities   • Finger clubbing and painful oedematous skin   • Other thoracic causes include bronchiectasis, mesothelioma, pleural fibroma, cardiac myxoma and bacterial endocarditis   • Squamous cell carcinoma is commonest cause   • Regresses following tumour resection

Adenocarcinoma

- Arises from bronchiolar epithelial glands
- Typically a peripheral nodule with spiculated margins
- More common in females

- Predominant lung cancer type in non-smokers
- Occasionally arises in scarred or fibrotic lung

Bronchoalveolar cell carcinoma

- 2–5% of all lung cancers
- Subtype of adenocarcinoma derived from type 2 pneumocytes and bronchiolar epithelium
- High prevalence within scarred or fibrotic lung
- Mucin-secreting tumour, which may present with bronchorrhoea
- Malignant cells may be carried to the contralateral lung
- Extrathoracic spread is unusual
- F-18-DG uptake is often low grade (i.e. false negative)

Imaging features

- Four recognised patterns of disease
  - Solitary pulmonary nodule (commonest pattern)
  - Unifocal area of consolidation mimicking pneumonia
  - Multifocal areas of consolidation with a ground-glass appearance
  - Multiple nodules, which may cavitate ('cheerio' sign)

Large cell carcinoma

- Large (majority > 7 cm), highly malignant, bulky necrotic tumour
- Locally invasive with early hilar and mediastinal adenopathy
- Often widely disseminated with metastases at presentation

Staging of non-small cell lung cancer

- Revised TNM staging system published in 2009
- Clinical staging uses information from non-invasive techniques such as CT and minimally invasive procedures such as endoscopic ultrasound, bronchoscopy and mediastinoscopy
- Pathological staging uses findings from surgically excised tissue and is the reference standard technique.

T staging

- T1: tumour diameter ≤ 2 cm (T1a) or 2–3 cm (T1b) and completely surrounded by lung
- T2: tumour 3–5 cm (T2a) or 5–7 cm (T2b) or invading either left or right main bronchus > 2 cm distal to carina or invading the visceral pleura
- T3: tumour > 7 cm or tumour invading either the main bronchus within 2 cm of the carina or invading non-vital structures such as chest wall, mediastinal pleura, pericardium or diaphragm
  - CT is unreliable for subtle chest wall invasion (65% accurate)
  - MRI and ultrasound are useful in equivocal cases
  - Localised chest wall pain is a good clinical indicator of invasion
  - Chest wall invasion can be treated with en-bloc resection
- T4: tumour invading a vertebral body or vital mediastinal structures such as the heart, trachea, great vessels or oesophagus or a malignant pleural effusion or satellite tumour nodules in the same lung as the primary tumour
  - CT is unreliable for subtle mediastinal invasion (65% accuracy)
  - Suggestive CT findings include tumour or mediastinal contact > 3 cm and tumour or vessel contact > 90% of circumference
  - Cytology analysis of aspirate from a malignant pleural effusion gives false-negative results in around one third of cases

N staging

- N1: ipsilateral positive hilar nodes
- N2: ipsilateral positive mediastinal nodes or subcarinal nodes
  - Boundary between N1 and N2 nodes is the superior pulmonary vein
  - Equivocal N2 nodes require PET scanning, endobronchial ultrasound sampling or mediastinoscopy sampling
  - Bulky N2 nodes may be treated with neoadjuvant therapy prior to surgery

- N3: contralateral positive mediastinal or hilar nodes or supraclavicular or neck nodes

M staging

- M0: no distant metastases
- M1a: contralateral lung metastases, pleural or pericardial dissemination
- M1b: distant metastases

Pancoast's tumour

- Tumour of the superior pulmonary sulcus
- Most commonly a squamous cell carcinoma
- Tumour invades lower brachial plexus and sympathetic chain
- Treatment is surgical resection if possible and radiotherapy

Clinical triad

- Ipsilateral Horner's syndrome
- Ipsilateral medial arm pain
- Wasting of small muscles of the hand

- MRI is superior to CT for staging Pancoast's tumours
- Sagittal post-contrast T1-weighted imaging (T1WI) is sequence of choice for assessing invasion into brachial plexus and subclavian vessels
- Pancoast's tumours are almost always associated with chest wall invasion
- Ipsilateral supraclavicular nodes, nerve root invasion and rib destruction are all potentially resectable
- Mediastinal nodes (N2) are considered non-resectable

CT-guided lung biopsy

- Ideally forced expiratory volume in 1 second (FEV_1) should be > 1.5 L
- Performed using a co-axial technique which minimizes the number of passes through the pleural
- Pneumothorax occurs in up to 40% of cases. Risk is highest with small central

lesions and lesions contiguous with the pleural surface
- Reported diagnostic accuracy in the region of 80–90% with an experienced operator
- Core biopsy is more accurate than fine-needle aspiration

PET–CT in non-small cell lung cancer

- PET–CT using F-18-DG is routinely performed in all patients considered operable candidates on CT criteria alone
- Limited role in T staging (though it can help to delineate tumour from collapse)
- More accurate than CT for N staging because size criteria (short axis node diameter > 1 cm) is unreliable
- CT has a sensitivity of approximately 70% for enlarged mediastinal nodes
- PET–CT has a sensitivity of approximately 90% for enlarged mediastinal nodes
- PET–CT shows metastases in approximately 20% of cases with a negative CT
- PET–CT is more accurate than CT and bone scintigraphy for extrathoracic disease including bone, adrenals, nodes and liver

Structures with normal PET uptake

- Myocardium
- Brown fat
- Thymus
- Strap muscles
- Extra-ocular muscles
- Vocal cords (if talking during the acquisition)

Lung metastases

- Most metastases occur via haematogenous spread, with tumour lodging peripherally in the pulmonary capillaries
- Majority are multiple
- Commonest primary sites are the breast, colon, kidneys and head and neck

Cavitating metastases

> **Causes of cavitating metastases**
>
> - Squamous cell carcinoma (commonest)
> - Cervical carcinoma
> - Colorectal carcinoma
> - Melanoma
> - Transitional cell carcinoma
> - Sarcomas
> - Any tumour after chemotherapy

Miliary metastases

- Rare
- Innumerable pulmonary nodules < 5 mm in diameter
- Indistinguishable from miliary tuberculosis
- Commonest primary tumours are the renal tumours, thyroid carcinoma, melanoma, choriocarcinoma and bone sarcoma

Calcified metastases

- Very rare except in osteosarcoma and chondrosarcoma
- Osteosarcoma metastases are associated with pneumothorax

> **Other recognised primary sites**
>
> - Breast
> - Thyroid
> - Colon and rectum
> - Ovary
> - Any tumour following chemotherapy

Endobronchial metastases

- Very rare
- Seeding of tumour cells in the bronchial submucosa
- Cause airways obstruction and distal collapse
- Commonest primary tumours are bronchial carcinoma, carcinoma of the breast, lymphoma and colorectal carcinoma

Lymphangitis carcinomatosis

- Permeation of pulmonary lymphatics by tumour cells
- Commonest primary tumours are bronchial, breast and stomach cancers
- Typically unilateral if from the bronchus and bilateral if from other sites

Imaging features

CXR
- Often normal
- May see reticulonodular shadowing and septal (Kerley B) lines
- Main differential diagnoses are pulmonary oedema and sarcoidosis

High-resolution CT (HRCT)
- Most sensitive imaging test
- Nodular interlobular septal thickening ('beaded septum' sign)
- Nodular bronchovascular bundle thickening

Lymphoma

Hodgkin's lymphoma

- Bimodal age peaks: 20–30 years and 70–80 years
- Presence of Reed–Sternberg cells (a type of T cell) is the diagnostic hallmark
- Nodular sclerosing subtype is the commonest histology
- Spreads contiguously along the lymphatic chain
- Commonly presents as non-tender cervical lymphadenopathy
- One third of patients present with fever (prolonged), weight loss and night sweats
- Alcohol-induced nodal pain is recognised
- > 80% have mediastinal adenopathy at presentation
- Lung parenchymal involvement is seen in 15% of cases; it is rare without adenopathy
- Thymic infiltration is seen in 30–50% of newly diagnosed Hodgkin's lymphoma

Non-Hodgkin's lymphoma

- Four times commoner than Hodgkin's lymphoma
- 90% are of B cell origin
- Diverse group subdivided into low, intermediate and high grade

- Some types are associated with infectious agents, e.g. *Helicobacter pylori* and gastric mucosa-associated lymphoid tissue (MALT)
- Increased risk in immunocompromised patients, e.g. post-transplant in a lymphoproliferative disorder
- Most present with lymphadenopathy and systemic symptoms
- One third present with extranodal involvement, e.g. in the gastrointestinal tract
- Potential for cure varies with histological subtype and stage
- 40% have intrathoracic disease
- Lung parenchymal involvement is seen in 5%, often without adenopathy

> **Parenchymal disease in Hodgkin's and non-Hodgkin's lymphoma**
>
> Wide range of imaging appearances
> - Multifocal non-segmental consolidation
> - Reticulonodular infiltrates
> - Multiple discrete pulmonary masses
> - Pleural effusions

Lymphoma staging: Ann Arbor

- Stage I: single lymph node region involvement only
- Stage II: two or more lymph node regions on same side of diaphragm
- Stage III: lymph node regions (including spleen) on both sides of diaphragm
- Stage IV: extranodal involvement, e.g. bone marrow, liver, lung
- E: extranodal disease
- A: absence of constitutional symptoms
- B: presence of constitutional symptoms
- X: bulky mass > 10 cm or mediastinal widening more than one third of CXR

Role of PET–CT in lymphoma

Diagnosis and staging
- > 90% sensitivity for detecting most types of lymphoma
- Less reliable with MALT and lymphocytic non-Hodgkin's lymphoma

- False positives from brown fat and from inflammatory and infective conditions

Assessing initial response to therapy
- Usually carried out after two or three cycles of chemotherapy
- A negative scan is a reliable indicator of treatment response

Post-therapy response
- Performed after completion of chemotherapy course
- Unlike CT, PET–CT can distinguish a fibrotic nodal mass from residual active disease
- A negative scan is associated with a low risk of recurrence
- A positive scan carries a high risk of recurrence
- False-positive scans are seen with thymic 'rebound' hyperplasia
- False-negatives scans are seen with granulocyte stimulating factor, which can cause intense marrow uptake, masking any residual disease

Long-term follow-up
- Higher sensitivity than CT and MRI in assessing recurrent disease

Leukaemia
- Infiltration is common but is rarely detected radiologically
- Leukostasis can obstruct the pulmonary vasculature in patients with high peripheral blast counts; this is seen as pulmonary oedema
- More typically, lung pathology is related to neutropenic infection

Castleman's disease
- Rare group of post-viral lymphoproliferative disorders
- Massive lymph node hyperplasia
- Large soft tissue mass, most often in the mediastinum
- Highly vascular, with intense contrast enhancement
- Rarely contains areas of calcification
- 10% have disseminated disease with skin lesions, splenomegaly and lymphocytic interstitial pneumonitis

1.2 Solitary pulmonary nodule and congenital lung disease

Solitary pulmonary nodule

- A discrete pulmonary mass < 3 cm in diameter
- Common incidental CXR finding
- Approximately 30% are malignant
- Common causes
  - Granuloma, e.g. tuberculosis, sarcoidosis (50%)
  - Bronchogenic carcinoma (30%)
  - Hamartoma (10%)
- Other causes (10%)
  - Metastases
  - Bronchocele
  - Round pneumonia
  - Round atelectasis
  - Fluid-filled abscess
  - Carcinoid tumour
  - Arteriovenous malformation
  - Progressive massive fibrosis
  - Developmental, e.g. sequestration, bronchogenic cyst

Morphological assessment

- 80% of nodules < 2 cm in diameter are benign
- Irregular, 'spiculated' margin suggests malignancy
- 80% of malignant nodules have well-defined margins
- Four recognised patterns of benign calcification: central nidus, diffuse solid, laminated and 'popcorn'
- Amorphous calcifications seen in 6% of lung cancers
- Intranodular fat (–40 to –120 HU) suggests a hamartoma
- Benign cavitation typically has a smooth, thin wall
- Malignant cavitation typically has a thick, irregular wall

Clinical assessment

- Only 1% of solitary pulmonary nodules in patients aged < 35 years are malignant
- Smoking history greatly increases risk of malignancy
- If there is a history of smoking-related cancer, then a solitary pulmonary nodule is more likely a lung primary
- If there is a history of melanoma or sarcoma, then a solitary pulmonary nodule is more likely a metastasis

Growth rate assessment

- Malignant lesions double in size between 30 days and 18 months
- Absence of growth over 2 years is reliable sign of a benign lesion
- Serial volume measurements are more accurate than diameter measurements

> **Three reliable signs of a benign lesion**
>
> - Fat density
> - Benign calcification pattern
> - No interval growth over 2 years

Imaging features

PET

- 85% of metabolically active solitary pulmonary nodules are malignant
- Standardised uptake value (SUV) > 3 is used as a reference
- High negative predictive value for lesions > 1 cm in diameter
- False positives
  - Tuberculosis
  - Histoplasmosis
  - Sarcoidosis

- Progressive massive fibrosis
- Rheumatoid nodules
- Intercurrent infection
- False negatives
  - Lesions < 1 cm in diameter
  - Carcinoid tumour
  - Bronchoalveolar cell carcinoma

Carcinoid tumour

- Neuroendocrine neoplasms of the lung (accounting for 1–2% of all lung cancers)
- Arise from Kulchitsky cells of the bronchial mucosa
- Highly vascular tumours supplied by bronchial arteries
- 90% are 'typical' and of low-grade malignancy
- 10% are 'atypical', with nodal and sclerotic bone metastases
- 80% arise centrally, 20% are seen as a peripheral solitary nodule
- Present clinically with haemoptysis (in 50% of cases) or recurrent pneumonia
- Can cause carcinoid syndrome (in 2–5% of cases) or Cushing's syndrome (in 2%)
- Can cause carcinoid syndrome in the absence of liver metastases

Imaging features

CXR or CT
- Well-defined perihilar mass with endobronchial component or well-circumscribed parenchymal nodule
- Atypical tumours may show mediastinal invasion
- 30% contain calcifications

F-18-DG PET
- Absent or low-grade uptake

MIBG or indium-111 octreotide scan
- More sensitive (60–90% sensitivity)

Hamartoma

- Commonest benign pulmonary neoplasm
- Composed of cartilage, epithelium and fat
- Peak incidence in fifth and sixth decades
- Associated with Carney's triad: gastrointestinal stroma tumour (GIST), paraganglioma, hamartoma
- Most exhibit slight growth if followed up over many years

Imaging features

CXR
- Well-circumscribed, lobulated pulmonary nodule
- 80% are located peripherally

CT
- 50% contain fat (–40 to –120 HU), which is diagnostic
- 30% contain 'popcorn' calcification, which is diagnostic

Arteriovenous malformation

- Capillary-free connection between pulmonary arterial and pulmonary venous systems
- 70% are associated with Osler–Weber–Rendu syndrome
- 30% of patients with Osler–Weber–Rendu syndrome have a pulmonary arteriovenous malformation
- Typically presents in middle age with exertional dyspnoea and haemoptysis
- A recognised cause of finger clubbing
- Extracardiac right-to-left shunt with risk of paradoxical embolism
- Risk of transient ischaemic attack is 40%, stroke 20% and brain abscess 10%
- Transarterial coil embolisation is treatment of choice if feeding artery measures > 3 mm in diameter
- Post-embolisation syndrome can occur (pleuritic pain, atelectasis and fever)

Imaging features

CXR
- Small lesions, often not visible
- Hypervascularity may be the only sign
- Well-defined lobulated oval mass (multiple lesions in one third of cases)
- Band shadow connecting mass to hilum
- Medial third of lower lobe is commonest location
- Decrease in size with Valsalva manoeuvre and erect posture

CT
- Enhancement of feeding artery and draining vein
- Rarely contains calcifications (pheboliths)

Congenital lung disease

Pulmonary agenesis, aplasia and hypoplasia

Pulmonary agenesis

- Complete absence of one or both lungs
- No trace of bronchial or vascular supply or parenchymal tissue
- Simulates a pneumonectomy on CXR, with a small ipsilateral hemithorax, an elevated hemidiaphragm and displacement of the mediastinum towards affected side
- CT confirms absence of ipsilateral pulmonary artery and bronchus

Pulmonary aplasia

- Absence of pulmonary vasculature and parenchyma
- There remains a rudimentary bronchus
- Similar CXR appearance to agenesis
- CT distinguishes from agenesis by showing rudimentary bronchus

Pulmonary hypoplasia

- An underdeveloped lung or lobe
- Most commonly secondary to a space-occupying lesion (e.g. diaphragmatic hernia) that stunts the growth of the lung *in utero*
- Affected lung is small with ipsilateral displacement of mediastinum

Scimitar syndrome

- Encompasses a variety of congenital abnormalities of the thorax which occur in combination
- Major components of scimitar syndrome
  - Hypoplastic lung and pulmonary artery
  - Partial systemic arterial supply (aorta or a branch)
  - Partial anomalous pulmonary venous drainage
- Draining vein most often empties into infra-diaphragmatic inferior vena cava (IVC)
- Hepatic veins, portal vein and right atrial drainage are described
- Associated with a spectrum of pulmonary anomalies, including tracheal stenosis, bilobed right lung and diaphragmatic hernia

- Almost exclusively involves the right lung
- Adult form is most often an incidental CXR finding
- Re-implantation of anomalous vein into the left atrium is only considered if left-to-right shunt fraction > 50%
- Horseshoe lung is a rare variant in which an isthmus of lung parenchyma extends from the right lung base across the midline behind the pericardium and fuses with the left lung base

Imaging features

CXR
- Small right hemithorax
- Rightward shift of heart and mediastinum
- Curvilinear tubular opacity coursing inferiorly from the right hilum towards the diaphragm (looks like a Turkish sword or scimitar)

Cystic adenomatoid malformation

- Malformation of terminal respiratory structures affecting part or whole of one lobe, sometimes two lobes, or even an entire lung
- Communicates with the tracheobronchial tree
- Supplied by a direct branch of the pulmonary artery and drains into pulmonary veins
- Usually diagnosed in neonates and infants
- Can rarely present in adulthood with recurrent chest infections or haemoptysis or (very rarely) malignant transformation (sarcomas and bronchoalveolar cell carcinoma have been reported)

Imaging features

CXR
- Multicystic parenchymal mass with air–fluid levels

Pulmonary sequestration

- Mass of non-functioning lung tissue not in normal continuity with the tracheobronchial tree and receiving a systemic arterial supply

- Almost always in lower lobes and more common in the left lung
- Divided into extralobular and intralobar types, depending on the pleural investment and pattern of venous drainage:

Extralobar sequestrations

- Discrete accessory lobe of non-aerated lung tissue invested in its own pleural envelope
- Majority are located immediately above or below left hemidiaphragm and have systemic venous drainage via the IVC or the azygous venous system
- Commonly associated with other congenital anomalies
- Presents in early childhood with shunt-induced respiratory distress

Intralobar sequestrations

- Commoner than the extralobar type
- Segment of non-functioning lung tissue, which is enclosed by the visceral pleura of an otherwise normal lung
- Systemic arterial supply is usually via a single large artery arising from the lower thoracic or upper abdominal aorta, though arterial supply from other arteries, including the coronary arteries, has been described
- Venous drainage is via the pulmonary veins into the left atrium
- Rarely associated with other congenital anomalies
- Usually presents in adulthood with recurrent pneumonias in a persistent location, caused by of insufficient drainage
- Haemoptysis is common as a consequence of high pressure within the feeding artery

Imaging features

CXR
- Lower lobe soft tissue mass
- Air–fluid levels (especially if infected)

CT angiogram
- Enhancement of mass
- Demonstration of anomalous feeding artery

Cystic fibrosis

- Autosomal-recessive pattern of inheritance
- Abnormally viscous secretions (elevated sweat test chloride level)
- Recurrent respiratory tract infections and bronchiectasis
- Bronchial wall thickening and mucus plugging
- Bullous lung disease (in 20–30% of cases); upper zone is predominantly affected
- Hyperinflation (in 80–90% of cases); lower zone is predominantly affected
- Liver disease is the second leading cause of death in CF
- Viscous secretions cause biliary stasis and periductal fibrosis
- A small percentage progress to multinodular stage cirrhosis

Imaging features

HRCT
- Air trapping ('mosaic attenuation')
- Tree-in-bud appearance (mucoid secretions or atypical mycobacterial infection)
- Bronchiectasis

Anatomy

Trachea

- Cartilaginous tube lined by ciliated columnar epithelium
- Extends from lower border of the cricoid cartilage (C6 level) to the carina (T5 level)
- Passes downwards and slightly posteriorly, often deviating to right
- Approximately 11 cm long and supported by around 20 incomplete cartilaginous rings
- Trachealis muscle bridges the gap between these rings
- Oval in cross-section with a flattened posterior margin
- Normal diameter < 23 mm in males and < 20 mm in females, measured at the level of aortic arch; diameter decreases with expiration
- Diameter normally increases with age
- Crossed by the left brachiocephalic vein, aortic arch, left common carotid artery and innominate artery
- The right vagus nerve descends on its right lateral aspect
- The left recurrent laryngeal nerve ascends on its posterolateral aspect
- Right-sided deviation on expiratory films is normal in children
- Deviation to the left may be seen with a right-sided aortic arch
- Normal carinal angle is approximately 65° (20° to the right and 45° to the left of the midline)

> ### Right paratracheal stripe
>
> - Separates the trachea from the right lung
> - Composed of paratracheal fat, lymph nodes, and visceral and parietal pleura
> - Normally < 3 mm thick (thicker in obese people)

Right main bronchus

- Shorter (around 2 cm long), wider and more vertical than the left main bronchus
- Azygous vein arches over it from behind to reach the superior vena cava (SVC)
- The right pulmonary artery lies anteriorly
- The first branch of the right main bronchus is to the upper lobe: the eparterial bronchus
- The right main bronchus continues as the bronchus intermedius (the interlobar artery is lateral)
- The bronchus intermedius divides into middle and lower lobe bronchi
- The middle lobe bronchus arises opposite the lower lobe apical segmental bronchus
- Usually terminates as four basal segmental bronchi

Left main bronchus

- Passes beneath the aortic arch
- The left pulmonary artery arches over it to lie posteriorly
- The first branch of the left main bronchus supplies both the upper lobe and the lingula
- The left main bronchus continues as the lower lobe bronchus, from which arises the lower lobe apical segmental bronchus
- Usually terminates as three basal segmental bronchi

Non-neoplastic tracheal disease

Tracheal bronchus

- Anatomical variant whereby an anomalous airway arises from the lateral wall of the trachea
- Majority are right-sided and arise within 2 cm of the carina
- Prevalence of 0.1–2% (more common in Down's syndrome)
- Displaced bronchus most often supplies the right apical segment; it less commonly supplies all three upper lobe segments
- Most often an incidental finding; may cause persisting lobar atelectasis in an intubated patient despite an adequately positioned endotracheal tube on CXR

Tracheobronchomegaly

- Atrophy of elastic and smooth muscle fibres of the trachea and main bronchi, which become markedly dilated
- Abrupt change to normal calibre at fourth or fifth bronchial divisions
- Associated with Ehlers–Danlos syndrome, Marfan's syndrome, cutis laxa and ankylosing spondylitis
- Can be acquired secondary to prolonged mechanical ventilation and inhalation of chemical irritants
- Most cases present in adult life with chronic cough, excessive sputum production, recurrent infections and expiratory stridor
- Y-shaped tracheal stents are used to maintain airway patency

Imaging features

CT
- Trachea and mainstem bronchial diameters > 3 standard deviations from mean
- Tracheal diameter > 3 cm, right main bronchus > 24 mm diameter, left main bronchus > 2 mm diameter
- Tracheobronchial diverticulosis and cystic bronchiectasis
- Collapse of central airways on expiration

Tracheobronchial stenosis

Causes

- Post-intubation or post-tracheostomy (commonest cause)
- Post-lung transplantation
- Tracheobronchial papillomatosis
- Tracheopathia osteoplastica
- Tuberculosis, sarcoidosis or amyloidosis
- Relapsing polychondritis or Wegener's granulomatosis
- Inflammatory bowel disease
- Post-traumatic, malignancy or idiopathic

Tracheobronchial papillomatosis

- Infection of tracheobronchial tree by human papilloma virus
- Occasionally caused by aerial dissemination of laryngeal disease (5–10%)

- Pulmonary spread is even more unusual (< 2%)
- Presents with hoarseness, inspiratory stridor, wheezing, recurrent pneumonia
- High-resolution CT shows diffuse airways nodularity
- Poor prognosis secondary to airways compromise
- Small risk of transformation into squamous cell carcinoma
- Pulmonary lesions are seen as multiple cavitating nodules

Relapsing polychondritis

- Idiopathic episodic inflammation of cartilaginous structures
- Predominantly affects the pinna, nose and upper airways
- Probably an autoimmune reaction against type III collagen
- Respiratory involvement occurs in 50% of cases
  - Associated with a poor prognosis
  - Can be life-threatening requiring tracheostomy
  - Causes tracheal thickening that spares the posterior wall and focal or diffuse stenosis of the trachea or bronchi
- Non-erosive polyarthropathy is common
- Associations include aortic aneurysm, aortic regurgitation and aortic dissection
- Nasal chondritis with saddle nose deformity if long-standing

Neoplastic tracheal disease

- Tracheal tumours account for 1% of all thoracic malignancies
- 90% of adult tracheal tumours are malignant
- Squamous carcinoma is the commonest histological type

Squamous cell carcinoma

- Majority located in distal trachea within 3 cm of the carina
- Presents with dyspnoea, cough and hoarseness
- Poor prognosis: 50% have mediastinal invasion at time of diagnosis
- Strong association with smoking

Adenoid cystic carcinoma (cylindroma)

- Slow growing malignant tumour, commonest in proximal trachea
- Tendency for submucosal extension and late recurrence
- Peak age is the fifth decade
- Equally common in males and females
- Better prognosis than squamous cell carcinoma
- Smoking is not a risk factor

Imaging features

CT
- Four recognised patterns:
  - Intraluminal soft tissue mass with extension through the tracheal wall
  - Diffuse or circumferential thickening of the tracheal wall
  - Soft tissue mass filling the trachea
  - Homogeneous mass encircling the trachea

Chronic obstructive pulmonary disease

- Includes asthma, chronic bronchitis and emphysema

Asthma

- Chronic inflammatory disorder of the airways caused by hyper-reactivity to a variety of stimuli
- Smooth muscle and mucus gland hypertrophy
- Airways obstruction, which reverses with bronchodilator agents
- Complications include pneumothorax, pneumomediastinum and allergic bronchopulmonary aspergillosis

Imaging features

CXR
- Bronchial wall thickening in up to 50% of patients

CT
- Bronchial wall thickening
- Air trapping (more pronounced on expiratory phase images)

Churg–Strauss syndrome

- Adult-onset asthma
- Peripheral blood eosinophilia
- Systemic vasculitis

Chronic bronchitis

- Chronic airways irritation from smoking causes mucous gland hypertrophy and hyper-secretion, and secondary infections maintain and promote the airways injury
- A clinical diagnosis: persistent cough with sputum production for at least 3 months in at least 2 consecutive years

Imaging features

CXR
- Thick-walled, mildly dilated bronchi
- Accentuation of peripheral vascular markings ('dirty chest')
- Areas of hyperinflation from small airways obstruction

Emphysema

- Permanent enlargement of air spaces distal to the terminal bronchioles, with destruction of alveolar walls and the elastic fibre network
- Imbalance of elastase–anti-elastase activity within the lung
- Tobacco smoke causes a neutrophil influx, with release of elastase and consequent proteolytic destruction of lung parenchyma. Anti-elastase enzymes act to limit the degree of destruction

Imaging features

CXR
- Hyperinflation: flat diaphragms, retrosternal air space > 2.5 cm
- Bullae: avascular radiolucent areas with thin curvilinear walls
- Pulmonary hypertension: enlarged central arteries and pruning

Scintigram
- Delayed wash-in and delayed wash-out of ventilation component

HRCT

Three main patterns: centrilobular (the commonest), panlobular and paraseptal

- Centrilobular pattern (commonest)
  - Low-attenuation areas located centrally, within the second pulmonary lobule
  - Spares the distal alveoli until late-stage disease
  - Upper lobe predominance
- Panlobular pattern
  - Low-attenuation areas throughout the entire second pulmonary lobule
  - Strong association with alpha 1-antitrypsin deficiency
  - Lower lobe predominance
- Paraseptal pattern
  - Low-attenuation areas in the subpleural regions
  - Strong association with spontaneous pneumothorax

Alpha-1 anti-trypsin deficiency

- Autosomal-recessive inheritance
- Most severe form is with the homozygous PiZZ genotype
- Deficiency of elastase inhibitor with progressive panlobular emphysema
- Disease process is accelerated by smoking
- Patients typically present in their 40s
- Can also cause childhood hepatitis and cirrhosis

Operative management of emphysema

- Bullectomy
- Excision of a large bulla or bullae to enable re-expansion of compressed adjacent lung
- Lung volume reduction surgery
- Removal of severely emphysematous portions of lung
- Outcome better with heterogeneous disease and upper lobe predominance
- Lung transplantation is reserved for end-stage disease

Bronchiectasis

- Irreversible dilatation of one or more bronchi
- Presents with purulent sputum production, recurrent chest infections and haemoptysis

Causes

- Acute or chronic necrotizing infection (commonest cause), e.g. tuberculosis, *Mycobacterium avium-intracellulare* complex
- Congenital: cystic fibrosis, dyskinetic cilia syndrome, Mounier–Kuhn syndrome, hypogammaglobulinaemia
- Allergic bronchopulmonary aspergillosis
- Pulmonary fibrosis 'traction bronchiectasis'
- Bronchiolitis obliterans
- Yellow nail syndrome
- Foreign body
- Idiopathic (in 40% of cases)

Dyskinetic cilia syndrome (Kartagener's syndrome)

- Structural abnormality of cilia and spermatozoa
- Recurrent sinus, ear and chest infections
- Male infertility
- Triad: dextrocardia or situs inversus, sinusitis and bronchiectasis

Imaging features

CXR

- Dilated, thick-walled bronchi as seen end-on ('ring shadows')
- Dilated thick walled bronchi as seen in profile ('tram lines')

HRCT

- Bronchial dilatation, with the internal diameter greater than the diameter of the adjacent artery
- Lack of peripheral bronchial tapering (seen within 1 cm of the pleura)

> **Morphological patterns of bronchiectasis**
>
> - Cylindrical: uniform bronchial dilatation
> - Varicose: beaded appearance ('string of pearls')
> - Cystic: central, clustered saccular dilatations

> **Swyer–James syndrome**
>
> - Severe respiratory infection in childhood, in which damage of respiratory bronchioles causes incomplete development of the alveolar buds
> - Unilateral hyperlucent lung with reduced volume on inspiration and air trapping on expiration
> - Matched perfusion and ventilation defect on ventilation–perfusion (V/Q) scan

Bronchiolitis obliterans

- Airflow limitation caused by submucosal inflammation or fibrosis of respiratory bronchioles
- Affected areas are under-ventilated, resulting in reflex vasoconstriction

Causes
- Post-infectious: respiratory syncytial virus, influenza, *Pneumocystis carinii* pneumonia
- Inhalation of toxic fumes, e.g. sulphur dioxide
- Connective tissue disease, e.g. rheumatoid arthritis
- Lung or bone marrow transplantation

Imaging features
CXR
- Usually normal, though may show mild hyperinflation

HRCT
- Well-defined areas of reduced lung opacity ('mosaic attenuation')
- Reduced vessel calibre and number in low-attenuation areas
- Findings more prominent on expiratory phase (because of air trapping)
- Bronchiectasis is commonly present as well

Lobar anatomy
- Wide variation in normal appearance

Right lung
- Oblique fissure separates the upper and middle lobes from the lower lobe
- Oblique fissure runs at 50° to the horizontal from the T4 level posteriorly to diaphragm anteriorly
- Only visceral pleura extends into oblique and horizontal fissures

Upper lobe
- Divided into anterior, posterior and apical segments
- Anterior segment lies adjacent to the horizontal fissure

Middle lobe
- Divided into medial and lateral segments
- Medial segment lies adjacent to right heart border

Lower lobe
- Apical segment can extend as high as T3
- Typically divided into four basal segments: anterior, lateral, posterior and medial

Left lung
- Left oblique fissure runs more vertically than the right, at 60° to the horizontal

Upper lobe
- Divided into apicoposterior and anterior segments

Lingula
- Divided into superior and inferior segments
- Lies adjacent to the left heart border

Lower lobe
- Typically apical segment and three basal segments: anterior, posterior and lateral

Fissures and junctional lines
- Horizontal fissure is seen in 50% of CXRs
- Azygous fissure is caused by failure of normal migration of the azygous vein, seen as a 'teardrop' in 0.5% of CXRs
- Superior accessory fissure separates apical segment of the right lower lobe from basal segments, seen parallel and inferior to the horizontal fissure in 5% of CXRs
- Inferior accessory fissure separates the medial basal segment of the right lower lobe from the basal segments, seen in 8% of CXRs

Posterior junctional line
- Normal landmark on CXR
- Posterior apposition of parietal and visceral pleura of both lungs
- Descends vertically from approximately T1 to the level of the arch of the aorta
- May occasionally form again below the arch

Anterior junctional line
- Normal landmark on CXR
- Anterior apposition of parietal and visceral pleura of both lungs as they come into contact anterior to the arch of aorta

Azygo-oesophageal line
- Normal landmark on CXR
- Invagination of the right lung into the recess between the azygous vein and the oesophagus
- Begins below the clavicles and descends inferiorly and to the left, ending at level of right ventricle

Posteroanterior radiographic appearances of lobar collapse

Right upper lobe
- Elevation of the right hilum and horizontal fissure
- Tracheal deviation to right
- Localized convexity at the right hilum indicates an underlying mass lesion (Golden's 'S' sign)

Left upper lobe
- Veil-like opacity in the left upper zone
- Elevation of the left hilum
- Sharply demarcated aortic arch (Luftsichel's sign)
- Splaying of vessels from compensatory lower lobe expansion

Middle lobe
- Depression of the horizontal fissure
- Hazy opacity in right mid-zone
- Loss of clarity of the right heart border

Lingula
- Loss of clarity of left heart border

Left lower lobe
- Triangular opacity behind cardiac shadow (sail sign)
- Loss of clarity of the medial hemidiaphragm

CXR

Conventional technique
- Focus–film distance of 180 cm
- Centred at T5 level

High-voltage technique
- Obscures fine rib detail
- Improves mediastinal penetration
- Shorter exposure time
- Similar dose to conventional technique (0.02 mSv)
- Air gap of 15 cm is used instead of grid to reduce scatter

- Better visualisation of some structures
  - Lung vasculature
  - Arch of the aorta
  - Trachea and main bronchi
  - Junctional lines
- Worse visualisation of some structures
  - Small pulmonary nodules
  - Pleural plaques

Pleural effusions

- Visible on a lateral decubitus X-ray when > 25 mL
- Visible on a PA CXR when > 300 mL
- More commonly left-sided in acute pancreatitis
- More commonly right-sided in Meigs' syndrome

1.4 Air space diseases

Cardiogenic pulmonary oedema

- Impairment of blood flow through the left heart chambers causing elevated left atrial pressure and pulmonary venous hypertension
- Causes include
  - Ischaemic heart disease
  - Arrhythmias, e.g. atrial fibrillation
  - Mitral stenosis or mitral regurgitation
  - Aortic stenosis or aortic regurgitation
  - Systemic hypertension
  - Constrictive pericarditis

Non-cardiogenic pulmonary oedema

- Defined as increased permeability of the pulmonary capillaries in the presence of a normal left atrial pressure
- Causes include adult respiratory distress syndrome (ARDS), neurogenic oedema and drug reactions

Pathophysiology

- Raised pulmonary venous pressure causes an imbalance between capillary hydrostatic and plasma oncotic pressures
- Radiological changes correlate with left atrial pressure
- This is measured indirectly via a Swan–Ganz catheter as the pulmonary capillary wedge pressure (PCWP)
- Normal PCWP is 8–10 mmHg

Imaging features

Evolution of CXR changes
- PCWP > 15 mmHg
  - Redistribution of blood flow to the upper zones
  - Seen on erect film as the diameter of vessels in the upper zone being the same as or greater than in the lower zone

- PCWP > 20 mmHg
  - Leakage of fluid into the interstitial spaces
  - Kerley B lines: perpendicular subpleural linear opacities
  - Kerley A lines: longer opacities radiating out from the hilum
  - Peribronchial cuffing: thickened oedematous bronchial walls
- PCWP > 25 mmHg
  - Fluid spills over into the pleural spaces, fissures and alveoli
  - Pleural effusions (usually bilateral and large)
  - Fluid in the horizontal and oblique fissures
  - Bilateral perihilar air space consolidation ('bats wings')

Atypical patterns of pulmonary oedema

- Unilateral: patient on side, re-expansion oedema
- Patchy: seen with emphysematous bullae
- Right upper lobe: mitral regurgitation jet

ARDS

- Life-threatening respiratory illness with 50% mortality
- Diffuse alveolar damage causes increased capillary permeability
- Later, type 2 pneumocyte proliferation and interstitial fibrosis develops
- Severe respiratory failure develops 12–24 hours after insult
- Patients require positive-pressure ventilatory support
- Mechanism of injury:
  - Direct, from inhaled toxic fumes or aspirated gastric contents
  - Indirect, e.g. sepsis, pancreatitis, burns, hypovolaemia

Imaging features

Evolution of CXR changes
- 0–24 hours: normal
- 24–48 hours: widespread patchy air space consolidation; massive consolidation with air bronchograms
- 3–14 days: slow resolution of air space changes; fine reticular pattern ('bubbly lung')

Features distinguishing ARDS from cardiogenic pulmonary oedema
- No pleural effusions
- No cardiomegaly

CT
- Early
  - Bilateral consolidation and ground-glass appearance
  - Predilection for gravity-dependent lung
- Late
  - Fibrosis (reticulation) and bronchial dilatation
  - Predilection for non-gravity-dependent lung
  - Extent of fibrosis correlates with duration of ventilation

Pulmonary haemorrhage
- Associated with a diverse range of conditions
- Severity ranges from subclinical to massive life-threatening haemoptysis
- Imaging features are those of patchy air space opacification
- Alveolar macrophages clear blood products quickly, and resolution of changes may be seen within a few days (unlike infection)
- Repeated episodes can induce a fibrotic response
- Causes include
  - Goodpasture's syndrome
  - Vasculitides, e.g. Wegener's granulomatosis, systemic lupus erythematosus
  - Drug, e.g. anticoagulants
  - Mitral stenosis
  - Idiopathic pulmonary haemosiderosis

Goodpasture's syndrome
- Autoimmune disease caused by antibodies against glomerular and alveolar basement membranes
- Pulmonary haemorrhage and glomerulonephritis

Imaging features
CXR
- Multifocal consolidation with air bronchograms

Other causes of pulmonary–renal syndrome
- Wegener's granulomatosis
- IgA nephropathy
- Henoch–Schönlein purpura
- Microscopic polyangiitis
- Systemic lupus erythematosus

Mitral stenosis
- Chronic disease causing pulmonary venous hypertension
- Frequently associated with atrial fibrillation due to left atrial enlargement
- Intra-alveolar haemorrhage is well recognised

Other lung manifestations of mitral stenosis
- Pulmonary oedema
- Pulmonary ossifications
- Pulmonary haemosiderosis

Idiopathic pulmonary haemosiderosis
- Rare cause of recurrent diffuse alveolar haemorrhage
- Most frequent cause of diffuse alveolar haemorrhage in children
- Presents with recurrent episodes of haemoptysis
- Associated with iron-deficiency anaemia
- Bronchoalveolar lavage shows haemosiderin laden macrophages
- Fibrotic response may be seen with recurrent episodes

Imaging features

CXR

- Patchy air-space opacities

Cryptogenic organising pneumonia

- Non-infectious illness with a subacute onset over several months
- Pathology shows small airways inflammation with buds of granulation tissue filling the bronchioles, alveolar ducts and alveoli
- Presents with dry cough, fever and dyspnoea
- 50% of cases are idiopathic
- 50% have an identifiable cause
  - Drug reaction, e.g. amiodarone, bleomycin, methotrexate
  - Connective tissue disease, e.g. rheumatoid arthritis
  - Post-lung transplantation
  - Radiotherapy injury
- Diagnosis is established via lung biopsy
- Characteristically responds rapidly to corticosteroids

Imaging features

CXR

- Non-specific
- Multifocal patchy air space consolidation

HRCT

- Non-specific
- Patchy ground-glass opacities
- Patchy bilateral air space consolidation

Causes of multifocal air space consolidation

- Infection, e.g. aspergillosis
- Pulmonary oedema
- Pulmonary haemorrhage, e.g. from a drug reaction
- Neoplasia, e.g. bronchoalveolar cell carcinoma, lymphoma
- Eosinophilic pneumonia
- Crytogenic organising pneumonia
- ARDS
- Alveolar proteinosis
- Amyloidosis

Alveolar proteinosis

- Idiopathic condition characterised by accumulation of periodic acid–Schiff (PAS)-positive phospholipid within the alveoli and interstitial spaces
- Caused by excess surfactant production from type 2 pneumocytes
- Antibodies against granulocyte macrophage colony-stimulating factor (GM-CSF)
- Associated with lymphoma, leukaemia and immunodeficiency
- Typically presents in middle age with progressive dyspnoea
- Secondary infections are common, especially with *Nocardia*
- Runs a variable clinical course: one third recover, one third remain stable, and in one third it is fatal
- Treat options include regular whole-lung lavage

Imaging features

CXR

- Bilateral symmetrical air space opacification
- Mimics cardiogenic oedema but no cardiomegaly and no effusions

HRCT

- 'Crazy-paving' pattern
  - Bilateral, patchy ground-glass opacities
  - Superimposed smooth, interlobular septal thickening

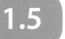

Diffuse lung disease

HRCT

Technical aspects

- Modality of choice for assessing parenchymal lung disease
- Narrow beam collimation (0.5–2 mm slice thickness)
- Edge-enhancing high-spatial resolution reconstruction algorithm
- Increased noise: poor for assessing mediastinal structures
- Performed in suspended full inspiration
- Expiratory imaging is used for evaluation of air trapping
- Prone imaging is used to distinguish dependent change from early fibrosis
- Incremental HRCT
  - Single slices at spaced intervals
  - 10–15% of radiation dose of conventional chest CT
- Volumetric HRCT
  - Contiguous spiral acquisition of entire thorax

Secondary pulmonary lobule

- Basic unit of lung structure marginated by connective tissue septa
- Polyhedral in shape and 1–2 cm in size (smaller centrally)
- Contains between 10 and 20 pulmonary acini
- Supplied centrally by a small bronchiole and pulmonary artery, which are surrounded by interstitial fibres and lymphatics
- A peripheral connective tissue septa extends between the lobules and contains both veins and lymphatics

Structures normally visible on HRCT

- Centrilobular artery
- Bronchi (not normally seen within 2 cm of pleura)
- Interlobular septa (only occasionally visible)
- Not centrilobular bronchiole and not pulmonary acini

HRCT signs

Halo sign

- Ground-glass attenuation surrounding a pulmonary nodule
- Usually caused by haemorrhage into surrounding lung

Causes

- Angioinvasive aspergillosis
- After biopsy or radiofrequency ablation
- Haemorrhagic lung metastases (from angiosarcoma or choriocarcinoma)
- Kaposi's sarcoma
- Wegener's granulomatosis
- Bronchoalveolar cell carcinoma
- Eosinophilic pneumonia
- Cryptogenic organising pneumonia
- Infection, e.g. tuberculosis, *Mycobacterium avium-intracellulare* complex, herpes simplex virus, cytomegalovirus, coccidioidomycosis

Mosaic attenuation

- Well-defined high- and low-attenuation areas in a lobular distribution
- Three main causes: small airways disease, vascular disease and parenchymal disease

Small airways disease

- Causes include asthma, bronchiolitis obliterans, cystic fibrosis and allergic bronchopulmonary aspergillosis
- Abnormal lung shows as lower-attenuation area
- More pronounced on expiratory phase imaging
- Reduced vessel calibre and number

Vascular disease

- Chronic thromboembolic pulmonary hypertension
- Abnormal lung shows as lower-attenuation area (owing to the relative hypoperfusion in these areas)
- Does not become more pronounced on expiratory phase imaging
- Reduced vessel calibre and number in low attenuation regions

Parenchymal disease

- Caused by any condition that produces ground-glass attenuation
- Abnormal lung shows as higher-attenuation area
- Vessel calibre and number is normal

Ground-glass opacification

- Hazy increase in lung opacity not obscuring the vessels
- Caused by alveolitis, partial air space filling or interstitial disease below the spatial resolution of HRCT (partial volume effect)

Causes

- Pulmonary oedema (heart failure, ARDS)
- Pulmonary haemorrhage
- Usual interstitial pneumonia (UIP), desquamative interstitial pneumonia (DIP), non-specific interstitial pneumonia (NSIP) or lymphocytic interstitial pneumonitis (LIP)
- Respiratory bronchiolitis associated with interstitial lung disease (RB-ILD)
- Infections, e.g. *Pneumocystis carinii* pneumonia, viral infection, mycoplasma infection
- Cryptogenic organising pneumonia
- Extrinsic allergic alveolitis
- Bronchoalveolar cell carcinoma
- Sarcoidosis
- Eosinophilic pneumonia
- Alveolar proteinosis
- Sickle cell disease

Interlobular septal thickening

- Represents interstitial fluid, fibrosis or cellular infiltration
- Causes of smooth septal thickening
  - Interstitial pulmonary oedema
  - Lymphangitis carcinomatosis (typically causes unilateral interlobular septal thickening)
  - Alveolar proteinosis
  - Lymphoma
- Causes of nodular septal thickening
  - Lymphangitis carcinomatosis
  - Sarcoidosis
  - Pneumoconiosis
  - Silicosis
  - Berylliosis

'Crazy-paving' pattern

- Ground-glass opacity with superimposed septal thickening
- Causes
  - Alveolar proteinosis
  - Infections, e.g. *Pneumocystis carinii* pneumonia, viral infection, mycoplasma infection, bacterial infection
  - Pulmonary oedema, e.g. from heart failure or ARDS)
  - Pulmonary haemorrhage, e.g. Wegener's granulomatosis, Goodpasture's syndrome, systemic lupus erythematosus
  - Bronchoalveolar cell carcinoma
  - Non-specific interstitial pneumonia
  - Cryptogenic organising pneumonia
  - Severe acute respiratory illness (SARS)
  - Lipoid pneumonia
  - Sarcoidosis

Centrilobular nodules

Causes

- Diseases involving the centrilobular bronchioles
  - Bronchiectasis
  - Bronchiolitis obliterans
  - Hypersensitivity pneumonitis
  - Endobronchial spread of tuberculosis
  - Bronchopneumonia
  - Cryptogenic organising pneumonia
  - Respiratory bronchiolitis associated with interstitial lung disease (RB-ILD)
  - Tracheobronchial papillomatosis
  - Diffuse panbronchiolitis
  - Bronchioalveolar cell carcinoma
  - Histiocytosis X
- Diseases involving the central perivascular lymphatics
  - Sarcoidosis
  - Lymphangitis carcinomatosis
  - Lymphocytic interstitial pneumonia
- Diseases involving the centrilobular arteries
  - Pulmonary oedema
  - Vasculitis

Tree-in-bud pattern

- Small, peripheral centrilobular nodules of soft-tissue attenuation connected to

multiple linear branching opacities
- Represents plugging of small airways with mucus, pus or fluid
- Can also occur with intravascular pulmonary tumour emboli
- Not visible on CXR

Causes

- Infections, e.g. tuberculosis, *Mycobacterium avium-intracellulare* complex, pyogenic infections, fungal infections, cytomegalovirus, other viral infections, *Pneumocystis carinii* pneumonia
- Bronchiectasis (of any cause)
- Bronchiolitis obliterans (of any cause)
- Diffuse panbronchiolitis
- Aspiration
- Allergic bronchopulmonary aspergillosis
- Connective tissue diseases, e.g. rheumatoid arthritis, Sjögren's syndrome
- Intravascular tumour emboli, e.g. from breast or stomach

Extrinsic allergic alveolitis

- Immunologically mediated disorder whereby inhalation of dust or other particulate antigens provokes a hypersensitivity reaction
- Includes pigeon fancier's lung (caused by avian proteins), farmer's lung (caused by spores of thermophilic actinomycetes) and malt worker's lung (caused by *Aspergillus clavatus*)
- < 50% of patients have serum IgG antibodies against a provoking antigen
- The presence of serum antibodies indicates exposure and not necessarily disease

Acute and subacute extrinsic allergic alveolitis

- Inhaled antigens reach the alveoli and provoke an inflammatory cell infiltrate via a type III hypersensitivity reaction
- Fever, rigors, cough and dyspnoea develop 6 hours after exposure and settle within 12–24 hours
- Repeated exposures cause a cell-mediated (type IV) reaction, with granuloma formation and obliterative bronchiolitis

- These changes are reversible with cessation of exposure

Imaging features

CXR
- Normal in 50% of cases
- Generalised haziness (ground-glass appearance) is common
- Multifocal consolidation is less common

HRCT
- Multiple, small, ill-defined nodules (< 5 mm in diameter)
- Centrilobular nodules and ground-glass appearance
- Air trapping on expiratory phase imaging
- Mid-zone predominance

Chronic extrinsic allergic alveolitis

- Prolonged (usually low-grade) exposure causes pulmonary fibrosis, with insidious onset of dyspnoea, type I respiratory failure and cor pulmonale

Imaging features

HRCT
- Pulmonary fibrosis with mid-zone-predominance

Sarcoidosis

- Idiopathic multisystem disease characterised by widespread development of non-caseating epithelioid granulomas
- 90% of patients have pulmonary involvement
- Granulomas are distributed along the lymphatics
- Most commonly presents in those aged 20–40 years
- More common in Afro-Caribbeans

Eponymous sarcoidosis syndromes

- Löfgren's syndrome (20% of cases of sarcoidosis)
  - Bilateral hilar lymphadenopathy
  - Erythema nodosum
  - Arthralgia
- Heerfordt's syndrome (5% of cases of sarcoidosis)

- Anterior uveitis
- Parotitis
- Eighth cranial nerve palsy

Investigations

- Serum angiotensin-converting enzyme: elevated in 60%, and level correlates with granuloma burden
- Serum calcium levels: elevated in 10%
- Bronchoalveolar lavage: increased CD4:CD8 ratio
- Gallium-67 scintigraphy: uptake in nodes and lung parenchyma
- Transbronchial lung biopsy: accuracy of 90%

Staging at time of presentation

- Stage 0: clear CXR (10% of cases)
- Stage 1: hilar nodal enlargement (50% of cases)
- Stage 2: hilar nodal enlargement and pulmonary infiltrates (30% of cases)
- Stage 3: pulmonary infiltrates alone (10% of cases)
- Stage 4: late-stage fibrosis
- The lower the stage at presentation the better the prognosis
- 60% of patients with stage 1 disease undergo spontaneous remission
- Poor prognostic factors include male sex, insidious-onset disease, lupus pernio, tracheal involvement and extrapulmonary manifestations
- Overall mortality 5–10%

Lymphadenopathy

- Hilar, paratracheal and bronchopulmonary nodes are most commonly involved
- Symmetrical, bilateral hilar adenopathy with a lobulated outer margin and well demarcated inner margin is classical CXR picture
- Degree of hilar adenopathy ranges from minimal to massive
- Asymmetric and unilateral hilar adenopathy are rare (< 5% of cases)
- Adenopathy usually resolves within the first year after diagnosis and almost never returns
- Classically nodes develop light 'eggshell' calcifications: seen in 3% of cases after 5 years and 30% after 10 years

Causes of bilateral hilar lymphadenopathy

- Sarcoidosis
- Lymphoma
- Metastases
- Tuberculosis
- Silicosis
- Berylliosis

Parenchymal disease

- 40% have parenchymal disease at the time of diagnosis
- A further 40% develop parenchymal changes; this usually occurs within the first year and is classically accompanied by nodal regression

Micronodular parenchymal disease

- Accounts for 75% of cases
- Mid-zone and upper zone predominance
- Multiple small (< 5 mm), well-defined nodules
- Nodules are located along
  - Bronchovascular bundles
  - Fissures
  - Subpleural regions
  - Interlobular septa ('beaded septum sign')
  - Centrilobular regions

Air space parenchymal disease

- Accounts for 20% of cases
- Multifocal bilateral, ill-defined air space disease
- Air bronchograms
- Mid-zone and upper zone predominance

Macronodular parenchymal disease

- Accounts for 5% of cases
- Bilateral multiple, ill-defined opacities of > 1 cm diameter
- Mid-zone predominance
- Rarely cavitated

Fibrotic stage (stage IV)

- Two thirds of parenchymal infiltrates resolve completely
- One third progress to pulmonary fibrosis over several years

- Fibrosis is usually predominant in the mid-zone and upper zone
- Bullae, cysts and traction bronchiectasis are common
- Mycetoma formation in upper lobe bullae is well recognised

Other thoracic manifestations

- Pleural effusion (in 2% of cases)
- Bronchial stenosis (in 2% of cases)

Cryptogenic fibrosing alveolitis

- Idiopathic pulmonary fibrosis with progressive dyspnoea, pulmonary hypertension and cor pulmonale
- Typical onset is in late middle age with mean survival of 3 years
- Finger clubbing and bilateral basal end-inspiratory crackles
- Commonest histological appearance is usual interstitial pneumonia (UIP)
  - Parenchymal inflammatory cell infiltrates, fibroblastic foci and areas of established fibrosis (temporal heterogeneity)
- Increased risk of bronchogenic carcinoma

Hamman–Rich syndrome

- Acute form of cryptogenic fibrosing alveolitis seen in 10% of cases
- Rapidly fatal, within a few months
- Histologically there is diffuse alveolar damage
- Multifocal air space consolidation
- Background fibrotic and ground-glass change

Imaging features

CXR
- Reticulonodular shadowing in the lower zone

HRCT
- Ground-glass opacity in a peripheral basal subpleural distribution
- Reticulation with honeycombing and traction bronchiectasis

- Enlarged 'reactive' mediastinal lymphadenopathy is common
- Pleural effusion is recognised but rare
- Ground-glass appearance is thought to represent active alveolitis, which may be corticosteroid-responsive in some cases
- Honeycombing represents irreversible established fibrosis

Connective tissue diseases

Rheumatoid arthritis

- Symmetrical deforming polyarthropathy of peripheral joints
- IgM rheumatoid factor-positive
- Extra-articular manifestations include a range of chest conditions

Pleural effusion

- Males nine times more commonly affected than females
- Associated with the presence of subcutaneous rheumatoid nodules
- Usually develops years after onset of the rheumatoid arthritis
- Typically small, unilateral and painless
- Exudate
  - Low glucose
  - Low pH
  - Lymphocyte-predominant
  - May contain rheumatoid factor
- Most resolve spontaneously

Interstitial fibrosis

- Males twice as commonly affected as females
- 20% of patients with rheumatoid arthritis develop it
- Lower-zone predominant
- Commonest histological pattern is usual interstitial pneumonia (UIP); it can mimic cryptogenic fibrosing alveolitis

Pulmonary nodules

- Pathologically the same as subcutaneous nodules
- Males twice as commonly affected as females
- Typically lobulated soft-tissue masses of 1–5 cm diameter
- Peripheral zone and mid-zone predominance

- 50% cavitate
- Rarely calcify

Caplan's syndrome

- Development of pulmonary nodules indistinguishable radiologically from rheumatoid nodules in patients with coal worker's pneumoconiosis and rheumatoid arthritis
- Background micronodular change suggests the diagnosis

> **Other chest manifestations of rheumatoid disease**
>
> - Bronchiectasis
> - Bronchiolitis obliterans
> - Drug toxicity, e.g. methotrexate pneumonitis

Systemic lupus erythematosus

- Multisystem autoimmune disease
- Anti-double-stranded DNA antibody-positive
- Females affected ten times more commonly than males
- Can be drug-induced by hydralazine, phenytoin or procainamide
- Antiphospholipid antibody and prothrombotic tendency occur in 30% of patients
- Butterfly facial rash, photosensitivity, Raynaud's phenomenon, non-erosive arthropathy, renal impairment, Liebmann–Sachs endocarditis
- Pulmonary disease is seen in 60% of patients

> **Pulmonary manifestations of systemic lupus erythematosus**
>
> - Pleural effusions (common)
> - Multifocal consolidation: vasculitic haemorrhage, atypical infection or lupus pneumonitis
> - Lower zone pulmonary fibrosis in < 5% of patients
> - Diaphragmatic elevation from myopathy

Polymyositis

- Inflammatory proximal myopathy
- Raised creatine kinase
- Electromyograph abnormalities
- 5% of patients have anti-Jo-1 antibodies, which are associated with lower zone pulmonary fibrosis
- Dermatomyositis has the features of polymyositis plus skin involvement
- Dermatomyositis is associated with an underlying malignancy

Scleroderma

Limited form of scleroderma

- Formerly called the CREST syndrome: calcinosis, Raynaud's phenomenon, oesophageal dysmotility, sclerodactyly, telangiectasias
- Anti-centromere antibodies are present

Diffuse form of scleroderma

- 90% develop lung fibrosis; non-specific interstitial pneumonia (NSIP) is the commonest pattern
- Increased incidence of bronchoalveolar cell carcinoma and adenocarcinoma
- Pulmonary arterial hypertension
- Gastrointestinal tract involvement (dilated small bowel 'hidebound')
- Acute renal failure and malignant hypertension secondary to an endarteritis obliterans
- Anti-Scl-70 antibodies are present

Imaging features

CXR

- Bilateral lower zone pulmonary fibrosis
- Dilated oesophagus with air–fluid level
- Apical surgical clips from sympathectomy
- Dilated sub-diaphragmatic small bowel loops
- Spontaneous pneumoperitoneum

Pulmonary vasculitides

Wegener's granulomatosis

- Necrotizing vasculitis of small and medium-sized arteries
- Positive for antineutrophil cytoplasmic antibodies (cANCA), specifically proteinase-3 (PR3)

- Multisystem disorder
- Males twice as commonly affects as females

Pulmonary disease

- Occurs in 95% of cases
- Multiple large (> 2 cm), peripheral nodules, which often cavitate
- Pulmonary haemorrhage, producing multifocal air space consolidation
- Tracheobronchial inflammation, causing subglottic tracheal stenosis
- Pleural effusion occurs in 25% cases, lymphadenopathy occurs but is rare

Renal disease

- Occurs in 90% of cases
- Rapidly progressive glomerulonephritis
- Commonest cause of death

Nasal and paranasal sinus disease

- Occurs in 80% of cases
- Bloody sinus discharge, epistaxis and collapse of nasal septum

Microscopic polyangiitis

- Small vessel vasculitis
- Positive for perinuclear antineutrophil cytoplasmic antibody (p-ANCA), specifically myeloperoxidase (MPO)
- Pulmonary haemorrhage, which produces multifocal consolidation

Churg–Strauss syndrome

- Triad of clinical features
  - Adult onset asthma
  - Peripheral blood eosinophilia
  - Systemic vasculitis

Imaging features

CXR
- Transient pulmonary infiltrates

HRCT
- Patchy, multifocal ground-glass opacities
- Peripheral ill-defined areas of consolidation

Behçet's disease

- Triad of clinical features
  - Oral ulceration
  - Genital ulceration
  - Iritis

- Other features
  - Associated with HLA-B51
  - Most prevalent in Turkish men
  - Positive pathergy reaction (pustule at site of a needle puncture)
  - Arterial and venous thromboses
  - Lung involvement in 5% of cases: pulmonary artery aneurysms, pulmonary infarcts and pulmonary haemorrhage

Drug-induced lung disease

- Numerous agents have the potential to cause pulmonary toxicity
- Wide range of histopathological processes including diffuse alveolar damage (DAD), non-specific interstitial pneumonia (NSIP), cryptogenic organizing pneumonia (COP), eosinophilic pneumonia and pulmonary haemorrhage
- Fibrosis in a basal distribution is a typical late-stage manifestation
- Clinically, cytotoxic drugs are the largest and most important group of causative agents

Agents commonly causing pulmonary drug toxicity

Cytotoxic agents
- Methotrexate
- Bleomycin
- Cyclophosphamide
- Doxorubicin

Non-cytotoxic agents
- Amiodarone
- Nitrofurantoin
- Sulfasalazine

Amiodarone-induced lung disease

- Tri-iodinated benzofuran with a long half-life (60 days)
- 5–15% of patients taking amiodarone develop pulmonary toxicity
- If detected early, the prognosis is good following discontinuation
- Drug metabolites are trapped by foamy macrophages, inducing a fibrotic reaction

Imaging features

CXR and HRCT

- Areas of peripheral high-attenuation consolidation
- Pleural inflammation and effusion are common
- Ground-glass opacities with septal thickening progressing to established fibrosis in chronic stage (basal predominance)
- High attenuation may also be seen within the liver and thyroid

Patterns of pulmonary fibrosis

- Predominantly upper zone
  - Sarcoidosis
  - Silicosis
  - Coal worker's pneumoconiosis
  - Histiocytosis X
  - Allergic bronchopulmonary aspergillosis
  - Radiation fibrosis
  - Tuberculosis
- Predominantly lower zone
  - Rheumatoid lung disease
  - Asbestosis
  - Scleroderma
  - Cryptogenic fibrosing alveolitis
  - Neurofibromatosis type 1
  - Drug-induced lung disease
  - Extrinsic allergic alveolitis (in the mid-zone and lower zone)

Interstitial lung diseases with preserved lung volumes

- Virtually all interstitial lung diseases cause a progressive reduction in lung volume, with the exception of four conditions, in which volumes are preserved or increased
  - Lymphangioleiomyomatosis
  - Pulmonary Langerhans' cell histiocytosis
  - Tuberous sclerosis
  - Neurofibromatosis type 1

Lymphangioleiomyomatosis

- Proliferation of interstitial smooth muscle bundles, which occlude the lymphatics, blood vessels and bronchioles
- Distal air trapping causes cyst formation and progressive destruction of lung tissue
- Subpleural cysts may rupture, resulting in pneumothorax
- Exclusively affects women, usually during the reproductive years
- A small percentage of cases are associated with tuberous sclerosis

Imaging features

CXR

- Normal or increased lung volumes
- Diffuse reticulonodular shadowing (caused by superimposition of cyst walls)
- Pneumothorax develops in approximately 70% of cases
- Pleural effusion (chylous, unilateral) develops in approximately 20% of cases

CT

- Multiple thin-walled cysts (most 2–5 mm in diameter)
- Typically cysts are round or polygonal in shape
- Symmetrical, uniform distribution
- Lung parenchyma between the cysts is normal

Pulmonary Langerhans' cell histiocytosis

- Isolated form of histiocytosis X
- Proliferation of atypical Langerhans' cells within lung parenchyma
- Presents in young adults; 90% are smokers
- Imaging features evolve and have a temporal heterogeneity
- Shows a mid-zone and upper zone predominance

Imaging features

CXR

- Often indistinguishable from lymphangioleiomyomatosis
- Normal or increased lung volumes
- Diffuse reticulonodular shadowing
- Pneumothorax develops in approximately 25% of cases

HRCT

- Bilateral small centrilobular nodules (1–10 mm in diameter)

- Irregularly shaped, thick- and thin-walled cysts
- Pneumothorax develops in 25% of cases
- Fibrosis seen with late-stage disease

Features suggesting Histiocytosis X over lymphangioleiomyomatosis

- Spares lung bases
- Cysts have irregular shapes
- Nodules seen in parenchyma between cysts

Tuberous sclerosis

- Lung involvement in 1–2% of cases
- Radiologically indistinguishable from lymphangioleiomyomatosis

Neurofibromatosis type 1

- Interstitial lung changes seen in 20% of cases

Imaging features

CXR
- Pulmonary fibrosis with a lower zone predominance
- Asymmetric bullae with an upper zone predominance
- 'Twisted ribbon' ribs
- High thoracic-curve scoliosis
- Paraspinal neurofibromas and lateral meningocele
- Subcutaneous neurofibromas

Amyloidosis

- Extracellular deposition of an insoluble fibrillar protein
- Takes up Congo red stain
- Amyloid light chain (AL) form
  - Derived from plasma cells and elevated in multiple myeloma
- AA – Amyloid-associated protein (AA) form
  - Synthesised in the liver and elevated in chronic inflammatory states
- AL form is predominant type to affect the lung

- Two main patterns of pulmonary disease, tracheobronchial and parenchymal, as well as a third form, reticulonodular infiltration
- Tracheobronchial form
  - Submucosal deposits are commonest pulmonary form
  - Circumferential nodular luminal narrowing with distal collapse
- Parenchymal form
  - Single or multiple pulmonary nodules mimicking malignancy
  - Larger lesions may cavitate or calcify
- Reticulonodular infiltration
  - Hilar and mediastinal adenopathy, which often calcifies

Alveolar microlithiasis

- Progressive, widespread calcium deposition within the alveoli
- Serum calcium levels are normal
- Often minimal early symptoms; an incidental imaging finding
- Many cases present in middle age with slowly progressive dyspnoea and eventual cor pulmonale from secondary fibrosis

Imaging features

CXR
- Scattered, dense micronodules ('sandstorm' appearance)
- Mid-zone and lower zone predominance

Scintigram
- Nodules show intense uptake on bone scan

Radiation-induced lung disease

- Common: occurs in up to 10% of patients receiving radiotherapy
- Radiographic changes are usually confined to the radiation portal
- Rarely produces more diffuse changes secondary to organising pneumonia
- Tangential beam commonly used for breast cancer typically causes a 2–3 cm strip of anterolateral fibrosis

Acute radiation-induced lung disease

- Transient pneumonitis develops 1–3 months after treatment
- Most patients are asymptomatic at this stage

Imaging features

CXR
- Non-segmental patchy consolidation and ground-glass changes
- Sharply defined linear interface with adjacent normal lung tissue
- Pleural effusions are uncommon
- Changes may resolve completely but most progress to fibrosis

Chronic radiation-induced lung disease

- Fibrosis develops 6–12 months after treatment

Imaging features

CXR
- Volume loss
- Linear scarring
- Traction bronchiectasis
- Sharply defined linear interface with adjacent normal lung tissue

PET
- Accurately detects residual or recurrent tumour within fibrosis

Silicosis and coal worker's pneumoconiosis

- Caused by inhalation of various inorganic dusts
- Particles lodge in respiratory bronchioles
- Silicosis caused inhaled dust containing silicon dioxide
- Coal worker's pneumoconiosis caused by inhaled coal dust particles
- Usually asymptomatic unless complicated by massive fibrosis
- Significant overlap in radiological appearances

Imaging features

CXR
- Micronodular opacities in the mid-zone and upper zone
- Pulmonary fibrosis in the upper zone
- Hilar adenopathy with 'eggshell' calcifications (in 5% of cases of silicosis; seen in coal worker's pneumoconiosis only if the coal dust contains silica particles)

HRCT
- Well-defined centrilobular micronodules

Causes of hilar 'eggshell' calcifications
• Silicosis
• Sarcoidosis
• Scleroderma
• Histoplasmosis
• Amyloidosis
• Tuberculosis
• Berylliosis
• Lymphoma (post-treatment)

Progressive massive fibrosis

- Late complication of coal worker's pneumoconiosis or silicosis
- Can cause severe dyspnoea and respiratory failure
- Large conglomerate fibrotic masses (no air bronchograms)

- Commences in lung periphery and migrates towards hila
- Mid-zone and upper zone predominance
- Typically bilateral and cavitating

Berylliosis

- Chronic exposure incites a granulomatous parenchymal reaction, which is indistinguishable from sarcoidosis
- Widespread micronodular shadowing, progressing to fibrosis
- Hilar and mediastinal lymphadenopathy

Asbestos-related lung disease

- Inhaled fibres are trapped in the lung, inciting a fibrogenic reaction
- Amphibolic fibres (crocidolite and amosite) are the main cause of clinically significant asbestos-related disease

Pleural plaques

- Commonest radiological manifestation of asbestos exposure
- Irritant effect from transpleural migration of asbestos fibres
- Usually occurs 20–30 years after exposure
- Clinically asymptomatic
- Discrete areas of fibrosis that usually arise from parietal pleura
- Visceral pleural plaques are less common
- Most often located along posterolateral chest wall and diaphragm
- Typically spare the apices and costophrenic angles
- Calcification occurs in 10–15% of cases
- CT is more sensitive than CXR for plaque detection
- Plaques have no relationship with mesothelioma

Causes of pleural calcification
• Asbestos-related pleural plaques
• Talc pleurodesis
• Haemothorax
• Tuberculous empyema

Pleural effusion

- Earliest manifestation of asbestos exposure (within 10 years)
- Benign haemorrhagic exudate of mixed cellularity
- Usually small (< 500 mL) and asymptomatic
- May be unilateral or bilateral
- Resolves over several months to leave residual pleural thickening

Diffuse pleural thickening

- Definition: smooth, uninterrupted pleural thickening (> 5 mm) that extends over at least 25% of the chest wall (50% if unilateral), or continuous sheet of pleural thickening (> 3 mm) that extends more than 8 cm in craniocaudal extent and more than 5 cm laterally
- Fibrosis of visceral pleura with fusion of the pleural layers
- Usually preceded by a benign pleural effusion
- Progressive restrictive ventilatory defect
- Features helping to distinguish it from pleural plaques
  - Ill-defined irregular margins
  - Involvement of interlobar fissures
  - Lack of sparing of the costophrenic angles or apices
  - Calcification rare

Causes of diffuse pleural thickening

Benign
- Asbestos-related
- Tuberculous empyema
- Haemothorax
- Talcosis
- Connective tissue diseases

Malignant
- Mesothelioma
- Metastatic adenocarcinoma
- Lymphoma

Round atelectasis

- Peripheral lobar collapse adjacent to an area of pleural thickening

- Round or oval subpleural opacity forming acute angle with pleura
- A history of asbestos exposure is common (in 70% of cases)
- Other causes include parapneumonic effusions, pneumothorax, uraemia, Dressler's syndrome, mesothelioma and cardiac failure

Imaging features

- Most commonly located posteriorly within the lower lobes
- Comet tail sign: crowding of bronchi and vessels entering lesion
- Shows enhancement post-contrast
- Air bronchograms seen within it in 60% of cases

Asbestosis

- Caused by prolonged heavy exposure with a lag of > 20 years
- Progressive dyspnoea and a restrictive ventilatory defect
- Finger clubbing and basal end inspiratory crepitations are typical
- Increased risk of developing bronchogenic carcinoma
- Basal subpleural curvilinear opacities are the earliest sign
- Established disease appears similar to fibrosing alveolitis with predominantly lower zone and mid-zone pulmonary fibrosis

Bronchogenic carcinoma

- Exposure to asbestos increases the risk of developing bronchogenic carcinoma 20-fold
- Synergistic effect with smoking: risk is increased 100-fold with both risk factors
- Amphibole fibres are more potent inducers than chrysotile
- Adenocarcinoma and squamous cell carcinoma are commonest tumour types
- Tumours are usually located peripherally and in the lower lobes

Malignant mesothelioma

- Malignant pleural tumour, which slowly encases the lung

- Commonest primary neoplasm of the pleura
- Accounts for < 1% of all thoracic neoplasms
- Latent period between exposure and disease is 30–40 years
- Most patients die within 1 year of diagnosis
- Tumour can arise from either pleural layer
- Frequently extends into the interlobar fissures, chest wall, mediastinum, diaphragm and underlying lung
- Haematogenous spread to involve liver and lung is recognised
- Can spread along the needle track of a percutaneous biopsy
- Mesothelioma can also arise from the peritoneum, pericardium and tunica vaginalis of the testis

Imaging features

CXR
- Unilateral pleural effusion is commonest finding
- Often there is an absence of mediastinal shift ('frozen hemithorax')

CT
- Markers of prior asbestos exposure are often absent
- Lobulated pleural based soft tissue mass encasing the lung
- Mediastinal lymphadenopathy is common

PET/CT
- Circumferential pleural uptake is characteristic
- Most accurate modality for detecting mediastinal nodal disease

Community-acquired pneumonias

Streptococcal pneumonia

- Commonest community-acquired pneumonia
- Risk factors include post-splenectomy, alcoholism, immunocompromise
- Infection begins in distal air spaces (lobar pneumonia)
- Typically unifocal peripheral consolidation with air bronchograms
- Resolves promptly with antibiotic treatment
- Only 1–2% of patients develop an empyema

Viral pneumonia

- Account for 10–15% of community-acquired pneumonia
- Influenza is the commonest virus affecting adults
- CXR may show a fine reticulonodular infiltrate
- Secondary bacterial infection is common (especially with *Staphylococcus aureus*)

Varicella-zoster virus

- Complicates chickenpox in 5% of adults (rare in children)
- Widespread nodular opacities appear 1–5 days after the skin rash
- These nodules occasionally persist and some eventually calcify

Causes of bilateral calcified lung nodules

- Varicella pneumonia
- Histoplasmosis
- Tuberculosis
- Mitral stenosis
- Alveolar microlithiasis
- Metastases (from osteosarcoma, mucinous adenocarcinoma, papillary thyroid tumours, testicular tumours, ovarian tumours or angiosarcoma)

Klebsiella pneumonia

- Rare cause of community-acquired pneumonia
- Typically affects elderly patients and alcoholics
- Classical CXR appearance is of a cavitating upper lobe consolidation with bulging of the adjacent fissure
- Commonly progresses to empyema
- Mortality is 30%

Severe acute respiratory syndrome (SARS)

- Transmissible respiratory illness caused by a coronavirus
- Incubation period is 2–10 days
- Presents with high fever, dry cough, dyspnoea and arthralgia
- 10–20% of patients require mechanical ventilation

Imaging features

- Extent of disease is underestimated with CXR
- HRCT shows a mixture of ground glass and consolidation
- 80% have air space opacification of varying extent at presentation
- A peripheral lower zone focal opacity is commonest pattern (40%)
- Extent of consolidation peaks 6 days after presentation and in those who recover has resolved by day 16
- Diffuse consolidation (14%) is associated with a high mortality
- Cavitation, lymphadenopathy, pleural effusions are not a feature

Atypical pneumonias

Mycoplasma pneumonia

- Common cause of non-bacterial pneumonia in young adults
- Presents initially with flu-like symptoms, which are followed by fever and dry cough

Imaging features

CXR
- Severity of findings are discrepant to clinical picture
- Reticulonodular opacities radiate out from hilum into lower lobe
- Progresses to confluent consolidation, which is bilateral in 40% of cases
- Pulmonary fibrosis and bronchiolitis obliterans are recognised

Extrapulmonary complications
- IgM cold agglutinins, causing haemolytic anaemia
- Erythema multiforme and Stevens–Johnson syndrome
- Meningoencephalitis
- Myocarditis

Legionella pneumophila
- Organism colonises air-conditioning systems and humidifiers
- Acquired by inhalation of the aerosol mist
- Mainly affects older adults, with a 20% mortality
- Patients can be critically ill with renal and hepatic failure
- CXR is non-specific with areas of consolidation

Other pneumonias

Aspiration pneumonia
- Caused by irritant effect of gastric contents combined with anaerobic infection
- Risk factors include reduced Glasgow coma scale, stroke and gastroesophageal reflux disease
- Affects the superior segment of the lower lobes and the posterior segment of the upper lobes
- Often progresses to abscess formation and empyema

Staphylococcal pneumonia
- Occurs as a superinfection following influenza virus or from septic emboli from tricuspid valve endocarditis related to intravenous drug use
- Consolidated areas have a propensity to cavitate

Pseudomonas pneumonia
- Infection develops in patients with pre-existing lung disease
- Delayed clearance of secretions predisposes to colonisation
- A common cause of recurrent pneumonia in cystic fibrosis
- Difficult to eradicate because of widespread drug resistance
- Multifocal consolidation on a background of chronic lung disease

Aspergillosis
- *Aspergillus* fungus causes a broad spectrum of disease in humans, ranging from hypersensitivity reaction to aggressive angioinvasion

Aspergilloma
- Colonisation of a chronic lung cavity, e.g. in tuberculosis or sarcoidosis
- Non-invasive process
- Most often occurs in lung apex
- Can cause severe haemoptysis requiring bronchial embolisation

Imaging features

CXR
- Thin-walled cavity containing a rounded gravity-dependent opacity
- Air crescent sign between the opacity and the cavity wall
- Fungal ball may contain calcifications

Invasive aspergillosis
- An often fatal infection in the severely immunocompromised
- Angioinvasion occurs, with haemorrhage and lung infarction
- Mortality is 60%

Imaging features

CXR
- Multiple, ill-defined patches of consolidation
- Lesions may cavitate in later stages of disease

HRCT
- Multiple nodules with surrounding ground-glass halos

- Lesions progress into more diffuse consolidation

Allergic bronchopulmonary aspergillosis

- Commonest cause of pulmonary eosinophilia in the UK
- Airway colonisation in patients with asthma or cystic fibrosis
- Recurrent hypersensitivity reactions with eosinophil influx
- Positive *Aspergillus* serum precipitins and elevated IgE levels
- Causes progression of asthma symptoms
- Expectoration of thick mucus plugs
- Complications of recurrent attacks
  - Central mucus plugging with distal collapse/consolidation/abscess
  - Central cystic bronchiectasis
  - Upper zone pulmonary fibrosis

Imaging features

CXR
- Recurrent transient upper zone pulmonary infiltrates

Pulmonary eosinophilia

- Blood eosinophilia ($> 0.4 \times 10^9$/L) and pulmonary infiltration

Causes:
- Asthma
- Allergic bronchopulmonary aspergillosis
- Vasculitides, e.g. Churg–Strauss syndrome, Wegener's granulomatosis
- Drug-induced disease, e.g. from non-steroidal anti-inflammatory drugs, sulphonamides
- Parasitic infestation, e.g. schistosomiasis, ascariasis
- Simple eosinophilic pneumonia (Löffler's syndrome)
- Acute eosinophilic pneumonia
- Chronic eosinophilic pneumonia
- Tropical pulmonary eosinophilia (filarial sensitivity)

Hydatid disease

- Principally caused by ingestion of *Echinococcus* tapeworm eggs excreted in the faeces of infected dogs
- The eggs hatch in the small bowel and penetrate the intestinal wall to reach the portal venous system, spreading primarily to liver
- In the liver they form cystic lesions, which grow slowly over many years
- Lung is involved in 5–15% of cases (with multiple lesions in 30% of these cases)
- Most patients are asymptomatic

Imaging features

- Seen as a well-defined, round or oval mass of uniform density
- Thin-walled water-attenuation lesion on CT
- Daughter cysts seen as curved internal septations
- Cyst calcification in the lung is rare
- Rupture into the pleural or pericardial cavity is recognised: a ruptured cyst may have a crumpled wall or air–fluid levels

Tuberculosis

- 97% of cases caused by *Mycobacterium tuberculosis*
- 3% caused by *Mycobacterium avium-intracellulare* complex or *Mycobacterium kansasii*
- Acquired via droplet inhalation
- At-risk groups are the elderly, alcoholics and immunocompromised patients

Primary tuberculosis

- Majority of cases are subclinical
- Commonest in infants and young children
- Inhaled organisms settle in alveoli

Imaging features

- Lobar or segmental consolidation (with a predilection for middle and lower lobes) with ipsilateral hilar lymphadenopathy
- Bilateral hilar adenopathy is an unusual feature

- Lymph nodes have low-attenuation centres and rim enhancement
- Painless unilateral pleural effusion in 25% and is often the only feature
- Infection is self-limiting in immunocompetent patients
- Consolidation resolves completely in 70% of patients and with a scar in 30%
- Ranke's complex may be seen: a calcified scar and calcified hilar nodes
- Failure to contain primary infection causes dissemination of disease (progressive primary) with miliary and systemic spread

Post-primary tuberculosis

- Re-infection or reactivation of primary tuberculosis
- Parenchymal consolidation (usually in apical segment of the upper lobe) progressing to cavitation (in 50% of patients) is the hallmark of reactivation TB
- Cavitation leads to haematogenous and endobronchial dissemination (tree-in-bud pattern)
- Tracheobronchial stenosis and bronchiectasis occurs in 10–40% of cases
- Pleural effusion is less common than in primary disease, occurring in 18% of cases
- Lymphadenopathy is unusual, occurring in 5% of cases
- Miliary disease more common than in primary tuberculosis

Causes of lung cavities

- Abscess: staphylocci, *Klebsiella*, septic emboli
- Granulomas: tuberculosis, histoplasmosis, sarcoidosis
- Bronchogenic carcinoma: squamous cell carcinoma, adenocarcinomoa
- Metastases, e.g. from squamous cell carcinoma in the head and neck
- Vasculitis: Wegener's granulomatosis, rheumatoid arthritis, systemic lupus erythermatosus
- Cystic bronchiectasis
- Pulmonary infarction

Other pulmonary manifestations

Miliary tuberculosis

- Occurs in 1–7% of all patients with tuberculosis (more commonly in secondary than primary disease)
- Represents widespread haematogenous dissemination of disease
- Typically seen in infants, the elderly and immunocompromised patients
- Multiple opacities of < 5 mm seen throughout both lungs (in 50% of cases)
- Very rarely associated with pleural effusion
- Also causes meningitis, hepatosplenomegaly and lymphadenopathy
- Delay in diagnosis is common because it can mimic a wide range of pathology
- Nodules resolve after treatment without scarring or calcification

Causes of miliary shadowing

- Tuberculosis
- Non-tuberculous infections: histoplasmosis, varicella
- Pneumoconiosis: silicosis, coalworker's pneumoconiosis
- Metastases, e.g. from melanoma, thyroid tumour, renal tumour, choriocarcinoma
- Sarcoidosis
- Ossifications, e.g. in microlithiasis, mitral stenosis
- Histiocytosis X
- Amyloidosis

Tuberculous empyema

- Associated with residual pleural thickening and calcification

Mycetoma formation

- Colonisation of an apical scar cavity with *Aspergillus*
- Haemoptysis is very common
- Air crescent sign on CXR

Tuberculoma

- Seen in both primary and post-primary tuberculosis
- Localised disease, which alternately activates and heals
- Well-defined nodule of 1–4 cm diameter with satellite lesions
- Commonest in right upper lobe
- Calcifications may be seen but cavitation is rare

HIV- and AIDS-related lung disease

- The HIV retrovirus impairs cellular immunity by targeting CD4$^+$ T-helper cells
- It also impairs humoral immunity, and patients develop a range of chest complications, including opportunistic infections and rare malignancies

CD4$^+$ T-cell count and pulmonary disease

< 400 cells/mm^3: pyogenic infection, tuberculosis
< 200 cells/mm^3: pneumocystis
< 100 cells/mm^3: Kaposi's sarcoma, cytomegalovirus
< 50 cells/mm^3: lymphoma, *Mycobacterium avium-intracellulare* complex

Bacterial pneumonia

- Often the cause of a first AIDS-related chest infection
- Occurs at relatively high CD4$^+$ T-cell counts
- *Streptococcus pneumonia* and *Haemophilus influenza* are the commonest pathogens
- Same radiological pattern as seen in immunocompetent patients

Opportunistic infections

Pneumocystis carinii pneumonia (now renamed Pneumocystis jiroveci)

- AIDS-defining illness occurring with CD4$^+$ T-cell counts < 200 cells/mm^3
- Reactivation of infection acquired in early life
- *Pneumocystis carinii* is a unicellular fungus that adheres to type 1 pneumocytes
- Proliferation causes a foamy exudate and interstitial thickening
- Presents with insidious onset of dry cough, fever and exertional dyspnoea
- Raised serum lactate dehydrogenase
- Gallium-67 uptake occurs before CXR changes
- Mortality of 10% from respiratory failure
- Radiology can suggest the diagnosis but confirmation is by silver stain of induced sputum

Imaging features

CXR
- Normal CXR at presentation in 20% of cases
- Classically CXR shows bilateral symmetrical perihilar reticular opacities
- 10% develop thin-walled cysts (pneumatoceles)
- One third of pneumatoceles rupture, causing pneumothorax

HRCT
- Diffuse ground-glass change with peripheral sparing

Atypical patterns of Pneumocystis carinii pneumonia

- Miliary nodules
- Larger nodules, which cavitate
- Focal air space consolidations
- Pleural effusion
- Lymphadenopathy
- Upper zone distribution (seen with patients on pentamidine aerosol prophylaxis)

Invasive aspergillosis

- An often fatal infection in the severely immunocompromised
- Angioinvasion occurs, with haemorrhage and lung infarction
- Mortality is 60%

Imaging features

CXR

- Multiple, ill-defined patches of consolidation
- Lesions may cavitate in later stages of disease

HRCT

- Multiple nodules with surrounding ground-glass halos
- Lesions progress into more diffuse consolidation

Tuberculosis

- Commonest worldwide manifestation of AIDS
- Radiological features depend on severity of immunosuppression

Early-stage disease

- Manifestations are similar to those of non-AIDS-related tuberculosis
- Reactivation can occur with CD4+ T-cell counts < 400 cells/mm^3

Late-stage disease

- Inability to mount a cell-mediated response (negative tuberculin test)
- Rapid progression of newly acquired infection
- Diffuse bilateral reticulonodular infiltrates

Mycobacterium avium-intracellulare complex

- Commonly isolated but rarely clinically significant
- Complication of end-stage disease (when CD4+ T-cell counts < 50 cells/mm^3)
- Usually causes extrathoracic disease, e.g. small bowel infiltration
- Pulmonary appearances are non-specific and similar to those of tuberculosis

Non-infectious pulmonary Disease

Kaposi's sarcoma

- Commonest AIDS-associated malignancy
- Causal agent is human herpes virus-8
- Almost all cases occur in homosexual or bisexual men
- Occurs in late-stage disease; pulmonary disease is rare in the absence of mucocutaneous lesions
- Bronchoscopy shows raised erythematous lesions along the tracheobronchial tree
- Occasionally lesions are large and cause collapse of distal airways

Imaging features

CXR

- Coarse linear opacities radiating from the hilum
- Multiple, ill-defined pulmonary nodules
- Pleural effusions (serosanguinous) in the majority of cases

HRCT

- Nodules with surrounding ground-glass halos
- Distribution along the bronchovascular bundles
- Lymphadenopathy in 30% of cases, which shows uniform enhancement

Lymphocytic interstitial pneumonia

- Diffuse interstitial infiltration by lymphocytes and plasma cells
- Rare in adults but commonest pulmonary complication in children
- Other associations include Sjögren's syndrome and primary biliary cirrhosis

Imaging features

CXR

- Reticulonodular pattern in the mid-zone and lower zone

HRCT

- Diffuse bilateral ground-glass appearance and centrilobular nodules
- Slowly progressive over several years

AIDS-related lymphoma

- High-grade non-Hodgkin's lymphoma of B-cell type
- Usually involves extranodal sites, e.g. the CNS
- Intrathoracic involvement is uncommon

Imaging features

CXR

- Hilar and mediastinal lymphadenopathy
- Interstitial infiltrates
- Rapidly enlarging parenchymal nodules, which may cavitate

Hilar and mediastinal adenopathy in AIDS

- Most cases are due to reactive nodal hyperplasia
- Other causes include tuberculosis, Kaposi's sarcoma and lymphoma

---

Pulmonary thromboembolism

Anatomy

- The pulmonary trunk is approximately 5 cm long and begins at the pulmonary valve (anterior to the aorta)
- It passes posteriorly and to the left to lie in the concavity of the aortic arch where it bifurcates into right and left pulmonary arteries
- The pulmonary trunk is covered by pericardium to its bifurcation
- The right pulmonary artery runs horizontally to the right, posterior to the ascending aorta and anterior to the right main bronchus; it is crossed anteriorly by the right superior pulmonary vein
- The left pulmonary artery arches over the left main bronchus to lie posterior to it and is crossed anteriorly by the left superior pulmonary vein; it is attached to the aortic arch by the ligamentum arteriosum
- Each main pulmonary artery subdivides into lobar arteries and then segmental arteries, which accompany the bronchi

Thromboembolic disease

- Majority of pulmonary emboli are caused by venous thromboembolism
- Non-thrombotic causes include fat emboli, amniotic emboli and septic emboli
- Pulmonary emboli account for 5–10% of deaths in hospital patients
- Mortality is 30% mortality if untreated (from recurrent pulmonary embolism)
- Mortality is 3% with anticoagulation and/or IVC filter placement

Pathophysiology

- More than 90% of pulmonary emboli arise from venous thrombosis within the deep leg or pelvic veins
- Emboli reach the right atrium, where they fragment and shower into the pulmonary arterial tree

- Most lodge peripherally, but large thrombi can lodge within the right heart or straddle the main pulmonary artery bifurcation (saddle embolus)
- Entrapment within a pulmonary artery causes cessation of distal blood flow and an increase in pulmonary vascular resistance
- There is continuing ventilation beyond the embolus as the airways remain patent and ventilated
- Large or multiple emboli can cause sudden death secondary to severe right ventricular strain and circulatory collapse
- Only around 10% of pulmonary emboli cause lung infarction because there is generally good collateral supply via the bronchial arteries

Clinical assessment

- Pulmonary embolism has a wide spectrum of clinical manifestations ranging from absence of symptoms to sudden death
- The classic triad of dyspnoea, haemoptysis and pleuritic pain is rare
- In the majority of patients a combination of clinical and laboratory findings is insufficient for reliable diagnosis of acute pulmonary embolism
- Scoring criteria that are based on clinical features, D-dimer and ECG findings can help in the decision about which patients should proceed to imaging investigations

D-dimer blood test

- By-product of clot fibrinolysis
- Considered raised if > 0.5 mg/L
- Negative result virtually excludes a pulmonary embolism
- Low specificity, because it is raised in many other conditions

Imaging features

CXR

- Main role is to exclude other diagnoses, e.g. pneumothorax
- Normal in around 15% of cases
- Non-specific signs (common)
  - Linear atelectasis (in 70% of cases)
  - Parenchymal opacity (in 60% of cases)
  - Pleural effusion (in 50% of cases); typically small and unilateral
  - Elevated hemidiaphragm (in 30% of cases)
- Specific signs (in < 10% of cases)
  - Oligaemia distal to embolus (Westermark sign)
  - Enlarged artery proximal to embolus (Fleischner sign)
  - Pleural-based wedge-shaped opacity (Hampton hump)—an infarction causing haemorrhagic congestion that is visible 12–24 hours after an embolic episode; it rarely undergoes cavitation, and it resolves over months from the periphery inwards ('melts away') to leave a residual linear scar or pleural thickening

Causes of an oligaemic lung

- Pulmonary embolism
- Pneumothorax
- Mastectomy
- Emphysema
- Foreign body
- Poland's syndrome (absent pectoralis)
- Macleod's syndrome

V/Q scan

- Assessment of pulmonary blood flow and alveolar ventilation
- Effective dose is approximately 2 mSv
- Ventilation component
  - Xenon-133 or krypton-81 are the most commonly used agents
  - Particle size 0.1–0.5 micrometres
  - Inhaled via aerosol in upright position
  - Performed before perfusion scan
  - Normal study shows homogeneous tracer accumulation
- Perfusion component
  - Albumin macroaggregates labelled with technetium-99m
  - 300,000 particles in a standard dose, each 10–30 micrometres in size
  - Intravenous injection given with the patient in the supine position to minimise gravitational gradient
  - The particles are microembolised in the pulmonary arterial capillary bed during first pass through the lungs
  - The particles obstruct about 0.2% of the pulmonary capillary bed
  - A half dose perfusion study is performed in pregnancy
  - Normal study shows homogeneous tracer distribution
  - Areas of absent perfusion are seen as photopenic defects
  - A normal perfusion scan excludes 95% of pulmonary emboli

Conditions in which a reduced number of particles should be used

- Right-to-left shunt
- Pregnancy
- Pulmonary hypertension

Interpretation

- Pulmonary embolus indicated by absent perfusion and normal ventilation (a V/Q mismatch)
- Reporting is based on the modified PIOPED criteria, derived from the Prospective Investigation of Pulmonary Embolism Diagnosis (PIOPED) study
  - A high-probability scan suggests > 80% likelihood of a pulmonary embolus
  - An intermediate scan suggests 20–80% likelihood of a pulmonary embolus
  - A low-probability scan suggests < 20% likelihood of a pulmonary embolus
- A high-probability scan in combination with high clinical pretest probability is > 90% accurate
- A low-probability scan in combination with low clinical pretest probability is > 90% accurate

- However 50–70% of V/Q scans are intermediate (non-diagnostic)
- Around 30% of patients with intermediate scans will have a PE
- Brain or kidney uptake is diagnostic of a right-to-left shunt
- The stripe sign is a perfusion defect with a peripheral zone of preserved perfusion and suggests a diagnosis other than pulmonary embolism
- Patients with persisting perfusion defects are at risk of developing pulmonary hypertension

Causes of V/Q mismatch

- Pulmonary embolism
- Emphysema
- Extrinsic arterial compression, e.g. tumour
- Primary pulmonary hypertension
- Pulmonary vasculitis
- Intralobar sequestration
- Pulmonary artery hypoplasia

Causes of a matched V/Q defect

- Pulmonary infarction
- Emphysema
- Pulmonary fibrosis

Causes of a reverse V/Q mismatch, in which perfusion exceeds ventilation

- Chronic obstructive pulmonary disease
- Bronchiectasis
- Consolidation or collapse
- Pleural effusion

Pulmonary angiography

- An invasive test, formerly the gold-standard imaging test for pulmonary embolism
- Quoted sensitivity and specificity of > 95%

- Main use is prior to *in situ* thrombolysis
- Arrhythmias are most common non-fatal complication (occurring in 5% of cases)
- Quoted mortality is approximately 0.5%
- Emboli seen as intraluminal filling defects

CT pulmonary angiography (CTPA)

- Multi-detector CT has replaced pulmonary angiography as the reference standard for diagnosing acute pulmonary embolism
- Quoted sensitivity and specificity > 95% down to segmental level
- Test bolus or bolus tracking technique to ensure optimal opacification of the pulmonary arterial tree
- Effective dose 3–6 mSv (equivalent to 1–2 years' background radiation)
- Cannot reliably exclude subsegmental emboli
- The presence of right ventricular dysfunction carries a worse prognosis and is an indication for thrombolysis or surgery

Imaging features
- Intraluminal filling defects surrounded by contrast
  - 'Polo mint' sign on axial section
  - 'Railway track' sign on coronal section
- Pulmonary infarct shows as a subpleural opacity and pleural effusion in most cases
- Right ventricular strain is seen with massive pulmonary embolism
  - Right ventricular dilatation (right ventricular cavity wider than left ventricular cavity)
  - Reverse bowing of the interventricular septum
  - Contrast reflux into the hepatic veins

Pitfalls in CTPA
- Causes of false-negative results
  - Inadequate contrast opacification
  - Subsegmental emboli
  - Partial volume and respiratory motion artefacts
- Causes of false-positive results
  - Inadequate contrast opacification
  - Lymph nodes adjacent to central pulmonary arteries

- Bronchial mucus plugging adjacent to peripheral branches
- Contrast mixing with unenhanced blood from the IVC (caused by patient inspiration)

CT venography

- Performed 3–4 minutes after administration of intravenous contrast
- 95% concordance with ultrasound for femoral vein thrombus
- Superior to ultrasound for iliac vein and IVC thrombi
- Improves sensitivity of venous thromboembolism diagnosis
- Increases radiation exposure by 2–4 mSv

Pulmonary embolism in pregnancy

- Pulmonary embolism is twice to four times as common in pregnancy
- Increased frequency caused by pressure effects on pelvic veins by the gravid uterus in combination with increased blood viscosity
- Second commonest cause of maternal death during pregnancy
- D-dimer levels are normally raised during pregnancy

Imaging features

V/Q scan
- Absorbed fetal dose is 0.4–0.6 mSv
- Approximately 70% of V/Q scans in pregnancy are normal
- Approximately 25% of V/Q scans in pregnancy are non-diagnostic
- Half-dose perfusion-only scintigraphy is commonly used

CTPA
- Absorbed fetal dose is 0.03–0.06 mSv
- Around 5–10% of CTPA examinations in pregnancy are non-diagnostic
- Lactating breasts are very radiosensitive, and CTPA carries a high effective dose (7.4 mSv per breast)

Deep vein thrombosis (DVT)

- Risk factors include immobility, pregnancy, malignancy, intravenous drug use and hypercoagulable states
- The left leg is more commonly affected than the right leg, owing to the compressive effect on the left iliac vein of the right iliac artery crossing it
- Below-knee DVT has a 20% risk of proximal extension if untreated
- Saphenous vein thrombosis has a risk of propagation into the deep venous system

Imaging features

Ultrasound
- > 90% sensitive for above-knee DVT
- Acute DVT
  - Dilated vein containing echo-poor thrombus
  - Non-compressible and absent colour flow
  - Non-occlusive thrombus may allow some compressibility
  - Adductor canal segment may normally be non-compressible
- Chronic DVT
  - Echo-bright thrombus in a contracted vein (although echogenicity is an unreliable sign in that both fresh and old thrombus can appear hypoechoic or hyperechoic relative to muscle)
  - Colour flow may be seen within the thrombus as a result of partial re-canalisation

Indirect signs of DVT

- Loss of phasicity (normal respiratory variation) when scanning distal to clot
- Loss of normal velocity increase with distal compression when scanning proximal to clot

Non-thrombotic pulmonary embolism

Septic emboli

- Most commonly arise from tricuspid valve endocarditis
- Typically patients are intravenous drug users
- *Staphylococcus aureus* is the commonest pathogen

Imaging features

CXR
- Multiple peripheral nodular opacities
- Mid- and lower zone predominance
- Frequently undergo cavitation
- Empyema is a well-recognised complication

Fat embolism

- Mechanical obstruction of the pulmonary capillary bed by fat globules, which incite a toxic endothelial reaction
- Closed fracture of a lower limb long bone is the commonest cause
- Occurs in 1–3% of patients with femoral neck fractures
- Occurs in up to 20% of patients following major pelvic trauma
- Other causes include liposuction and pancreatitis
- Symptom lag > 24 hours
- Symptoms include dyspnoea, agitation and petechial rash

Imaging features

CXR
- Lag > 24 hours
- Bilateral patchy infiltrates
- Clears in 7–14 days, or may progress to ARDS
- Not associated with pleural effusion or pneumothorax

Amniotic fluid embolism

- Rare obstetrical emergency
- Amniotic fluid enters the maternal circulation through small tears in the uterine veins during labour
- This triggers a massive anaphylactic reaction with disseminated intravascular coagulation
- Abrupt onset of dyspnoea, cyanosis and hypotension
- Mortality is 80%, secondary to cardiopulmonary collapse

Imaging features

CXR
- Widespread bilateral air space consolidation

IVC filters

- Prevent pulmonary embolism by trapping thrombus from the pelvic and leg veins
- Endovascular placement under fluoroscopic guidance via a femoral or right internal jugular vein approach
- Most filters are permanent and placed in the IVC
- Indications for filter placement
  - DVT or pulmonary embolism with a contraindication to anticoagulation
  - DVT or pulmonary embolism with a complication from anticoagulation
  - Pulmonary embolism while on anticoagulation
  - Prophylaxis in high-risk patients, e.g. following pulmonary thromboendarterectomy

Indications for supra-renal filter placement

- Renal vein thrombosis
- IVC thrombus extending above the renal veins

Complications

- Failure: ongoing pulmonary embolism in 3% of patients
- IVC thrombosis in 10%
- Embolisation of the filter

Pulmonary arterial hypertension

- Mean pulmonary artery pressure > 25 mmHg at rest and > 30 mmHg with exercise
- Causes include idiopathic pulmonary hypertension, chronic thromboembolic pulmonary hypertension, longstanding left-to-right shunts and pulmonary veno-occlusive disease

Imaging features

CXR
- Enlarged proximal pulmonary arteries
- Peripheral pruning of vessels
- Right ventricular enlargement

CT
- Main pulmonary artery diameter > aortic diameter at corresponding level
- Right-sided cardiac chamber enlargement
- Right ventricular hypertrophy (free wall > 3 mm)
- Tricuspid regurgitation (shows as reflux of contrast into hepatic veins)
- Laminated (often partially calcified) thrombus lining the central pulmonary arteries

Idiopathic pulmonary arterial hypertension

- Smooth muscle hypertrophy of small pre-capillary pulmonary arteries (plexiform lesion)
- Mean age of presentation is 36 years, with a slight female preponderance
- Presents with progressive dyspnoea and signs of right heart strain
- 5-year survival rates around 55% with vasodilator infusions

Imaging features

CXR
- Findings suggestive of pulmonary hypertension at time of presentation in 90% of cases

V/Q scan
- Mottled appearance or low probability for pulmonary embolism

CT
- General features of pulmonary hypertension
- Lungs may be clear or have multiple centrilobular ground glass opacities

Intra- and extracardiac shunts

- Chronically raised blood flow induces intimal hyperplasia and a plexiform arteriopathy
- Pulmonary pressure (if untreated) may exceed systemic blood pressure, with partial or complete shunt reversal (Eisenmenger's syndrome). This is heralded by cyanosis and is considered inoperable

Causes
- Atrial septal defects: ostium secundum, ostium primum, sinus venosus
- Ventricular septal defects: perimembranous, muscular
- Partial anomalous pulmonary venous drainage (often associated with sinus venous type atrial septal defect)
- Patent ductus arteriosus
- Truncus arteriosus

Chronic thromboembolic pulmonary hypertension (CTEPH)

- 3–4% of patients with acute PE are thought to develop CTEPH
- Those with proximal disease affecting 5 or more segmental vessels may be candidates for thromboendarterectomy surgery

Imaging features

V/Q scan
- Multiple segmental and subsegmental perfusion defects

CT
- Multiple stenoses, webs and occlusions
- Laminated central thrombi are also common; approximately 10% are calcified
- Mosaic attenuation pattern on lung windows in 80–100% patients
- Bronchial artery hyperplasia, pericardial effusion and peripheral lung infarcts

Left heart disease

- Any longstanding condition that impedes pulmonary venous return can lead to pulmonary arterial hypertension
- Imaging findings are those of pulmonary venous hypertension with upper zone venous diversion and interstitial oedema
- Left atrial enlargement may be evident with mitral stenosis
- Causes
  - Mitral stenosis
  - Left ventricular failure
  - Left atrial myxoma
  - Fibrosing mediastinitis

Pulmonary veno-occlusive disease

- Intimal fibrosis of the pulmonary venules
- Associated with cytotoxic drugs and the ingestion of herbal teas
- Focal areas of oedema and haemorrhage

Imaging features

CT
- Interstitial oedema with septal thickening predominates
- Normal left atrial and pulmonary vein dimensions
- May be associated ground-glass opacities

Pulmonary capillary haemangiomatosis

- Uncontrolled capillary proliferation
- Treatment with vasodilator therapy can be fatal

Imaging features

CT
- Centrilobular 'fluffy', ground–glass nodules predominate
- Interlobular septal thickening may also be seen

Post-thoracotomy

- Lung resections are performed via a posterolateral incision through the fifth or fifth intercostal space

Pneumonectomy

- Fluid slowly fills the vacant hemithorax

Imaging features

- Rising air–fluid level over weeks to months
- Rate of fluid accumulation is very variable
- Tracheal and mediastinal shift towards the surgical side
- Bronchopleural fistula
  - Caused by dehiscence of the bronchial stump, infection or recurrent tumour
  - Drop in an existing air–fluid level
  - Air in a previously obliterated space
  - Mediastinal shift away from the surgical side
  - Aspiration of pneumonectomy space fluid into the contralateral lung
- Empyema
  - Reported incidence of 1–5%
  - CT is modality of choice for assessment
  - Expansion of post-pneumonectomy space, mediastinal shift towards the opposite side, straightening of the normally concave mediastinal border, and irregular, thick, enhancing residual pleura

Lobectomy

- The remaining lobes hyperinflate, the diaphragm elevates and the mediastinum shifts towards the surgical side
- Fluid slowly fills any remaining space with a rising air–fluid level over several weeks

Lines and tubes

Endotracheal tube

- Correct position is in mid-trachea, 5 cm above the carina

- A lower positioned tube may descend into the right main bronchus with neck flexion (causing right lung hyperinflation and carrying the risk of pneumothorax)

Complications of positive pressure ventilation

- Pneumothorax
- Pneumomediastinum
- Subcutaneous emphysema
- Pneumoperitoneum

Tracheostomy

- Should lie centrally in the trachea with the tip a few centimetres above the carina
- A small amount of surgical emphysema is expected
- Large-volume emphysema suggests tube leak or tracheal injury
- Long-term complication is tracheal stenosis

Central venous pressure line

- Used to monitor right atrial pressure
- Tip should be around the junction of the SVC and the right atrium
- Rarely, the tip may fracture, with embolisation

Swan–Ganz catheter

- Monitors pulmonary artery pressure
- Tip should lie 5 cm beyond pulmonary trunk in left or right pulmonary artery

Lung transplantation

Indications

- Accepted therapy for many forms of end-stage lung disease
- Single lung transplantation is the more commonly performed

- Indications include chronic obstructive pulmonary disease and interstitial lung disease e.g. lymphangioleiomyomatosis
- Double lung transplantation is performed in pulmonary hypertension and cystic fibrosis
- Contraindicated in malignancy or with active extrathoracic infection

Early complications

- Reperfusion oedema
  - A re-implantation response
  - Non-cardiogenic pulmonary oedema
  - Begins in the first 48 hours after transplant and resolves by day 10
  - Caused by a combination of surgical trauma, ischaemia and denervation of transplanted lung
  - CXR shows perihilar haziness of the transplanted lung
  - Diagnosis of exclusion (not due to infection, oedema or rejection)
- Acute rejection
  - Very common: 80% have an episode in the first 3 months after transplant
  - Non-specific symptoms (fever, tachypnoea and dyspnoea)
  - CXR shows non-specific features: septal lines and pleural effusions
  - Transbronchial biopsy shows perivascular lymphocytic infiltrate
  - HRCT shows multifocal patchy areas of ground-glass attenuation
  - Treated by increasing the degree of immunosuppression
- Infection
  - Commonest cause of perioperative mortality
  - Occurs in up to 50% of lung transplant recipients
  - Denervated lung has impaired mucociliary drainage
  - Commonest organisms are *Pseudomonas*, *Aspergillus* and cytomegalovirus
  - Patients are given prophylactic antibacterial, antifungal and antiviral drugs

- Airway anastomotic dehiscence
  - Potentially fatal complication affecting < 2% of patients
  - Blood supply to the bronchi is via the bronchial artery and is impaired by low cardiac output states, leading to ischaemia
  - Bronchial stenosis is a recognised late complication

Late complications

- Chronic rejection
  - Pathologically the features are those of bronchiolitis obliterans, with a submucosal inflammatory process of the terminal bronchioles
  - Eventually leads to fibrosis and permanent obliteration
  - HRCT shows mosaic attenuation (air trapping)
- Post-transplant lymphoproliferative disorder
  - Occurs in approximately 5% of patients after a lung transplant (higher than for any other organ)
  - Associated with Epstein–Barr virus
  - Occurs at a mean of 4 months' postoperatively
  - Ranges in severity from low to aggressive high-grade non-Hodgkin's lymphoma
  - CT shows multiple pulmonary nodules and mediastinal adenopathy

Post-cardiac surgery

- Most operations performed via a midline sternotomy
- Left lateral thoracotomy used for mitral valvotomy or coarctation of the aorta
- Majority have a small left pleural effusion and basal atelectasis
- Phrenic nerve damage can cause hemidiaphragm paralysis
- Thoracic duct damage causes a chylous pleural effusion
- Mediastinitis is uncommon, occurring in < 1% of patients
- Late autoimmune pericarditis is recognised (Dressler's syndrome)

- Leading cause of death in children and young adults in the UK
- Majority of cases caused by road traffic accidents

Fractures

Rib fractures

- Commonest skeletal injury resulting from blunt chest trauma
- Complications include pneumothorax and pulmonary contusions
- First to third rib fractures
  - Markers of high-velocity injury
  - Associated with brachial plexus and subclavian vessel injury
- Eighth to 11th rib fractures
  - Associated with hepatic, splenic and renal injuries
  - Splenic injury is associated with rib fractures in 40% of cases
  - In children there is a strong association with non-accidental injury
- Flail chest
  - Two fracture sites on each of three or more consecutive ribs
  - Free-floating segment moves paradoxically with respiration
  - Associated with massive underlying lung contusion
  - Impairs mechanics of ventilation and requires ventilatory support

Sternal fracture

- Uncommon injury usually caused by a direct blow
- Displaced fractures associated with myocardial contusion
- Anterior mediastinal haematoma is a common finding

Thoracic spine fracture

- Commonest at the mobile thoracolumbar junction region
- Usually a hyperflexion injury or an axial compression (burst) injury
- Associated with spinal cord injury in 40% of cases

Imaging features

CXR
- Haematoma seen as a bulge in the left paraspinal line

Pleural space

Haemothorax

- Blood in the pleural space
- Usually from intercostal venous or arterial bleeding

Imaging features

CXR
- Detected on frontal CXR when > 250 mL
- Concave upward sloping of costophrenic angle (meniscus sign)

CT
- High-attenuation fluid (35–70 HU)

Thoracic duct

- Drains lymph from the abdomen and lower limbs
- Arises from the cisterna chyli behind the right crus of the diaphragm
- Enters the thoracic cavity through the aortic hiatus
- Ascends anterior to the vertebral column between the azygous vein and the aorta
- The posterior intercostal arteries and the hemiazygous vein cross behind it
- At the level of the carina (T5) it deviates to the left of the oesophagus
- Ascends into the neck and passes behind the left subclavian vessels
- Arches anteriorly over the left lung apex to drain into the left internal jugular vein at its junction with the subclavian vein

Chylothorax

- Can occur following chest trauma or in patients with lymphangioleiomyomatosis

Imaging features

CXR
- Low-attenuation fluid (negative HU value)

Pneumothorax

- Occurs in 30–40% of cases of major chest and abdominal trauma
- Usually caused by a rib fracture or penetrating injury
- Chest drain indicated if clinical signs of tension are present
- Unilateral oedema (re-expansion) is well recognised
- If pneumothorax does not respond to the insertion of a chest drain, consider a malpositioned drain, a tracheobronchial injury or a bronchopleural fistula

Causes of pneumothorax

Spontaneous pneumothorax:
- Rupture of a subpleural bleb
- Paraseptal emphysema
- Infections, e.g. *Pneumocystis carinii* pneumonia
- Cystic lung disease e.g. lymphangioleiomyomatosis
- Osteosarcoma metastases

Traumatic pneumothorax:
- Rib fracture with laceration
- Chest compression injury

Iatrogenic pneumothorax:
- Central line insertion
- Lung biopsy

Imaging features

Erect CXR
- Thin line of visceral pleura with absent peripheral lung markings
- Appearances become more pronounced on expiratory film

Supine CXR
- Deep costophrenic sulcus sign

Tension pneumothorax

- Progressive build-up of air due to a one-way valve mechanism
- Compression of SVC leads to rapid circulatory collapse

Imaging features

CXR
- Contralateral mediastinal shift
- Depression of ipsilateral hemidiaphragm
- Widening of intercostal spaces

Pulmonary contusion

- Commonest lung injury in blunt chest trauma (occurring in 30–70% of cases)
- Capillary haemorrhage into alveolar and interstitial spaces
- Radiographically apparent within 6 hours of injury
- Haemoptysis is most frequent clinical symptom

Imaging features

CXR
- Non-segmental air space consolidation

CT
- Parenchymal opacification with subpleural sparing
- Imaging hallmark is rapid resolution (usually within 72 hours)

Diaphragm

Anatomy

- Dome-shaped sheet separating the thoracic and abdominal cavities
- Peripheral fibromuscular bands converge on to a central tendon
- Thoracic surface lined by parietal pleura
- Abdominal surface lined by peritoneum except over the bare area
- Anteriorly attaches to the xiphisternum, laterally to the lower six costal cartilages and posteriorly to the crura and arcuate ligaments
- Medial arcuate ligament is a fascial thickening over the psoas muscle
- Lateral arcuate ligament is a fascial thickening over the quadratus lumborum muscle
- The crura are attached between vertebral bodies L1 and L3
- The median arcuate ligament lies between the two crura – the aorta, azygous vein and thoracic duct pass behind it at the T12 level

- Openings
  - Oesophagus at the T10 level
  - IVC at the T8 level
- The right phrenic nerve passes through the IVC hiatus. Lymphatics and branches of the left phrenic nerve pierce the diaphragm
- A small posterolateral defect (Bochdalek hernia) and areas of marked thinning (eventration) occur in up to 5% of the population

Diaphragm rupture

- Occurs in 1–8% of patients who survive major chest or abdominal trauma
- Blunt trauma causes a sudden rise in intra-abdominal pressure
- Left-sided tears are seen in 70% of cases, right-sided tears in 30% (because of the protective effect of the liver)
- The posterolateral region is commonest location
- Defects are usually large (> 10 cm) in blunt trauma; penetrating trauma usually causes small focal tears (< 2 cm)
- Associated with splenic, liver and thoracic spine injuries
- Potentially devastating complications if not repaired
- Negative pressure pulls abdominal contents into the thoracic cavity
- Visceral strangulation has a > 50% mortality

Imaging features

CXR
- Unreliable for evaluation of diaphragmatic injury
- May see intra-thoracic abdominal viscera or the tip of a nasogastric tube in the chest

CT
- Multiplanar reconstructions improve detection
- Collar sign
- Constriction of stomach or other viscera by the defect
- Dependent viscera sign
- Stomach or spleen contacting posterior chest wall (on axial sections)

MRI
- T1 sequence: a dark line with bright fat on either side is normal

- Tears seen as a defect in this low-signal line

Mediastinal injury

Blunt traumatic aortic injury

- Shearing injury caused by sudden deceleration (usually as a result of a road traffic accident)
- 90% of tears occur at the relatively 'fixed' isthmus; 4–5% occur at the arch of the aorta; 5–9% occur in the ascending aorta; 1–3% occur at the diaphragmatic hiatus
- 80–90% of cases involve laceration through all three layers of the aortic wall, resulting in exsanguination and death at the scene
- The incomplete type of injury may not be recognised in clinically stable patients and may evolve into a pseudoaneurysm with a high risk of late rupture; CT has lead to improved detection of these injuries
- Endovascular repair is the current gold standard for pseudoaneurysm
- Occasionally may present years later with incidental CXR finding of a calcified mediastinal mass
- Imaging involves demonstration of aortic wall abnormality (direct sign) or indirect evidence such as a mediastinal haematoma
- A mediastinal haematoma which does not abut the aorta or great vessels usually represents venous bleeding

Imaging features

CXR
- A normal CXR has a high negative predictive value (98%) for aortic injury but does not exclude it
- Indirect signs of mediastinal haematoma
  - Superior mediastinal widening
  - Indistinct aortic arch outline
  - Trachea and oesophageal deviated to the right
  - Depression of the left main bronchus
  - Widened left paraspinal stripe
  - Widened right paratracheal stripe
  - Left apical pleural cap

CT
- Aortic wall contour abnormality or defect
- Adjacent mediastinal haematoma

- Intraluminal clot at the site of intimal disruption
- Pseudoaneurysm or aortic dissection (rare)
- Pericardial haematoma and coronary artery extension may be seen if the ascending aorta is involved

Aortogram
- Reserved for problem solving in equivocal cases and for guiding endovascular stent graft placement

Tracheobronchial tear

- Uncommon injury, occurring in 1–3% of cases of major blunt chest trauma
- Associated with high rib fractures and multiple organ injury
- Bronchial tear more common than tracheal injury
- Right main bronchus is the most commonly injured site
- 80% of cases occur within 2.5 cm of the carina
- Signs of pneumomediastinum, pneumothorax and surgical emphysema
- May be indicated by a pneumothorax that fails to respond to chest tube placement
- Lung collapses peripherally as a result of disruption of the normal central attachments holding it to the mediastinum ('fallen lung' sign)

1.11 Mediastinum

Anatomy

- Extends from thoracic inlet to diaphragm. Divided into two parts
  - Superior mediastinum
  - Inferior mediastinum, which is further divided into anterior, middle and posterior sections

Superior mediastinum

- From thoracic inlet to an imaginary line drawn between the T4 vertebral body and manubriosternal junction
- Contents
  - The arch of the aorta and its branches
  - The SVC and the brachiocephalic veins
  - The trachea
  - The oesophagus
  - The thoracic duct and lymph nodes
- Causes of a superior mediastinal mass
  - Goitre
  - Cystic hygroma
  - Lymphoma

Imaging features

CXR
- Widened paratracheal stripe
- Tracheal deviation
- Negative cervicothoracic sign: a mass extending above the clavicle with no lung tissue between the mass and the neck

Thyroid masses

- Normal thyroid extends to just below level of cricoid cartilage
- Thyroid goitres and rarely carcinomas can extend retrosternally
- Anaplastic carcinoma is the commonest type of thyroid mass to do this
- Extension is usually anterior to the brachiocephalic vessels
- Rarely can extend behind the oesophagus
- Tracheal deviation is common
- Tracheal and oesophageal compression is recognised

Imaging features

CT
- Mediastinal thyroid mass
  - Continuous with the thyroid gland above
  - High attenuation on non-contrast scan (because of the high iodine content of the thyroid)
  - May contain punctuate calcifications
  - Displays marked contrast enhancement

Anterior mediastinum

- Space between sternum and pericardium
- Contents are the thymus, internal mammary vessels and lymph nodes
- Causes of an anterior mediastinal mass
  - Thymic lesions
  - Teratoma
  - Thyroid goitre/tumour
  - Terrible lymphoma

Normal thymus

- Bi-lobed gland with an arrowhead appearance
- Undergoes fatty replacement or involution with age
- Normally visualised on CT in < 50% of people over the age of 40 years
- Normal anteroposterior diameter in adults < 13 mm
- CT shows homogeneous soft tissue attenuation
- MRI shows a mildly high T1 signal and a very high T2 signal

Thymic hyperplasia

- Gland retains its normal shape
- Gland retains homogeneous CT attenuation and MRI signal
- Causes
  - Hyperthyroidism
  - Acromegaly

- Addison's disease
- Rebound after chemotherapy, burns or a course of corticosteroids

Thymoma

- Commonest tumour of the anterior mediastinum
- Peak age 50 years
- Often an incidental CXR finding (in 50% of cases)
- Paraneoplastic symptoms are common
  - Myasthenia gravis (in 50% of cases)
  - Hypogammaglobulinaemia (in 10% of cases)
  - Pure red cell aplasia (in 5% of cases)

> **Thymic lesions in myasthenia gravis**
>
> - 20% will have a thymoma
> - 65% will have thymic hyperplasia
>
> CT is routinely performed in all patients with myasthenia gravis

Benign thymoma

- Accounts for two thirds of thymomas
- Tumour does not breach the thymic capsule

Imaging features

CT
- Well-defined, lobulated mass distorting the normal thymic contour
- 30% contain areas of necrosis and haemorrhage
- 7% contain thin peripheral capsular calcifications
- Surrounding fat plane is preserved
- Displays mild contrast enhancement

Invasive thymoma

- Accounts for one third of thymomas
- Tumour breaches the thymic capsule and spreads contiguously through the mediastinum and into the pleural space, where it disseminates via drop metastases
- Trans-diaphragmatic spread can occur via the retrocrural space to involve the upper abdominal organs and retroperitoneum

Imaging features

CT
- Ill-defined mass encasing or invading mediastinal structures
- Drop metastases seen as areas of nodular pleural thickening

Thymic cyst

- Congenital cyst
  - Arises from remnants of the thymopharyngeal duct
  - CT shows a thin-walled, unilocular cyst of water attenuation
  - Can appear more solid if there is a high protein content
  - MRI shows a low T1 signal and a high T2 signal
- Acquired cyst
  - Seen in thymic tumours and in HIV-positive patients
  - Multilocular cyst with variable wall thickness

Thymolipoma

- Rare benign tumour composed of fat and thymic tissue
- Can reach a large size, with compression of adjacent structures

Thymic carcinoma

- Rare aggressive malignancy
- Very locally invasive with early lymphatic and distant spread
- Heterogeneous, ill-defined mass with mediastinal adenopathy and pleural and pericardial effusions

Thymic carcinoid

- Neuroendocrine tumour arising from the (APUD) cell line
- Associated with multiple endocrine neoplasia (MEN) type 1
- Carcinoid syndrome is very rare
- 40% secrete ACTH, causing Cushing's syndrome
- Large heterogeneous invasive mass

Germ cell tumour

- Mediastinum is the commonest extragonadal site

- Arises from mediastinal cell rests
- Accounts for 10% of anterior mediastinal masses
- Commonest between the second and fourth decades
- Teratoma is the commonest subtype

Teratoma

- Tissue elements from more than one germ cell layer
- Majority are benign (< 3% become malignant)
- Rarely rupture into the pleural or pericardial space

Imaging features: CT
- Multicystic mass with enhancing septae
- 60% contain fat (fat-fluid level is diagnostic)
- Commonly contains foci of calcification

Ectopic parathyroid adenoma

- 20% of parathyroid adenomas are ectopic
- Anterior mediastinum is a common site
- Preoperative localisation via MRI or technetium-99m MIBI scan, with a combined accuracy of > 90%

Imaging features

MRI
- Well-defined, rounded mass of 1–2 cm diameter
- High T2 signal ('light bulb' sign)

Technetium 99m MIBI
- Adenoma shows tracer accumulation

Middle mediastinum

- Contents
  - The heart
  - The great vessels
  - Lymph nodes
  - The oesophagus
  - The trachea
  - The bronchi
- Causes of a middle mediastinal mass
  - Lymphadenopathy
  - Aortic arch vascular anomalies
  - Azygous vein anomalies
  - Mediastinal bronchogenic cyst
  - Oesophageal tumours, duplication cyst
  - Pericardial cyst

Imaging features

CXR
- Filling in of AP window
- Displaced azygo-oesophageal recess

Bronchogenic cyst

- Arises from abnormal budding of the ventral foregut
- Lined by ciliated columnar respiratory epithelium
- Mediastinal bronchogenic cyst
  - Accounts for two thirds of bronchogenic cysts
  - Most often in a subcarinal or right paratracheal location
  - Can cause stridor, dysphagia and intractable cough
  - Can rarely compress the main stem coronary artery
- Intrapulmonary bronchogenic cyst
  - Accounts for one third of bronchogenic cysts
  - Predilection for the lower lobes
  - Commonly present with secondary infection

Imaging features

CXR
- Rounded, fluid-density mass near the carina

CT
- Sharply marginated mass with a smooth border
- 50% show water attenuation, 50% higher attenuation (because they contain protein or blood)
- 1–2% have calcified walls or milk of calcium within cyst fluid
- May display a thin rim of mural enhancement

MRI
- Variable T1 signal, uniformly high T2 signal

Pericardial cyst

- See below (Section 2.14)

Posterior mediastinum

- Space between the posterior aspect of the heart and the vertebral column

- Contents
  - Descending thoracic aorta
  - Parasympathetic chain
  - Nerve roots
  - Lymph nodes
  - Vertebrae
- Causes of a posterior mediastinal mass
  - Neurogenic tumour
  - Lymphoma
  - Paraspinal abscess
  - Bochdalek's hernia
  - Extramedullary haemopoiesis

Imaging features

CXR
- Widened paratracheal stripe
- Positive cervicothoracic sign: a mass extending above the clavicle with lung tissue between the mass and the neck

Neurogenic tumours

Schwannomas and neurofibroma
- Benign nerve sheath tumour that grows along parent nerve
- 50% of neurofibromas occur in patients with neurofibromatosis type 1
- Rounded mass orientated along axis of intercostal nerve
- May have an intraspinal component ('dumbbell-shaped')
- MRI shows a high-signal T2 rim with a low-signal centre ('target' sign)

Sympathetic ganglia tumour
- Ganglioneuroma (in young adults) and neuroblastoma (in children)
- Oval, paraspinal mass vertically orientated along the spine

Parasympathetic tumour
- Extra-adrenal phaeochromocytoma
- Commonest in the aortopulmonary window and paravertebral region
- MRI shows heterogeneous mass lesions that enhance avidly

Paraspinal abscess
- Develops from spread of osteomyelitis in a vertebral body
- Most commonly caused by tuberculosis
- Rim enhancement with non-enhancing central pus collection

- Associated vertebral body destruction and disc space narrowing

Extramedullary haemopoiesis
- Haemopoietic activity occurring at sites other than bone marrow
- Seen in severe anaemia or extensive marrow infiltration
- Commonly involves the liver, spleen and lymph nodes
- Can cause well-defined bilateral paravertebral masses

Mediastinitis

Acute bacterial mediastinitis
- Life-threatening condition with a 50% mortality
- Most commonly caused by oesophageal perforation
- Rarely a complication of cardiac surgery or from direct spread of retropharyngeal infection

Imaging features

CXR
- Widened mediastinal outline
- Pneumomediastinum and subcutaneous emphysema
- Air–fluid levels with abscess formation

CT
- Extraluminal mediastinal air and peri-oesophageal fluid collections

Oesophageal perforation

Distal (iatrogenic or due to foreign body, malignancy, Boerhaave's syndrome)
- Left-sided pleural effusion
- Normal mediastinal outline

Proximal (due to blunt chest trauma)
- Right-sided pleural effusion
- Widened mediastinum

Contrast swallow studies show extraluminal contrast extravasation and are 90% accurate for detecting a perforation

Fibrosing mediastinitis

- Progressive hilar and mediastinal infiltration by fibrous tissue
- Idiopathic, or secondary to tuberculosis, histoplasmosis, sarcoidosis, radiotherapy, drug reaction, retroperitoneal fibrosis
- Causes progressive encasement of mediastinal structures, with narrowing of the trachea, main bronchi, SVC, pulmonary veins, pulmonary artery, left atrium and brachiocephalic veins
- Often presents with symptoms of airway compromise or SVC obstruction

Imaging features

CXR
- Non-specific, may show calcified hilar and mediastinal nodes

CT
- Localised or diffuse soft-tissue mediastinal mass
- Commonly contains calcifications
- Obliterates fat planes and compresses adjacent structures

Pneumomediastinum

- Causes
  - Asthma (commonest cause)
  - Oesophageal perforation
  - Intraperitoneal or retroperitoneal free air, which can track superiorly
  - Bronchial perforation

Imaging features

CXR
- Streaky translucencies, best seen along the left heart border
- Subcutaneous emphysema in the neck
- Continuous diaphragm sign
- Air outlines thymus ('thymic sail' sign) seen in children

Venous pathology

Anatomy

- The azygous vein commences anterior to the L2 vertebral body as a branch of the IVC or a continuation of the right ascending lumbar vein

- It then ascends to the right of the aorta and the thoracic duct, entering the thorax behind the median arcuate ligament
- The right second to 12th intercostal veins drain into it (the right first intercostal vein drains directly into the right brachiocephalic vein)
- The right posterior intercostal arteries cross behind it
- At the T5 level the azygous vein arches anteriorly over the right main bronchus to drain into the SVC
- The hemiazygous vein commences anterior to the L2 vertebral body as a branch of the left renal vein or left ascending lumbar vein
- It ascends to the left of the aorta and the thoracic duct
- At the T9 level it crosses laterally, draining into the azygous vein
- The accessory hemiazygous vein receives the left fourth to eighth intercostal veins (the left first to third intercostal veins drain directly into the left brachiocephalic vein) and descends on the left side of the vertebral column
- At the T8 level it crosses laterally draining into the azygous vein

SVC obstruction

Causes of SVC obstruction

Malignant (80% of cases)
- Bronchogenic carcinoma
- Lymphoma
- Mesothelioma

Benign (20% of cases)
- Central venous catheters
- Fibrosing mediastinitis
- Constrictive pericarditis
- Ascending aortic aneurysm

- Presents with upper extremity swelling and dyspnoea, and dilated chest wall collateral veins
- Blood drains to right heart via azygous vein and other collaterals
- Treatment of malignant causes is with

radiotherapy, chemotherapy or placement of self-expanding stents
- Benign causes are more difficult to traverse with stents

Persistent left SVC
- Commonest congenital venous anomaly
- Failure of obliteration of the left anterior cardinal vein
- Occurs in 0.5% of the general population but in up to 4% of patients with congenital heart disease
- 90% connect to the right atrium via the coronary sinus
- 10% connect to the left atrium (right-to-left shunt)

Azygous continuation of IVC
- Associated with total anomalous pulmonary venous drainage, polysplenia and rarely asplenia
- Suprarenal portion of the IVC is absent

- Venous blood reaches heart via the azygous or hemi-azygous veins
- Hepatic veins drain directly into right atrium

Imaging features

CXR
- Dilated azygous vein
- Widened paravertebral stripes

CT
- Dilated azygous veins and azygous arch

Causes of azygous vein enlargement (> 1 cm)
• Inspiration
• Right heart failure
• Portal hypertension
• Constrictive pericarditis
• SVC or IVC obstruction
• Azygous continuation of IVC

1.12 Aorta

Anatomy

Thoracic aorta

- Composed of the aortic root and ascending, arch and descending parts
- Originates at the aortic valve (which lies posterior to pulmonary trunk)
- The coronary arteries arise from the three sinuses of Valsalva above the valve cusps
- Left coronary ostia from left sinus, right coronary from right sinus. The posteriorly placed non-coronary sinus does not normally give rise to a coronary artery
- The left coronary artery arises from the left sinus and the right coronary artery from the right sinus. No vessel arises from the non-coronary cusp (the most posterior cusp)
- The thoracic aorta arches posteriorly from right to left over the pulmonary trunk, left main bronchus and left pulmonary artery
- The origin is invested in a pericardial sheath with the pulmonary trunk
- The aortic arch lies at the level of T4 and gives off the innominate, left common carotid and left subclavian arteries (variations are common)
- These are crossed anteriorly by the left brachiocephalic vein
- The left superior intercostal vein passes anterior to arch as it drains into the left brachiocephalic artery (the 'aortic nipple' on CXR)
- The aortic arch becomes the descending aorta at the isthmus where the ligamentum arteriosum attaches, making this part of aorta prone to deceleration injuries
- The descending aorta courses inferiorly through the posterior mediastinum with the spinal column to its right and the lung to its left
- The descending aorta gives off nine pairs of posterior intercostals arteries (the third to 12th intercostal arteries)

- The upper two pairs arise from the costocervical trunk of the subclavian artery
- The anterior intercostal arteries arise from the internal mammary arteries
- The descending aorta passes through diaphragm behind the median arcuate ligament at T12 to become the abdominal aorta

Abdominal aorta

- Retroperitoneal course from the hiatus to the bifurcation at L4
- Midline unpaired branches
  - Coeliac artery (at T12 level)
  - superior mesenteric artery (at L1 level)
  - inferior mesenteric artery (at L3 level)
- Lateral paired branches
  - Inferior phrenic arteries (at T12 level)
  - Middle adrenal arteries (at L1 level)
  - Renal arteries (at L2 level)
  - Gonadal arteries (at L3 level)
  - Lumbar arteries (two pairs)

Congenital anomalies of the aortic arch

Left aortic arch branch patterns

- Together account for up to 99% of cases
- Classical pattern (innominate, left carotid, left subclavian arteries) (70% of cases)
- Left common carotid common artery origin with the innominate artery (12% of cases)
- Left common carotid artery arises from the innominate artery (bovine arch) (9% of cases)
- Left vertebral artery arises directly from the arch (5% of cases)
- Aberrant right subclavian artery (0.4–2% of cases)
- Common origin of left common carotid and subclavian arteries (1% of cases)
- Separate origin of right common carotid and subclavian arteries (1% of cases)

Right aortic arch branch patterns

- Together account for up to 1–2% of cases
- Mirror-image branching (in order: left innominate artery, right common carotid artery, right subclavian artery (65% of cases)
- Aberrant left subclavian artery (in order: left common carotid artery, right common carotid artery, right subclavian artery, aberrant left subclavian artery (35% of cases)

Double aortic arch

- A rare anomaly

Left arch with aberrant right subclavian artery

- Right subclavian artery arises as last branch of the aortic arch
- Associated with congenital heart defects in 10–15% of cases
- Usually asymptomatic, can rarely cause 'dysphagia lusoria'

Imaging features

CXR
- Right paratracheal opacity
- Opacity posterior to trachea on lateral CXR

CT
- Last and most posterior vessel to come off aortic arch
- Origin is commonly dilated (Kommerell's diverticulum)
- Traverses the mediastinum
  - Posterior to oesophagus in 80% of cases
  - Between oesophagus and trachea in 15% of cases
  - Anterior to trachea in 5% of cases

Double aortic arch

- Most common and serious vascular ring
- Complete vascular ring around trachea and oesophagus
- Presents in neonates or children with respiratory distress and stridor
- The descending aorta is left-sided in 75% of cases
- The ascending aorta divides into separate right and left arches, which pass on either

side of the trachea; the right arch is higher than left
- Each arch gives a single subclavian and common carotid artery
- The subclavian arteries arise posterior to the carotids
- The right arch crosses behind the oesophagus to join the left arch as the descending thoracic aorta

Imaging features

CT and MRI
- Four vessels evenly spaced around trachea – four artery' sign on axial image

Contrast swallow
- Lateral view shows posterior indentation
- Frontal view shows bilateral indentations ('reverse S-shape')

Coarctation of the aorta

- Eccentric luminal narrowing caused by infolding of the aortic wall
- Most commonly a focal narrowing distal to the origin of the left subclavian artery
- Blood flow to the descending aorta via intercostal collateral vessels
- Rarely a long segment of tubular hypoplasia, which presents in neonates with heart failure and congenital cardiac anomalies

> ## Associations in tubular hypoplasia type
>
> - Bicuspid aortic valve
> - Intracardiac malformations
> - Turner's syndrome (45XO)
> - Berry aneurysms

Imaging features

CXR
- 'Figure three' sign of pre- and post-stenotic dilatation
- Inferior rib notching (of third to ninth ribs) from dilated intercostal collaterals
- Unilateral, right-sided rib notching in the right aortic arch with coarctation proximal to an aberrant left subclavian artery

- Unilateral left-sided rib notching in the left aortic arch with coarctation proximal to an aberrant right subclavian artery

CT angiogram
- Modality of choice for follow-up after stent insertion

MRI (modality of choice pre-stent and postsurgery)
- Modality of choice before and after stent insertion
- Clearly depicts extent of coarctation, quantifies the shunt and shows the collateral vessels
- Complications include re-coarctation and aneurysm formation

Pseudocoarctation

- Elongation of the ascending aorta ('high aortic arch')
- Arch buckles at ligamentum arteriosum insertion
- No pressure gradient across buckle
- No rib notching
- Anteromedial deviation of aorta and oesophagus
- Associated with hypertension, bicuspid aortic valve, patent ductus arteriosus, atrial septal defect, ventricular septal defect and a single ventricle

Aortic dissection

- Caused by an intimal tear; blood dissects into the tunica media, creating a false lumen
- Central tearing chest pain radiating between the scapulae
- Asymmetric peripheral pulses and blood pressures (in 60% of cases)
- Stanford classification
  - Type A (70% of cases): involves the ascending aorta with or without involvement of the arch
  - Type B (30% of cases): begins distal to the origin of the left subclavian artery and involves only the descending aorta

Risk factors

- Hypertension (60–90% of cases)
- Pregnancy
- Coarctation
- Bicuspid aortic valve
- Adult polycystic kidney disease
- Marfan's syndrome
- Ehlers–Danlos syndrome
- Vasculitis, e.g. systemic lupus erythematosus, rheumatoid arthritis, Takayasu's arteritis

Type A dissection
- High early mortality if not treated promptly
- Requires surgical intervention (surgical mortality is 10–35%)
- Endovascular approach is a new treatment option being trialled
- Complications
  - Dissection extension into the coronary arteries (causes myocardial infarction)
  - Dissection extension into the common carotid arteries (causes stroke)
  - Rupture into the pericardial sac (causes cardiac tamponade)
  - Aortic valve disruption (causes acute aortic regurgitation in 60% of cases)

Type B dissection
- Best treated initially with blood pressure control
- Often become aneurysmal over time, requiring endovascular stenting or surgery
- Endovascular or surgical intervention is needed if the dissection becomes symptomatic secondary to distal compromise, i.e. mesenteric, renal or limb ischaemia

Imaging of dissection
CXR
- Normal in 25% of cases
- Mediastinal widening in 60% of cases
- Ill-defined aortic arch contour
- Inward displacement of intimal calcification (> 1 cm)

Multidetector CT
- > 95% accurate
- Modality of choice in the acute setting
- Contrast-enhanced acquisition shows dissection as two opacified channels separated by an intimal flap
- ECG-gating is technique of choice for assessing extension into the aortic root and coronary arteries
- Features of false lumen
  - Larger than true lumen
  - Anterior in the ascending aorta, posterolateral in the descending aorta
  - Rarely thrombosed in the acute setting
  - Delayed enhancement compared with true lumen
  - Partial luminal thrombosis is an adverse prognostic sign on follow-up of type B dissection

MRI
- T1 spin-echo shows blood as black; flap seen as a high-signal line
- Post-gadolinium (superior to black blood sequence): contrast is bright, flap seen as dark line

Transoesophageal echocardiogram
- > 90% accurate
- High resolution imaging which clearly depicts the intimal flap
- Aortic valve, ascending and descending aorta are well seen
- Aortic arch and branches often obscured by trachea – 'blind spot'

Arch aortogram
- Traditional technique but currently only used prior to endovascular repair

CT pitfalls in aortic dissection

False negatives
- Insufficient contrast enhancement of aortic lumen
- Too slow an injection rate, poor timing of contrast bolus

False positives
- Streak artefacts
  - Contrast in the SVC
  - Contrast in left brachiocephalic vein (left arm injection)
  - Pacemaker leads, surgical clips
  - Curvilinear aortic motion artefacts (ECG-gating improves this)
- Structures adjacent to ascending aorta
  - Aortic valve cusps
  - Superior pericardial recess
  - Residual thymic tissue
- Structures adjacent to descending aorta
  - Left superior intercostal vein
  - Left inferior pulmonary vein
  - Ductus diverticulum
  - Kommerell's diverticulum
  - Atelectatic lung
  - Aneurysm with intraluminal thrombus

Variants of aortic dissection

Intramural haematoma
- Haemorrhage of the vasa vasorum into the media layer
- Can progress to an intimal tear and the classic dissection pattern
- Non-contrast CT shows a crescent of high attenuation within the aortic wall
- Cannot be diagnosed with aortography
- Requires emergency surgical repair if it involves the ascending aorta
- Usually managed conservatively if it involves the descending aorta; it can disappear following antihypertensive treatment
- Differential diagnosis is thrombosed false lumen of dissection (intramural haematoma does not spiral around aorta)

Penetrating atherosclerotic ulcer
- Atherosclerotic lesion with ulceration penetrating the intima layer and haematoma formation within the media
- Occurs in elderly patients with hypertension and atherosclerosis
- Most commonly involves the descending thoracic aorta
- CT shows a focal ulcer with subintimal haematoma
- May progress to transmural rupture (in 40% of cases) or aortic dissection
- Usually treated with an endovascular aortic stent graft

Thoracic aortic aneurysm

- Aetiology
  - Atherosclerosis
  - Cystic medial necrosis (in Marfan's syndrome or Ehlers–Danlos syndrome)
  - Infective (bacteria or syphilitic)
  - Aortopathy (bicuspid aortic valve)
- Fusiform dilatation (saccular dilatations are mycotic or traumatic)
- Most commonly involves the distal arch or the descending aorta
- Progressive dilatation with aortic regurgitation, rupture
- Predisposes to aortic dissection
- Local compressive effects produce dysphagia and stridor
- Surgical or endovascular repair is indicated if diameter > 5.5 cm
- Risk of rupture if diameter > 6 cm is 10% per year

Imaging features

CXR
- Mediastinal mass with curvilinear calcifications

CT
- Mural thrombus and calcifications

Mycotic (non-syphilitic) aneurysm

- Infective destruction of intima and media
- Bacterial seeding via the vasa vasorum
- Risk factors include septicaemia from bacterial endocarditis, intravenous drug use and immunosuppression
- Majority occur in the ascending aorta near the sinus of Valsalva
- High risk of rupture

Takayasu's arteritis

- Chronic, granulomatous, large-vessel vasculitis
- Most common in young Asian females
- Intimal proliferation leading to stenoses and occlusions
- Diminished or absent pulses
- Mainly affects the aorta and its major branches
- May also involve the pulmonary, coronary and renal arteries

Imaging features

Catheter angiogram
- Patchy stenoses and occlusions

CT and MRI
- Enhancing mural thickening and luminal narrowing

Abdominal aortic aneurysm (AAA)

- True aneurysm involving all three layers of the arterial wall
- Affects 5% of men and 1% of women over the age of 65
- Defined as aortic diameter > 3 cm or double the normal size
- Elective repair considered if diameter > 5 cm
- 90% arise below the origin of the renal arteries (infra-renal)
- 80% have occlusion of the inferior mesenteric artery and lumbar arteries
- Majority contain mural thrombus, which may protect it from rupture
- Endovascular repair is standard technique in majority (65%) of cases

CT signs of AAA rupture

- Adjacent retroperitoneal haematoma (typically left sided)
- Active extravasation of contrast agent

Signs of impending AAA rupture

- Diameter > 7 cm
- Growth > 5 mm in 6 months
- Abdominal pain
- Crescent of high attenuation within wall

Aortoenteric fistula

- Late complication of AAA or aortic reconstructive surgery (about 10 years postoperative)

- Most fistulas involve the third part of the duodenum
- Present with abdominal pain, haematemesis and melena

Imaging features

CT
- Intraluminal and periaortic extraluminal gas
- Contrast extravasates into the bowel, and therefore contrast agent should not be administered before CT scanning

Inflammatory aneurysm

- AAA with surrounding inflammation and fibrotic adhesions
- Caused by an exaggerated immune response to atherosclerosis
- Associated with hypertension, smoking and diabetes
- Accounts for 5–10% of all AAAs
- Majority are infra-renal
- Males affected more often than females
- Median age of 60
- Raised ESR
- Majority are symptomatic, causing fever, back pain and weight loss
- Low risk of rupture compared with atheromatous aneurysm
- Adhesions most often involve the duodenum, IVC or left renal vein
- 10–20% have obstructive uropathy from ureteric involvement

Imaging features

Ultrasound
- Sonolucent halo surrounding aorta

CT
- Thick enhancing tissue rind around aneurysm, with or without calcification
- Adjacent inflammation subsides following surgical repair

Endovascular aneurysm repair (EVAR)

- An alternative to surgical repair of AAA
- Requires favourable vascular anatomy

- > 50% of patients with AAA are suitable for EVAR
- Endograft is used to exclude blood flow from the aneurysm sac
- Procedure performed via bilateral femoral artery cut-downs
- Graft is preloaded on a special delivery system
- Deployed under fluoroscopic guidance above and below the sac
- EVAR has a lower 30-day mortality (1.6%) than surgical repair (4.6%)
- At 4 years it has a high re-intervention rate (up to 40%)
- EVAR is more expensive than conventional surgical repair

EVAR exclusion criteria

- Neck angulation > 60°
- Neck length < 15 mm
- Iliac arteries diameter < 6 mm

Complications
- Endoleak (blood leak into old aneurysm sac)
  - Type 1: persistent perigraft channel (because of ineffective seals at top and bottom); requires urgent intervention
  - Type 2: retrograde flow into sac via the inferior mesenteric artery or lumbar arteries; usually managed conservatively
  - Type 3: a major defect in graft fabric (mechanical failure); treated with an additional graft
  - Type 4: a minor leak seen through porous graft fabric; usually managed conservatively
  - Type 5: sac increasing in size but no endoleak visible (endotension)
- Other complications
  - Graft thrombosis
  - Graft kinking
  - Graft infection
  - Shower embolism
  - Colonic necrosis

Peripheral vascular disease

- Usually results from atherosclerosis; multiple risk factors including genetics, smoking and diet
- Atherosclerosis is an arterial disease but may also effect veins exposed to arterial pressures
- Involvement of vessels is usually segmental and progressive
- Can cause stenoses, occlusions and aneurysms
- Clinical presentation is with intermittent claudication, rest pain or ulcer disease
- Commonest cause of claudication is aortoiliac disease, and the treatment of choice is balloon angioplasty followed by stenting
- Femoropopliteal occlusive disease is more common than iliac disease, and the treatment of choice is angioplasty
- Angioplasty for infrapopliteal disease is usually reserved for ischaemic foot ulcers or rest pain
- In multilevel vascular occlusive disease, treatment should commence at the highest level lesion to improve 'in-flow'
- High angioplasty success rates are achieved by treating short segment disease with good 'run-off', i.e. 3 cm for iliac arteries and < 10 cm for femoral arteries
- Stenoses longer than 10 cm give less favourable results
- 20% of patients with claudication who undergo angioplasty eventually require amputation

Diagnostic angiography

Digital subtraction angiography

- Access is via puncture of the common femoral artery (or the brachial, radial or popliteal artery if the common femoral artery is not suitable), followed by wire and catheter insertion: Seldinger's technique
- Contrast is injected via the catheter by hand or pump, and images are acquired
- Computer subtracts an initial non-contrast 'mask' image from a subsequent contrast-enhanced image
- Contrast resolution is superior to screen-film arteriography as bone, soft tissue and gas shadows are removed
- 1024×1024 matrix has a spatial resolution of three line pairs per millimetre
- Patients must remain still and hold their breath for imaging of the thoracoabdominal and pelvic vessels
- Buscopan is routinely used to prevent peristalsis
- Very slight movements can be corrected using 'pixel shifting'
- Contrast volumes and flow rates vary depending on the territory being assessed
  - Aortic arch: 25–40 mL at 15–20 mL/second
  - Abdominal aorta: 25 mL at 12–15 mL/second
  - Coeliac artery or superior mesenteric artery: 15 mL at 8–10 mL/second
- Demonstration of common iliac vessel bifurcation is best achieved with contralateral oblique views, e.g. right anterior oblique view for left iliac arteries
- Demonstration of femoral vessel bifurcation is best achieved with ipsilateral oblique views, e.g. left anterior oblique view for left femoral arteries
- Demonstration of distal vessels of the foot is best achieved by using biplane arteriography (lateral and posteroanterior projections)
- Pseudo-occlusions can be produced by excessive plantar flexion and external compression
- Peripheral vasodilators may be used to vasodilate for pressure gradient recordings

Catheters

- High flow with side holes for central vessels
- Low flow with end hole for selective vessels
- Higher flow rates can also be achieved using a shorter catheter with a larger diameter

Types
- Pigtail, for the aorta and pulmonary artery
- Cobra, for mesenteric, renal and contralateral iliac arteries
- Simmons, for the mesenteric arteries and arch vessels
- Microcatheters, for coaxial subselection
- Straight, for runoff vessels

Imaging features

MR angiogram
- Contrast-enhanced MR angiography is a widely used technique for peripheral vascular and carotid imaging
- It is faster and has a better signal-to-noise ratio than time of flight angiography; however, it tends to overestimate stenosis severity
- Uses T1-shortening effects of gadolinium-based contrast agents
- Most metallic stents (except the Nitinol type) exhibit artefacts that preclude MR angiographic evaluation of in-stent patency
- Imaging using contrast kinetics is used in evaluating run-off vessels and vascular malformations
- Increasing incidence of nephrogenic systemic fibrosis from free gadolinium has lead to emergence of new non-contrast enhanced sequences such as steady state free precession (bright blood imaging) and ECG-gated flow spoiled (fresh blood imaging)

Peripheral vascular ultrasound
- Normal peripheral arterial waveform is triphasic
- Stenosis causes an increase in velocity and spectral broadening
- A significant stenosis causes at least a doubling of velocity
- Loss of triphasic waveform downstream of flow can be used to make an indirect inference about upstream stenosis or occlusions

CT angiogram
- The current method of choice for imaging the thoracoabdominal aorta, common femoral arteries and carotid arteries
- Used both in planning and in surveillance of abdominal aortic aneurysm repair
- Can assess in-stent stenosis in vessels > 3 mm in diameter
- Increasingly used in assessing peripheral vascular disease. Isotrophic high spatial resolution is achievable with 16-detector scanners and above, which enables assessment of pedal vessels
- Presence of calcium causes blooming artefact and makes accurate quantification of stenoses difficult

Endovascular ultrasound
- Expensive and needs larger arteriotomy; not commonly used
- Miniature ultrasound probe is attached to a catheter tip and positioned in the target vessel lumen using a guide wire
- Catheter is slowly slid backwards as images are acquired
- Can be used to assess atheromatous plaque volume and morphology, the effects of angioplasty and stenting, and in planning endovascular treatments
- Can underestimate intimal flaps by re-opposing them to the wall

General principles of percutaneous angioplasty and stenting

- French size refers to outer circumference in catheters, inner circumference in sheaths
- Angiograms are initially performed to act as a 'road map'
- Stenotic lesion is crossed using a wire
- Heparin in a single dose of 5000 IU is routinely administered

- Angioplasty balloon catheter of an appropriate size is railroaded over wire and across the stenosis
- The balloon or stent diameter is chosen to be 5–10% oversized
- Balloon is inflated for 30 seconds to 1 minute (for up to 2 minutes if there is resistance)
- Residual stenosis < 20% is considered a technical success
- Higher grades of residual stenosis or angioplasty complications are indications for stent placement
- Non-covered, self-expanding or balloon-mounted stents are commonly used
- Stents re-occlude acutely via in-stent thrombosis and subacutely by the process of neointimal hyperplasia

Iliac artery angioplasty and stenting

- Iliac artery percutaneous transluminal angioplasty (PTA) is technically successful in around 95% of patients
- Short (< 3 cm), non-calcified stenotic segments are more effectively treated than occlusions
- Percutaneous transluminal angioplasty and stenting is the treatment of choice for iliac artery disease, with outcomes similar to surgery
- The addition of stenting improves long-term patency rates (90% patent at 1 year versus 75%; 80% patent at 4 years versus 65%)
- Success rates of angioplasty and stenting for stenoses below the inguinal ligaments are lower than for those in the iliac arteries

Femoropopliteal angioplasty and stenting

- Common femoral artery disease is best treated by endarterectomy but if necessary it can be done via a contralateral approach
- Superficial femoral artery disease is treated as per the TransAtlantic InterSociety Consensus (TASC) guidelines, and angioplasty is best
- Subintimal angioplasty can be performed in long occlusions in patients with ulcer

disease to help in healing because the duration of patency is shorter
- Self-expanding stents with improved flexibility are sometimes used for calcified or long lesions

Guide to approximate balloon and stent sizes

- Aorta: 12–15 mm
- Renal arteries: 4–6 mm
- Common iliac arteries: 8–10 mm
- External iliac arteries: 7–8 mm
- Common femoral and superficial femoral arteries: 5–6 mm
- Popliteal arteries: 4–5 mm
- More distal vessels: 2–3 mm

Choose a diameter of 10% more than the vessel diameter

Intra-arterial thrombolysis

- Indications are an 'acute white leg' caused by emboli from a distant source or an *in situ* thrombus
- Contraindications (absolute) are surgery in previous 6 weeks, a recent stroke and a known bleeding disorder
- Alteplase or recombinant tissue plasminogen activator (rt-PA) is used
- Side effects include bleeding, allergic reaction, nausea and vomiting, and reperfusion injury with compartment syndrome in legs or arms

Delivery technique

- Routine angiographic approach: place multi-hole catheter in thrombus or clot
- Inject a bolus dose (5–10 mg) of alteplase with short bursts in length of clot to give an extra mechanical effect
- Re-site the catheter into the clot and continue slow rate infusion with check angiograms every 4–6 hours
- If bleeding occurs, stop the infusion and call for help
- If check angiogram shows clearance, look for a local cause such as stenosis or occlusion, and treat appropriately

- In cases of popliteal aneurysm, surgery or endovascular stent graft are indicated
- If no local cause is found, assess for a central distal cause such as from the aorta or perform an echocardiogram to look for a cardiac cause

Complications of PTA and stenting

- Puncture: haematoma, pseudoaneurysm, arteriovenous fistula, infection
- Contrast-related: renal failure, allergic reaction
- Catheter-related: embolism, stroke, dissection
- Therapy-related: haemorrhage
- Mortality is 0–1.2%
- Stent infection is rare

Femoral artery pseudoaneurysm

- A false aneurysm, i.e. an aneurysm that does not involve all three layers of the artery wall
- High-pressure leak contained by adjacent tissues and haematoma
- Occurs in < 1% of diagnostic angiograms and in 3–5% of interventional procedures; higher risk with large-bore catheters
- Ultrasound-guided compression or thrombin injection can be used to treat narrow-necked aneurysms

Imaging features

Ultrasound
- Echo-poor 'sac' seen adjacent to the femoral artery
- The sac may contain internal echoes (because of partial thrombosis)
- Swirling blood flow seen within the sac using colour Doppler with inflowing and outflowing half-moons ('ying–yang' sign)
- Communicating 'neck' links parent artery to the sac

Acute limb ischaemia

- Secondary to embolisation of plaque debris, which tends to lodge at arterial bifurcations or areas of pre-existing narrowing

- Presents with the 'five Ps': pain, paraesthesia, pulselessness, pallor, perishing with cold
- High risk of limb loss without emergency treatment
- Treatment is with surgery (thrombectomy or bypass grafting) or using intra-arterial thrombolysis (involving an infusion for up to 48 hours)

Renal failure induced by contrast material

- Increased risk with pre-existing renal insufficiency or diabetes
- Risk can be reduced by using non-ionic contrast media or carbon dioxide contrast and by pre-procedural hydration

Contrast reactions and treatment

Urticaria

- Supportive treatment if scattered or transient
- For a protracted reaction consider antihistamine (intramuscularly, orally or intravenously)
- If profound consider adrenaline (1:1000) 0.1–0.3 mg intramuscularly

Bronchospasm

- Oxygen by mask (6–10 L/minute)
- Beta-2-agonist metered dose inhaler (two or three deep inhalations)
- If normotensive, give adrenaline (1:1000) 0.1–0.3 mg intramuscularly
- If hypotensive, give adrenaline (1:1,000) 0.5 mg intramuscularly

Laryngeal oedema

- Oxygen by mask (6–10 L/minute)
- Adrenaline (1:1000) 0.5 mg intramuscularly, repeated as needed

Hypotension with bradycardia (vasovagal reaction)

- Elevate patient's legs
- Oxygen by mask (6–10 L/minute)
- Atropine 0.6–1.0 mg intravenously, repeated if needed after 3 minutes (up to a maximum of 3 mg in total)
- Intravenous fluids rapidly (normal saline or lactated Ringer's solution)

Generalised anaphylactoid reaction

- Call for resuscitation team
- Suction airway if needed
- Elevate patient's legs if hypotensive
- Oxygen by mask (6–10 L/minute)
- Adrenaline (1:1,000) 0.5 mg intramuscularly
- Histamine-1 (H1) blocker, e.g. diphenhydramine 25–50 mg intravenously

Contrast medium extravasation

- Elevate affected limb
- Apply ice packs to affected area
- If symptoms do not resolve quickly, admit and monitor
- If skin or soft tissues are threatened consider surgical treatment

Pulse oximetry monitoring

- Causes of a low reading
  - Low PaO_2
  - Cold extremities
  - Hypotension
  - Dyshaemoglobinaemia
  - Skin pigmentation, e.g. jaundice
  - Nail varnish
  - Motion

Pharmacology

Lignocaine

- Indication: local anaesthesia
- Mechanism of action: reversible blockage of nerve conduction
- Dose: 10 mg/mL (1%); maximum dose: 20 ml
- Cautions: allergy, impaired cardiac conduction
- Contraindications: hypovolaemia, complete heart block
- Side effects: confusion, respiratory depression, convulsions, hypotension and bradycardia

Midazolam

- Indication: conscious sedation
- Mechanism of action: facilitates action of gamma-aminobutyric acid(GABA), the major inhibitory neurotransmitter; half-life of 2 hours
- Dose: slow intravenous injection (approximately 2 mg/minute) 5–10 minutes before procedure; initially 2 mg increased in steps of 1 mg
- Cautions: cardiac or respiratory disease, myasthenia gravis
- Contraindications: unstable myasthenia gravis, severe respiratory depression, acute pulmonary insufficiency
- Side effects: hypotension, arrhythmias, convulsions, confusion, urinary retention, injection site reactions

Glyceryl trinitrate

- Indication: local vasodilatation
- Mechanism of action: relieves smooth muscle spasm (both venous and arterial)
- Dose: 100–200 µg boluses; intra-arterial infusion rate, 15–20 µg/minute
- Cautions: monitor blood pressure
- Contraindications: hypotension, severe aortic stenosis, recently taken nitrate-based medication for erectile dysfunction

Glucagon

- Indication: reduces intestinal peristalsis
- Mechanism of action: smooth muscle relaxation (cyclic AMP-mediated)
- Dose: 1 mg
- Cautions: insulinoma, phaeochromocytoma (may induce a hypoglycaemic or hypertensive crisis)

Buscopan (hyoscine butylbromide)

- Indication: antispasmodic agent, reduces intestinal motility
- Mechanism of action: antimuscarinic agent
- Dose: 20 mg/mL; maximum dose: 160 mg
- Contraindications: myasthenia gravis, paralytic ileus, pyloric stenosis, prostatic enlargement
- Side effects: antimuscarinic

Atropine

- Indication: treatment of bradycardia
- Mechanism of action: inhibits acetylcholine
- Dose: 0.6–1.2 mg intravenously; maximum dose: 3 mg
- Contraindications: closed-angle glaucoma
- Side effects: anticholinergic

Peripheral vascular anatomy

Iliac artery

- The aorta bifurcates into the right and left common iliac arteries
- Within the pelvis each common iliac artery divides into the internal and external iliac arteries
- The internal iliac artery supplies the organs of the pelvis and buttock
- Reduced blood flow via the internal iliac artery leads to buttock claudication in patients with poor collateralization; it can also present as erectile dysfunction
- The external iliac artery gives off the deep circumflex iliac artery and the deep external pudendal artery

Femoral artery

- The external iliac artery exits the pelvis to become the common femoral artery as it crosses beneath the midpoint of the inguinal ligament
- The femoral vein lies medial to the common femoral artery; the femoral nerve lies laterally to the common femoral artery
- The common femoral artery descends superficially in the femoral triangle and gives three superficial branches: the inferior epigastric artery, the external pudendal artery and the circumflex iliac artery
- After a short distance it gives a deep branch, the profunda femoris artery, which leaves through the floor of the triangle
- The profunda femoris artery has medial and lateral circumflex femoral branches and deep perforating branches supplying adductor and flexor compartments
- The common femoral artery continues as the superficial femoral artery
- At the apex of the femoral triangle the superficial femoral artery enters the adductor canal anterior to the femoral vein and winds medially round the thigh
- It becomes the popliteal artery at the adductor hiatus

Popliteal artery

- The popliteal artery descends in the floor of the popliteal fossa deep to the popliteal vein
- It has several genicular branches, which serve as collateral pathways when the femoral artery is occluded
- It divides at the lower border of popliteus muscle into anterior tibial and tibioperoneal trunks

Run-off vessels

- The anterior tibial artery descends anterior to the interosseous membrane deep to the tibialis anterior and extensor digitorum muscles; it passes in front of the ankle joint to become the dorsalis pedis artery
- The tibioperoneal trunk divides after a few centimetres into the posterior tibial and peroneal arteries
- The posterior tibial artery descends between deep and superficial muscle compartments then passes behind the medial malleolus deep to the flexor retinaculum, dividing into the medial and lateral plantar arteries
- The peroneal artery descends close to the fibula. It supplies branches to the lateral compartment before dividing into calcaneal and lateral malleolar branches

Non-atherosclerotic Pathology

Buerger's disease

- Not common among Caucasians
- Non-necrotising panarteritis of the small and medium-sized peripheral arteries, in which there is luminal occlusion by highly cellular thrombus
- Strong association with smoking
- < 2% of cases occur in women
- Presents with claudication symptoms in young patients

Imaging features

Angiography
- Multifocal stenoses and occlusions of the calf and forearm arteries
- 'Corkscrew' collaterals are characteristic

Raynaud's syndrome

- Episodic pain affecting the fingers, toes and extremities with phasic colour changes (white, blue, red)
- Primary Raynaud's is a cold-induced spasm of smooth muscle in the arterial wall
- Secondary Raynaud's is a stenotic process that produces arterial occlusion
- Causes of secondary Raynaud's syndrome
  - Atherosclerosis (the commonest cause)
  - Thoracic outlet syndrome, e.g. a cervical rib
  - Connective tissue diseases, e.g. scleroderma
  - Vasculitis, e.g. Takayasu's arteritis, systemic lupus erythematosus
  - Drugs, e.g. methysergide
  - Buerger's disease
  - Trauma, e.g. 'vibration white finger'
  - Polyvinyl chloride exposure

Popliteal artery entrapment syndrome

- Caused by an anomalous anatomic relationship between the popliteal artery and surrounding musculotendinous structures
- Arterial compression by these structures occurs with plantar flexion and causes intermittent claudication symptoms
- Compression most often caused by the medial head of the gastrocnemius muscle, less commonly by the popliteus muscle or a deep fibrous band
- Usually affects healthy young men 20–40 years of age
- Aneurysmal dilatation can lead to thrombosis with distal embolisation and acute limb ischaemia

Imaging features

Doppler, MR angiogram and catheter angiogram
- Medial deviation or angulation of the artery in the popliteal region
- Mid-portion narrowing, which is most marked in plantar flexion
- Occasionally post-stenotic dilatation

- Medial head of the gastrocnemius muscle arises laterally on femoral condyle

Polyarteritis nodosa

- Pan-mural necrotizing vasculitis affecting small and medium-sized arteries, thought to be a result of immune complex deposition
- Can be associated with hepatitis B and HIV infection
- Clinical symptoms of ischaemia from arterial branch occlusions
- Renal involvement in 70–80% of cases
- Central nervous system involvement in 10% of cases
- Treatment is with systemic corticosteroids; aneurysms of polyarteritis nodosa may resolve over time as remission occurs
- Prophylactic treatment of large aneurysms by covered stents or catheter embolisation is considered to prevent rupture

Imaging features

Angiogram
- Multiple visceral organ arterial ectasias and microaneurysms
- Arterial occlusive lesions (in > 90% of cases)

Causes of small and medium-sized vessel vasculitis

- Polyarteritis nodosa
- Behçet's syndrome
- Churg–Strauss syndrome
- Microscopic polyangiitis
- Kawasaki's disease
- Rheumatoid vasculitis
- Systemic lupus erythermatosus vasculitis
- Wegener's granulomatosis

Causes of large vessel vasculitis

- Giant cell arteritis
- Takayasu's arteritis

Vascular calcifications

- Causes
  - Atherosclerosis
  - Diabetes
  - Chronic renal failure
  - Hyperparathyroidism
  - Hyperlipidaemia
  - Haemochromatosis ('bronze diabetes')

Acute gastrointestinal haemorrhage

Upper gastrointestinal bleeding

- Proximal to the ligament of Treitz
- Accounts for 75% of cases
- Peptic ulcer disease accounts for > 50% of cases
- Other common causes are varices and Mallory–Weiss tears
- Presents with haematemesis and melaena
- Upper gastrointestinal endoscopy identifies bleeding source in 90% of cases

Lower gastrointestinal bleeding

- Distal to the ligament of Treitz
- Accounts for 25% of cases
- Diverticular disease is the commonest cause
- Other common causes are angiodysplasia, neoplasia and colitis
- Haemorrhoids account for 10% of cases
- Haematochezia (red blood per rectum)
- Sigmoid or colonoscopy identifies bleeding source in 90% of cases, but colonic preparation is essential

Diagnosis and management

- 80% of gastrointestinal bleeds will cease spontaneously
- In the remaining 20% intervention is required
- Endoscopy should be the first-line diagnostic and therapeutic procedure and can identify a bleeding source in > 90% of cases
- Gastrointestinal bleeding is typically intermittent, and imaging tests are sensitive only when there is evidence of active haemorrhage, such as tachycardia or systolic blood pressure < 100 mmHg

Imaging methods to identify bleeding source

Radionuclide scintigram
- Colloid sulphur or labelled red blood cell scan
- Detects bleeding at rates as low as 0.1 mL/minute
- Can image for up to 24 hours after injection

CT angiogram
- No oral contrast agent
- Thin-section, three-phase (pre-, arterial and venous) scan
- Detects bleeding at rates as low as 0.3 mL/minute
- Hyperdense intraluminal contrast extravasation

Mesenteric angiogram
- Detects bleeding as low as 0.5 ml/minute
- Better sensitivity with carbon dioxide contrast, vasodilators and anticoagulants
- Contrast blush or intraluminal extravasation

Embolisation

- Deliberate occlusion of a vessel
- Various agents are used
- Permanent agents
  - Coils (provide a large thrombogenic surface)
  - Detachable balloons
  - Absolute alcohol
  - Glue
- Temporary agents
  - Autologous clot
  - Gelfoam
  - Polyvinyl alcohol (a particulate agent that causes thrombosis)
- Coils should be slightly bigger than the lumen of the target vessel
- Unintentional distal embolisation of systemic vessels is more common at the end of the procedure than the beginning

Acute gastrointestinal haemorrhage

- Selective coil embolisation is the preferred method
- Has a high technical success rate for cessation of bleeding
- Complications include failure and bowel infarction needing surgery

Varicocele embolisation

- 90% of varicoceles are left-sided
- Embolisation is used for symptom relief or associated infertility
- Access is via the right common femoral vein or the internal jugular vein
- Left testicular vein drains into left renal vein
- Right testicular vein drains into the IVC, which is more difficult to access
- Coils are deployed distal to the first joining branch at level of inguinal canal
- If coils are too small they will embolise into pulmonary arteries
- Testicular vein spasm is a frequent problem

Uterine fibroid embolisation

- Widely accepted as a first-line treatment for symptomatic fibroid disease as an alternative to hysterectomy or myomectomy
- Not suitable to treatment of pedunculated fibroids
- Requires bilateral uterine artery embolisation (via the first or second branches of the anterior division of the internal iliac arteries) to induce ischaemic infarction
- Polyvinyl alcohol is typically used (particle size 300–500 micrometres)
- Angiographic endpoint is to-and-fro flow within the uterine artery
- Complete embolisation of both arteries is undesirable, since this will cause uterine necrosis

Complications

- Postoperative pain (severe for up to 24 hours)
- Post-embolisation syndrome
- Sepsis

- Failure (in 10% of cases)
- Premature menopause
- Hysterectomy

Bronchial artery embolisation

- The bronchial arteries originate directly from the descending aorta, most commonly between the T4 and T6 levels
- Classically there are two arteries on the left and one on the right, but variations are numerous
- They supply the tracheobronchial tree
- The left main bronchus marks their origin in most cases
- A descending thoracic aortogram is performed prior to selective bronchial angiography
- Polyvinyl alcohol (particles > 250–300 micrometres, to avoid passage into spinal vessels and the bronchopulmonary anastomosis causing spinal cord and lung infarction) is the agent of choice

Complications

- Chest pain (commonest)
- Dysphagia, caused by occlusion of oesophageal branches
- Spinal cord ischaemia, caused by occlusion of radicular branches

Hepatic artery chemoembolisation

- Used in the treatment of hepatocellular carcinoma, carcinoid and some liver metastases
- Lipoidal emulsified with cisplatin or doxyrubicin, or polyvinyl alcohol is used
- Deprives tumour of its nutrient source, causing ischaemic necrosis
- Hepatic arteriography and portography are mandatory to evaluate vascular anatomy and patency prior to treatment
- Portal vein thrombosis is not a contraindication *per se* but selective arterial embolisation must be performed in this setting
- Non-target organ complications include ischaemic cholecystitis, splenic infarction, bowel ischaemia, pulmonary embolism and spinal cord ischaemia

Renal artery stenosis

- Accounts for 2–5% of all cases of hypertension
- Haemodynamically significant when > 70% luminal narrowing
- Causes reduced perfusion pressure at the glomerulus, which stimulates renin production leading to a rise in angiotensin and thus a rise in blood pressure
- Causes hypertension refractory to drug treatment
- Atherosclerosis is the cause in 70% of cases
  - Commonest site is within 2 cm of the ostium
  - Stents are used because there is a high recurrence rate with angioplasty alone
  - Quoted risk of renal artery rupture is 1%
- Fibromuscular dysplasia is the cause in 30% of cases
  - Mid- and distal vessel disease
  - Good results with balloon angioplasty alone
  - Indications for intervention are hypertension that is resistant to best medical therapy, flash pulmonary oedema and acute or acute-on-chronic renal failure in patients with single kidney

Imaging features

Ultrasound
- Unilateral small kidney
- MR angiography peak systolic velocity > 180 cm/second
- Ratio of peak systolic renal velocity to aortic velocity > 3.5
- 'Parvus tardus' interlobar artery Doppler waveform (acceleration time > 0.07 second); this has a high specificity but a low sensitivity for renal artery stenosis

MR angiogram and catheter angiogram
- Atherosclerosis (proximal stenosis)
- Fibromuscular hyperplasia (focal disease)
- Can affect vessels at all levels, with a stenotic or 'beaded' appearance and aneurysm formation

Carotid imaging

Anatomy
- The common carotid artery (CCA) bifurcates at the C4 level into the internal carotid artery (ICA) and the external carotid artery (ECA)
- The ECA has no branches in the neck

Branches of the ECA
- Superior thyroid artery
- Ascending pharyngeal artery
- Lingual artery
- Facial artery
- Occipital artery
- Posterior auricular artery
- Temporal artery
- Maxillary artery (first branch is the middle meningeal artery, terminal branch is the sphenopalatine artery)

Atherosclerotic ICA stenosis
- Stenosis between 70% and 99% has been shown in the North American Symptomatic Carotid Endarterectomy Trial (NASCET) to benefit from endarterectomy surgery
- Methods of assessing stenosis are Doppler ultrasound, MR angiography, CT angiography and catheter angiography

Carotid Doppler ultrasound

Features of a normal ECA waveform
- ECA arises anteromedial to the ICA and has side branches in the neck
- Demonstrates the 'temporal tapping' phenomena
- Has a high resistance waveform, i.e. low end-diastolic flow
- Waveform has a characteristic notch and may dip below the baseline (diastolic flow reversal)

Features of a normal ICA waveform
- No side branches in the neck
- No 'temporal tapping' phenomena
- Has a low resistance waveform, i.e. high end-diastolic flow

Features of a normal CCA waveform
- Intima–media thickness, measured just proximal to carotid bulb, is normally < 0.8 mm

- Thickening is recognised as an independent risk factor for cardiovascular events
- CCA waveform is higher resistance than the ICA waveform but lower than the ECA waveform
- Can normally dip below the baseline

Criteria for diagnosing ICA stenosis

- Direct signs
  - Peak systolic velocity in the ICA > 230 cm/second
  - ICA/CCA peak systolic velocity gradient > 4
- Indirect signs
  - Spectral broadening of ICA waveform ('filling in' under the curve)
  - ECA waveform shows increased diastolic flow ('ICA-like')

Limitations of ultrasound

- Operator-dependent and not reproducible
- Calcified plaques interfere with Doppler interrogation
- Inability to visualise ICA lesions near skull base
- Inability to interrogate origins of the great vessels
- Problems distinguishing high-grade stenosis from occlusion

MR angiography

- Contrast-enhanced MR angiography is technique of choice
- This is an accurate non-invasive technique for evaluating the extracranial carotid vessels
- Can image their origins at the aortic arch
- Has a tendency to overestimate the degree of stenoses

Residual 'trickle' flow in high-grade stenosis

- Residual flow: suitable for surgery
- Absent flow: unsuitable for surgery

CT angiography

- Non-invasive but involves radiation and iodinated contrast

- Accurate assessment is possible because it can evaluate plaque composition
- Improved spatial resolution for depicting dissection, intramural haematoma and aneurysm
- Postoperative complications following carotid endarterectomy are best imaged by CT angiography, including in-stent stenosis

Catheter angiography

- Definitive imaging test for distinguishing between high-grade stenosis and occlusion of the ICA
- Carries an approximately 1% risk of stroke

Carotid dissection

- Accounts for 10–25% of strokes in younger adults (< 45 years age)
- Increased risk with fibromuscular dysplasia, Ehlers–Danlos syndrome, Marfan's syndrome and homocystinuria
- Most commonly occurs spontaneously or following minor, unrecalled trauma. Less commonly caused by major trauma or penetrating injuries
- Presents with headache, stroke or an ipsilateral painful Horner's syndrome

Imaging features

MR angiogram, CT angiogram and catheter angiogram

- Commonest location is the cervical ICA at C1–C2 level
- Tapered narrowing of vessel over a few centimetres
- Lumen typically reconstitutes within the bony carotid canal
- Intracranial extension is rare

Carotid stenting

- Endovascular procedure that is an alternative to carotid endarterectomy
- Currently used in high or low surgically inaccessible sites, for recurrence after carotid endarterectomy and in postoperative and post-radiotherapy necks
- Especially suited for patients with significant medical co-morbidities who are considered too high an anaesthetic risk
- Shortened hospitalisation and convalescence times

- Similar 30-day stroke risk to that of carotid endarterectomy (approximately 5%)
- Distal embolic protection devices (filters) have been developed to reduce the risk of stroke further
- Can also be used (with a covered stent) to treat carotid dissection and blow-out with bleeding

Subclavian steal syndrome

- Narrowing (partial steal) or occlusion (complete steal) of the proximal subclavian (or brachiocephalic) artery
- Blood flows in a retrograde direction down the ipsilateral vertebral artery to supply the distal subclavian artery, diverting flow away from the vertebrobasilar circulation
- Can cause syncopal episodes, vertigo and ataxia, classically induced by exercising the arm on the affected side

Imaging features

Ultrasound
- Normal vertebral artery waveform is low resistance with forward (antegrade) flow throughout the cardiac cycle
- Partial steal
  - Antegrade flow in the vertebral artery during diastole
  - Retrograde flow in the vertebral artery during systole
  - Exercising the arm on the affected side exaggerates waveform change
  - Brachial artery has a monophasic waveform (normally triphasic)
- Complete steal
  - Retrograde flow throughout the cardiac cycle

Trans-jugular intrahepatic portosystemic shunt

- Creation of a path and placement of a covered stent (the preferred type) or a bare metal stent between the hepatic vein and the portal vein to reduce portal venous pressure
- Can also create the path between the IVC and the portal vein

- Used as a measure in patients with portal hypertension and repeated variceal bleeding
- Low mortality rate (1%) compared with surgical shunting
- Complications
  - New or worsening hepatic encephalopathy (in 5–35% of cases)
  - Shunt thrombosis (rate is 50% at 1 year); treated via thrombolysis (acutely) or stenting
  - In-stent stenosis, needing routine surveillance (6-monthly Doppler studies and yearly angiography)

Percutaneous nephrostomy

- Provides temporary drainage of the urinary tract as well as access for a variety of pyeloureteric procedures
- Indications
  - Acute hydronephrosis
  - Pyonephrosis (infected obstructed system)
  - Palliation for malignant obstruction
  - Ureteric stricture dilatation, stenting or stone removal
- Ultrasound-guided puncture is a safe and reliable technique
- The posterior calyces in the mid- and lower poles are the best target
- However, access via the lower pole gives an acute angle of entry into the renal pelvis and can make further tracking of stents difficult
- 'Brödel's bloodless line' of incision lies at the junction of the anterior two thirds and the posterior one third of the kidney
- The colon is retrorenal in 2% of patients, more often on the left side and in relation to the lower pole
- Pus requires at least an 8 F catheter to ensure adequate drainage
- Upper pole calyx puncture is only needed for nephrolithotomy
- Ureteric stenting is indicated when long-term drainage is required and should be performed only once any infection has abated

Anatomy

Cardiac chambers

- Normal heart lies obliquely with its apex to the left (levocardia)

Right atrium

- Forms the right border of the heart on frontal CXR
- Receives systemic venous return via the SVC and the IVC
- The sinoatrial (SA) node lies at the junction of the SVC and the right atrium
- The crista terminalis separates the atrial appendage from the right atrium and it contains internodal tracts connecting the SA node with atrioventricular (AV) node
- The atrial appendage is broad-based with a ridged muscular wall
- The fossa ovalis (closed foramen ovale) lies in the interatrial septum
- The coronary sinus drains into the smooth posterior wall of the right atrium
- The tricuspid valve has three cusps, each attached to papillary muscles of the ventricular wall by the cordae tendinae
- A muscular fold (conus) separates the tricuspid valve from the pulmonary valve

Right ventricle

- Forms the anterior wall of the heart
- Thin-walled, heavily trabeculated, crescent-shaped cavity
- Convexity of the interventricular septum normally bulges into it
- Pulmonary valve (which has three cusps) is the most anterior and the most superior heart valve
- Identified also by the muscular infundibulum

Left atrium

- Forms the posterior border of the heart on lateral CXR
- Not seen on a frontal CXR unless enlarged
- Receives paired superior and inferior pulmonary veins
- Tubular appendage projects anteriorly from its left superior border

- The mitral valve is bicuspid; the anterior cusp separates the left ventricular inflow and outflow tracts

Left ventricle

- Forms the left border of the heart on frontal CXR
- Thick-walled, finely trabeculated, cone-shaped cavity
- Circular in cross-section
- The mitral valve is in fibrous continuity with the aortic valve
- Above each of the three aortic valve cusps is a sinus of Valsalva

Coronary artery anatomy

Left coronary artery

- Arises perpendicular to the aorta above the left coronary cusp
- Mainstem courses behind the pulmonary trunk for 1–3 cm then bifurcates into the left anterior descending (LAD) and left circumflex (LCx) vessels
- LAD runs in the anterior interventricular groove giving off diagonal and septal perforator branches, which supply the anterolateral wall of left ventricle and the anterior two thirds of the interventricular septum
- LCx runs posteriorly under the left atrial appendage in the left atrioventricular groove and gives off obtuse marginal branches
- LCx supplies the posterolateral wall of the left ventricle
- LCx gives rise to the posterior descending artery in 10% of people

Right coronary artery

- Arises perpendicular to aorta above the right coronary cusp
- Courses to the right and descends in the right atrioventricular groove
- First branch is the conal artery, supplying the SA node
- Supplies the right ventricle, the inferior wall of the left ventricle and the posterior third of the interventricular septum

- Gives rise to the posterior descending artery in 70% of people

> ### Coronary dominance: vessel giving rise to the posterior descending artery and the AV nodal branch
>
> - 70% are right coronary artery-dominant
> - 20% have a co-dominant system
> - 10% are left coronary artery-dominant

Coronary artery anomalies

- 1–2% of people have an anomaly of the coronary arteries
- A huge number of variations have been described
  - High take-off above sinotubular junction (commonest anomaly)
  - Trifurcation of left main stem, giving a ramus intermedius branch
  - Single coronary arising from left, right or posterior cusps
  - Separate origin of LAD and LCx vessels

> ### 'Malignant' coronary artery anomalies (< 1% of cases)
>
> - Inter-arterial course: left or right coronary aretery arising from the contralateral sinus and running between both outflow tracts; carries a risk of exercise-induced arterial compression and is linked with sudden cardiac death in young adults
> - Coronary artery arising from pulmonary artery: 90% die in the first year of life
> - Coronary artery fistula: can cause ischaemia

Cardiac chamber enlargement

Left atrial enlargement

Causes
  - Mitral stenosis, mitral regurgitation
  - Aortic stenosis, hypertension, coarctation of the aorta
  - Hypertrophic cardiomyopathy
  - Atrial fibrillation (if long-standing)
  - Left atrial myxoma
  - Ventricular septal defect (not atrial septal defect)
  - Patent ductus arteriosus

Imaging features

CXR
- Straightening of left heart border
- Elevated left main bronchus (splayed carina)
- Double right heart border

> ### Conditions simulating left atrial enlargement
>
> - Partial pericardial defect
> - Pulmonary stenosis (dilated left pulmonary artery)
> - Persistence of a left SVC
> - Coronary artery fistula
> - Corrected transposition

Left ventricular enlargement

- Causes
  - Ischaemic heart disease, hypertension
  - Aortic regurgitation or aortic stenosis
  - Cardiomyopathy
  - Coarctation of the aorta
  - Ventricular septal defect
  - High output states, e.g. hyperthyroidism, severe anaemia, Paget's disease, pregnancy, arteriovenous fistulas (anywhere)

Imaging features

CXR
- Left, downward displacement of the apex
- Rounding of the left cardiac border

Right atrial enlargement

- Causes
  - Tricuspid regurgitation (e.g. pulmonary hypertension)
  - Ebstein's anomaly
  - Atrial septal defect
  - Arrhythmogenic right ventricular cardiomyopathy

Right ventricular enlargement

- Causes
  - Left heart failure (pulmonary venous hypertension)
  - Pulmonary arterial hypertension
  - Left to right shunts
  - Outflow tract obstruction, e.g. pulmonary stenosis

Imaging features

CXR
- Elevation of cardiac apex ('coeur en sabot')

Cardiomyopathy

Hypertrophic cardiomyopathy

- Asymmetric hypertrophy of interventricular septum is the commonest subtype
- Other subtypes include apical, mid ventricular and symmetric hypertrophic cardiomyopathy (difficult to distinguish from athletic and hypertensive heart disease)
- 50% hereditary, 50% sporadic
- Associated with sudden cardiac death from arrhythmias and exercise-induced outflow tract obstruction (termed hypertrophic obstructive cardiomyopathy)

Imaging features

Echocardiogram and MRI
- Asymmetrical septal hypertrophy (commonest subtype)
- Increased left ventricular mass
- Small left ventricular cavity with obliteration in systole
- Low left ventricular end systolic volume ('hyper-dynamic circulation' with elevated ejection fraction) in > 70% of cases
- Mitral valve systolic anterior motion or prolapse

Restrictive cardiomyopathy

- Infiltrative process of ventricular myocardium
- Causes include amyloidosis, sarcoidosis and haemochromatosis
- Diastolic dysfunction ('stiff myocardium')
- Clinically mimics constrictive pericarditis

Imaging features

MRI
- Diffuse myocardial signal and perfusion abnormality

CT
- Cardiac CT is useful in differentiating calcified pericardium from restrictive cardiomyopathy

Dilated cardiomyopathy

- Causes include alcohol, post-viral changes and pregnancy
- Ventricular dilatation and global hypokinesis
- CT coronary angiography is useful in excluding coronary ischaemia

Arrhythmogenic right ventricular dysplasia

- Fibrofatty replacement of right ventricular myocardium
- Autosomal-dominant condition typically affecting young males
- Presents with ventricular arrhythmias and right heart failure

Imaging features

MRI
- High T1 and T2 signal in the right ventricular wall, which suppresses with fat saturation imaging
- Focal or global dyskinesia of the right ventricular wall
- Delayed enhancement of right ventricular wall, outflow tract and papillary muscles

Cardiac myxoma

- Commonest benign cardiac tumour
- Can arise from any endocardial surface
- Majority attached to interatrial septum
- 80% occur in left atrium and are usually pedunculated
- 20% occur in right atrium and are usually sessile
- 20% are calcified (more common in the right atrium than the left)
- Clinically may mimic mitral stenosis, with a mid-diastolic murmur
- Can cause embolic phenomenon (stroke, pulmonary embolus)

Imaging features

MRI
- Intraluminal filling defect with a lobulated contour
- Large tumours may be seen to prolapse through the mitral valve on cine sequences
- Usually heterogeneous contrast enhancement (distinguishes a myxoma from thrombus)

Congenital heart disease

Fetal circulation
- Oxygenated blood leaves the placenta via a solitary umbilical vein
- Travelling in the umbilical cord, oxygenated blood reaches the umbilicus and then runs in the falciform ligament to the porta hepatis
- Here the porta hepatis joins the intrahepatic left portal vein, and most blood passes via the ductus venosus into the left hepatic vein and the IVC
- Blood entering the right atrium is directed by a valve towards the foramen ovale, through which the blood enters the left atrium
- Some blood enters the pulmonary artery but high lung resistance diverts most of it via the ductus arteriosus to the descending aorta
- Each internal iliac artery gives an umbilical artery, which passes deoxygenated blood back to the placenta in the umbilical cord

Cyanosis without pulmonary plethora
- Tetralogy of Fallot
- Ebstein's anomaly
- Tricuspid atresia

Tetralogy of Fallot
- The four features of the tetralogy
  - Pulmonary stenosis
  - Right ventricular hypertrophy
  - Large ventricular septal defect
  - Aortic valve overriding the ventricular septum

- Pulmonary stenosis is progressive; cyanosis develops around 3 months of age
- Child often adopts a squatting posture, which forces blood through the tight pulmonary valve
- Multiple associations, e.g. coronary artery and valvular anomalies

Treatment
- Blalock–Taussig shunt (from the subclavian artery to the ipsilateral pulmonary artery)
- Surgical closure of the ventricular septal defect (VSD) and patch repair of the pulmonary stenosis

Imaging features
CXR
- Boot-shaped heart
- Elevated apex (because of right ventricular hypertrophy)
- Small pulmonary trunk
- Right aortic arch in 25% of cases
- Pulmonary oligaemia

Ebstein's anomaly
- Displacement of the tricuspid valve deep into right ventricular cavity
- Proximal right ventricle is 'atrialised' but contracts synchronously with remainder of the ventricle
- Impaired ventricular function with cyanosis and oligaemia
- Severe tricuspid regurgitation and massive right atrial dilatation
- Associated with other structural and conduction defects
- Wolf–Parkinson–White syndrome is a common cause of death
- 50% mortality in first year of life

Imaging features
CXR
- Box-shaped heart
- Dilated azygous vein

Tricuspid atresia
- Complete agenesis of the tricuspid valve
- Fibrous tissue occupies the cleft between the right atrium and the right ventricle
- Obligatory right-to-left atrial septal defect (ASD) or patent foramen ovale to sustain life

- Most also have a small VSD allowing some left-to-right flow through a hypoplastic right ventricle to the pulmonary artery
- Severe cyanosis at birth
- Rarely there may be pulmonary plethora (if the VSD is large)

Imaging features

MRI or echocardiogram
- Large right atrium and hypoplastic ventricle

Surgical shunt procedures

- Blalock–Taussig shunt in infancy
- Glenn anastomosis after infancy (from the IVC to the pulmonary artery)
- Fontan operation (external graft from right atrium to pulmonary artery)

Cyanosis with pulmonary plethora

- Transposition of the great arteries
- Total anomalous pulmonary venous connection
- Truncus arteriosus
- Tricuspid atresia with a large VSD
- Tingle (single) ventricle

Transposition of the great arteries

- Systemic and pulmonary circulations are in parallel
- Aorta arises from the right ventricle, the pulmonary artery from the left ventricle
- Cyanosis at birth with pulmonary plethora
- Shunt-dependent, i.e. relies on ASD, VSD or patent ductus arteriosus (PDA) to sustain life
- Treated with prostaglandin E1 to stop closure of the ductus arteriosus
- 90% mortality in first year of without surgical intervention

Imaging features

CXR
- 'Egg-on-side' appearance of the heart
- Right ventricular hypertrophy
- Narrow vascular pedicle—pulmonary trunk lies posteriorly

Congenitally corrected transposition

- Atrioventricular and ventriculoarterial discordance
- Ventricles are transposed with morphological right ventricle supplying systemic circulation
- Aortic root lies anteriorly with respect to the pulmonary outflow tract
- May present with left ventricular failure in adulthood, owing to failure of the systemic ventricle
- Acyanotic lesion

Total anomalous pulmonary venous connection

- Pulmonary veins all drain to the systemic veins or the right atrium
- The SVC is the commonest site for the connection
- Complete left to right shunt: shunt dependant (ASD or PFO)
- The pulmonary vein may be obstructed, causing low cardiac output

Imaging features

CXR
- 'Figure-of-eight'-shaped heart

Scimitar syndrome

- Partial anomalous pulmonary venous connection
- Associated with a hypogenetic right lung
- Anomalous vein seen adjacent to the right side of the heart
- Most commonly drains to the subdiaphragmatic IVC
- Occurs almost exclusively on the right side

Truncus arteriosus

- Failure of septation of the embryonic truncus arteriosus
- A single vessel drains both ventricles,

supplying the systemic, pulmonary and coronary circulations
- Moderate cyanosis and pulmonary plethora

Imaging features

CXR
- Truncus is larger than a normal ascending aorta

Acynotic congenital heart condisions with pulmonary plethora

- ASD
- VSD
- PDA

Left-to-right shunt

- Has the potential to increase pulmonary blood flow, leading to plexogenic arteriopathy and pulmonary hypertension if untreated
- Large shunts (e.g. VSD, PDA) cause pulmonary hypertension within the first few years of life
- Smaller shunts (e.g. ASD) will often not present until adulthood
- Shunt reversal occurs when pulmonary resistance rises above systemic resistance (Eisenmenger's syndrome); pulmonary vessels become pruned and central pulmonary arteries and conus remain enlarged, and left atrial size decreases in VSD. Patients are cyanosed

Imaging features

CXR
- Enlarged pulmonary conus
- Enlarged left and right pulmonary arteries
- Enlarged pulmonary vessels (plethora)
- Enlarged left atrium in VSD; normal left atrium in ASD

Pericardium

Anatomy

- Fibroserous sac consisting of visceral and parietal layers
- Envelops the four cardiac chambers, the first few centimetres of the ascending

aorta, and the pulmonary trunk as far as its bifurcation
- Pericardial cavity normally contains 20–50 mL of serous fluid
- Inner visceral layer is adherent to myocardium or epicardial fat
- Outer parietal layer is attached inferiorly to the diaphragmatic tendon
- Normal pericardium is seen on CT and MRI as a thin (< 2 mm) linear band
- Superior pericardial recess lies posterior to ascending aorta
- Normal aortopulmonary window contains fat

Congenital absence of the pericardium and pericardial sac defect

- Complete absence (10% of cases) is benign condition with a normal life span
- Partial absence (90% of cases)
  - More common on the left side and in males
  - Associated with bronchogenic cyst, VSD, PDA, ASD, tetralogy of Fallot, diaphragmatic hernia and pulmonary sequestration
  - Herniation through the defect can cause arrhythmia and sudden death

Imaging features

CXR
- Radiolucent cleft in the aortopulmonary window
- Straight left heart border (bulging left atrium through defect)
- Absence of left pericardial fat pad
- Increased distance between the heart and sternum on lateral view

CT
- Lung tissue interposed between the aorta and pulmonary trunk
- Pulmonary trunk deviated to the left

Pericardial effusion

- > 50 mL of fluid in the pericardial cavity
- Causes
  - Infection (viral, bacterial, tuberculous)
  - Heart failure
  - Uraemia
  - Hypothyroidism

- Connective tissue disorders
- Malignancy (of breast or lung, or lymphoma)
- Myocardial infarction (Dressler's syndrome)
- AIDS
- Trauma

Imaging features

CXR
- Enlargement of the cardiopericardial shadow
- Clear cardiac margins ('pencil line')
- 'Water bottle' heart

CT
- Water attenuation with simple effusions
- Higher attenuation with blood, malignancy, infective conditions and hypothyroidism
- Nodular enhancing pericardium suggests malignant involvement

MRI
- Low T1 signal, high T2 signal seen with simple effusions
- High T1 signal is characteristic of blood, commonly heterogenous

Cardiac tamponade

- Haemodynamically significant cardiac compression from pericardial contents causing impaired diastolic filling and reduced stroke volume
- Requires urgent pericardiocentesis (echo- or CT-guided)
- Can be caused by rapid accumulation of as little as 100 mL of fluid
- Pulsus paradoxus (inspiratory drop in blood pressure)

Imaging features

Echocardiogram, MRI and ECG-gated CT
- Diastolic right ventricular/atrial collapse

Constrictive pericarditis

- Fibrous pericardial thickening, which prevents normal diastolic ventricular expansion
- Kussmaul's sign (paradoxical rise of jugular venous pressure on inspiration)

- Clinically mimics restrictive cardiomyopathy
- Commonest causes are radiation therapy and cardiac surgery
- Can be secondary to any cause of pericarditis

Imaging features

CXR
- Small or normal-sized heart
- Linear pericardial calcifications in > 50% of cases
- Dilated azygous vein

CT/MRI
- Pericardial thickening (> 4 mm) and calcifications
- Narrow tubular right ventricular cavity
- Contrast reflux into the hepatic veins, coronary sinus and IVC

Pericardial cyst

- Unilocular, mesothelial-lined cyst
- Outpouching of parietal pericardium
- Does not communicate with the pericardial space
- Usually an asymptomatic incidental finding
- Right cardiophrenic angle is the commonest location

Imaging features

CXR
- Lobulated mass at the cardiophrenic angle

CT
- Round, thin-walled, water-attenuation cyst
- The wall may calcify

MRI
- Low T1 signal, high T2 signal

Nuclear cardiology

- SPECT scans provide a three-dimensional display of radionuclide distribution
- Images acquired over a 180° arc from right anterior oblique to left posterior oblique views
- More accurate than older planar imaging technique

Radiopharmaceutical agents

Thallium-201

- Intravenous injection at maximal heart rate ('stress study')
- Decays to mercury-201 by electron capture
- Emits both gamma-rays and X-rays
- 90% is cleared from the blood after its first circulation
- 4% is taken up by the heart at rest and 10% during maximal exercise
- Enters cardiac myocytes via the sodium–potassium ATPase pump
- Distribution through the myocardium is proportional to perfusion
- Images are acquired immediately after injection
- Booster injection and repeat imaging at 2–4 hours for a 'rest study'
- Repeat imaging at 24–48 hours to assess hibernating myocardium

Limitations of thallium

- High radiation dose (18-22 mSv)
- Low signal-to-noise ratio in obese patients

Technetium-99m

- Labelled with perfusion tracer, e.g. sestamibi
- Passive diffusion into cardiac myocytes
- No redistribution; retained in myocardium for up to 48 hours, and hence the need for separate rest and stress imaging
- Stress study is done first for ischaemia; rest study is done first to assess viability
- Lower dose (8 mSv) than thallium but not as good as thallium for assessing viability

Stress imaging

- Myocardial stress response is critical in patient assessment
- Perfusion defects are only seen at rest with > 90% stenosis
- Heart rate achieved should ideally be > 85% maximum predicted
- Dynamic exercise (treadmill) or pharmacological stress whereby adenosine, dipyridamole or dobutamine are used to induce coronary artery vasodilation and tachycardia
- Imaging can be with SPECT or MRI (and more recently CT perfusion imaging has been described)
- Sensitivity for detecting > 70% coronary stenosis
  - ECG stress test: 65% sensitivity
  - Myocardial perfusion imaging: 80–90% sensitivity

Patterns of abnormality

- Reversible defect
  - Perfusion defect at stress but normal at rest
  - Implies inducible ischaemia
- Fixed defect
  - Perfusion defect at stress that persists at rest
  - Implies myocardial scar tissue, e.g. old myocardial infarction
- Lung uptake
  - A little lung uptake is a normal finding but a lung–myocardial uptake ratio > 0.5 signifies impaired left ventricular function
  - Lung uptake is also seen with bronchogenic carcinoma and lymphoma

False positive cardiac SPECT

- Cardiomyopathies
- Coronary spasm
- Infiltrative disease e.g. sarcoidosis

False negative cardiac SPECT

- 'Balanced' triple-vessel disease
- Inadequate stress

Cardiac MRI

Clinical applications

- Congenital heart disease
- Myocardial viability assessment
- Cardiomyopathy

- Valvular assessment (including prosthetic)
- Pericardial disease

Basic sequences

Spin-echo sequence (black blood)

- Double inversion recovery pulse suppresses signal from moving blood
- Mainly used for anatomical and morphological overview
- Can be used to assess for aortic dissection and coarctation
- Parameters can be adjusted to obtain both T1WI and T2WI
- Fat saturation sequences are useful for diagnosing arrhythmogenic right ventricular dysplasia

Gradient-echo sequence (bright blood)

- Rapid acquisition using balanced steady-state free, precession (SSFP) sequence with low flip angles
- Image contrast depends on ratio of T2/T1 times
- Excellent inherent contrast between myocardium (dark) and luminal blood (bright)
- Used to create cine-images for assessing wall motion abnormalities, valvular function and turbulent flow (signal loss)

Basic scanning method

- Phased array cardiac surface coil
- ECG gating and/or respiratory gating
- R wave chosen as gating signal reference point

MR coronary artery angiography

- ECG trigger delayed to acquire images in end-diastole
- SSFP sequence with respiratory (navigator) gating
- No contrast media required
- Limited by poor spatial resolution (1–2 mm) at 1.5 Tesla

- Mainly used to identify coronary artery anatomical variants and to assess for proximal vessel patency

Myocardial perfusion imaging

- Dynamic first-pass imaging following a gadolinium contrast bolus
- Rapid image acquisition (high temporal resolution) is achieved via echoplanar sequences and segmented k-space filling
- Normal myocardium shows a uniform 'contrast blush'
- Delayed 'wash-in' is seen in areas of relative hypoperfusion
- Stress images are acquired using intravenous vasodilators (adenosine) to induce vasodilation and increase oxygen demand
- With significant stenosis (> 70%), flow cannot be sufficiently increased, which causes hypoperfusion in an arterial territory
- Study is later repeated at rest for comparison
- MR perfusion imaging is similar to PET and catheter angiographic studies in terms of detecting myocardial ischaemia

Delayed enhancement imaging

- Technique of choice for distinguishing viable myocardium from non-viable myocardium
- Accurately sizes regions of myocardial necrosis
- More sensitive than SPECT, PET and dobutamine stress echocardiography for detection of subendocardial infarcts (improved spatial resolution)
- Myocardial scar tissue shows delayed uptake of contrast, which washes out more slowly than in normal myocardium
- Delayed images acquired 10–20 minutes after gadolinium administration
- An inversion recovery pulse is used to null the myocardial signal and make gadolinium accumulation stand out

Myocardial infarction

- Subendocardial or transmural delayed hyperenhancement corresponding to an epicardial arterial territory

- < 25% thickness: good functional recovery likely with revascularisation
- > 75% thickness: poor functional recovery likely with revascularisation

Hibernating myocardium

- This is contractile dysfunction caused by chronic hypoperfusion
- Absence of delayed hyperenhancement
- Shows good functional recovery with revascularisation

Delayed enhancement in other pathologies

- Many non-ischaemic pathologies are associated with delayed gadolinium enhancement
- The pattern typically does not correspond to an arterial territory which helps with distinction

Hypertrophic cardiomyopathy

- Patchy hyperenhancement within hypertrophied regions
- Correspond to areas of minor infarcts or fibrosis
- Junction of the right ventricular free wall and the interventricular septum is a typical site
- High levels of enhancement correlate with a worse prognosis

Sarcoidosis

- Cardiac involvement seen in 20–30% of cases
- May initially cause a restrictive picture; a dilated picture more typical of late-stage disease
- Mid-myocardial wall hyperenhancement seen in affected areas, most often along the interventricular septum and basal inferolateral wall

Myocarditis

- Non-specific, patchy mid-myocardial wall hyperenhancement
- Diffuse involvement, which decreases during healing phase

Amyloidosis

- Infiltration of fibrillar proteins causing a restrictive cardiomyopathy

- Hyperenhancement is globally diffuse, and typically subendocardial

Cardiac CT

- Mainly used for non-invasive coronary artery evaluation

Coronary CT angiography

- High negative predictive value for exclusion of haemodynamically significant coronary artery disease in selected patient groups
- Calcified coronary artery plaque burden is a predictor of future cardiovascular events, but absence does not rule it out
- The amount of calcium underestimates the true extent of atherosclerotic disease
- Technique
  - Performed using ECG gating
  - Non-contrast study is usually performed first for assessment of coronary artery calcium burden
  - Target heart rate is 50–60 beats per minute (intravenous beta-blockers are administered to achieve this rate)
  - Intravenous contrast bolus is injected at a fast rate (5–6 mL/second), followed by a saline chaser to reduce SVC and right heart streak artefacts
  - Data are continuously acquired over one or more heart beats
  - Reconstructed using various post-processing algorithms
  - Phase of least cardiac motion (end-diastole) is selected at around 70% of the R–R interval
  - Review is made using axial source images, maximum intensity projections (MIPs) and multiplanar reformats (MPRs)
  - Isotropic voxel dimensions (equal size in the x, y and z axes) allow reconstruction in any plane without loss of image quality
  - Volume-rendered images are not diagnostic but help in obtaining a bird's eye view of grafts and other anomalies

Image resolution

- Cardiac CT requires high temporal and spatial resolution to 'freeze' cardiac motion and resolve the coronary vessels

Temporal resolution

- 64-slice CT: approximately 160 milliseconds
- Dual-source CT: approximately 80 milliseconds
- Electron beam CT: approximately 70 milliseconds
- This compares with MRI at 30–40 milliseconds and fluoroscopy at 1–10 milliseconds

---

Factors to improve temporal resolution

- Increased gantry rotation time
- Multiple segment reconstruction (in which data are selected from several cardiac cycles instead of from a single cycle; this requires retrospective ECG gating)

Spatial resolution

- 64-slice CT: approximately 0.4 mm, versus MRI (1–2 mm)

Factors to improve spatial resolution

- Thinner detector width
- Decreased reconstruction interval (the degree of overlap between reconstructed axial images; decreasing the reconstruction interval increases overlap and improves resolution)
- Small field of view
- Low pitch

Cardiac CT dose reduction

- Typical effective CT calcium scoring dose is 1–3 mSv
- Typical effective CT angiography dose is 5–15 mSv (equivalent to 500 CXRs)
- Effective dose using ECG-gated dose modulation is 3–10 mSv
- This compares with diagnostic coronary catheter angiography at 3–6 mSv

ECG-gated dose modulation

- A method of reducing dose by 10–40%
- Uses ECG gating to reduce the tube current during parts of the cardiac cycle that are not used in image reconstruction, e.g. systole

Heart valve imaging

- Echocardiography is the first-line test
- Cardiac MRI is also a reliable means of assessment and provides accurate assessment of transvalvular gradients
- Cardiac CT is the best means of assessing valvular calcification. Although it cannot directly assess the gradient across a valve it can be used to provide indirect assessment of function via orifice area measurement

Chapter 2

Musculoskeletal system and trauma

Ossification centres

- Clavicle
  - Membranous ossification with the secondary ossification centre appearing at the sternal end
- Scapula
  - Coracoid (17 years), acromion (15–18 years), scapula (20 years)
- Humerus
  - Greater tuberosity (1 year), lesser tuberosity (2 years), humeral head (5 years)
- Elbow
  - CRITOL: capitellum (1 year), radial head (3 years), internal epicondyle (5 years), trochlea (9–11 years), olecranon (9–11 years), lateral epicondyle (9–11 years)
  - Epiphyses fuse together and with the shaft at 17 years
- Hand
  - Capitate and hamate (4 months), triquetral (3 years), lunate (4 years), trapezium, trapezoid and scaphoid (6 years), pisiform (11 years)
  - Metacarpal heads fuse before the bases
- Femur
  - Proximal femur (6 months to 1 year), greater trochanter (3–5 years), lesser trochanter (8–14 years), distal femur (at birth)
- Tibia
  - Proximal tibia (at birth)
- Feet
  - Calcaneus and talus (6 months), cuboid (at birth), navicular (3 years)

Important muscle attachments

- These muscle attachments are best remembered by the patterns of avulsion injuries encountered in practice
- Pelvis
  - Ischial tuberosity: hamstrings
  - Anterior superior iliac spine: sartorius, tensor fascia lata
  - Anterior inferior iliac spine: rectus femoris (straight head)
  - Groove above the anterior acetabular rim: rectus femoris (reflected head)
  - Symphysis and inferior pubic ramus: adductors, gracilis
- Femur
  - Greater trochanter: gluteus medius, gluteus minimus
  - Lesser trochanter: iliopsoas
- Knee
  - Lateral tibial plateau: second fracture, bony avulsion injury of the iliotibial band and the lateral collateral ligament (anterior oblique band)
  - Fibular head: lateral collateral ligament, long head of biceps femoris (conjoint tendon)
  - Anterior tibial intercondylar area: anterior cruciate ligament
  - Posterior tibial intercondylar area: posterior cruciate ligament
  - Inferior pole of patella: patellar tendon
- Ankle and foot
  - Calcaneus, posterior surface: Achilles tendon
  - Base of fifth metatarsal: peroneus brevis
- Humerus
  - Greater tuberosity: supraspinatus, infraspinatus and teres minor
  - Lesser tuberosity: subscapularis
- Elbow
  - Medial epicondyle: common flexor origin
  - Lateral epicondyle: common extensor origin

Accessory bones

- Accessory navicular (os tibiale externum, os naviculare): seen in 5% of the population, found on the medial aspect of the foot
- Os trigonum: found just posterior to the talus
- Os vesalianum: found near the base of the fifth metatarsal
- Os acromiale: failure of fusion of the

acromion, seen in 10% of the population over 25 years of age

Joints of the upper limb

Shoulder joint

- A synovial ball-and-socket joint

Rotator cuff

- Four muscles comprise the rotator cuff; it is deficient in the inferior aspect
  - Supraspinatus: from the supraspinous fossa of the scapula to the greater tuberosity of the humerus
  - Infraspinatus: from the infraspinous fossa of the scapula to the greater tuberosity of the humerus
  - Teres minor: from the lateral border of the scapula to the greater tuberosity of the humerus
  - Subscapularis: form the anterior surface of the scapula to the lesser tuberosity of the humerus

Bursas

- There are two bursas associated with the shoulder joint
  - The subacromial–subdeltoid bursa
  - The subscapular bursa, which normally communicates with the joint space (unlike the subacromial–subdeltoid bursa)

Elbow joint

- Synovial hinge joint
- The capitellum articulates with the radial head and the trochlea articulates with the semilunar notch (trochlear notch) of the ulna
- There are two fat pads, anterior and posterior
  - The anterior is seen in 15% of the population
  - Elevation of the posterior fat pad is always abnormal
- The anterior humeral line intersects the mid-third of capitellum; the longitudinal axis of the radius should pass through the centre of capitellum

Wrist joint

- Synovial ellipsoid joint

- Between distal end of the radius and the scaphoid, lunate and triquetral bones
- Contents of the carpal tunnel: nine tendons (four flexor digitorum superficialis tendons, four flexor digitorum profundus tendons and one flexor pollicis longus tendon) and the median nerve
- The ulnar nerve and artery course through Guyon's canal, at the volar aspect of the pisiform

Carpals

- Proximal row: scaphoid, lunate, triquetral and pisiform
- The pisiform is a sesamoid bone in the tendon of the flexor carpi ulnaris
- Distal row: trapezium, trapezoid, capitate and hamate

Articulation of the carpals

- Scaphoid articulates with the trapezium and trapezoid distally, the capitate and lunate medially
- Capitate articulates with seven bones: the scaphoid and lunate proximally, the second, third and fourth metacarpal distally, the trapezoid on the radial side, and the hamate on the ulnar side
- Hamate articulates with the fourth and fifth metacarpals distally, the trapezium medially, and the capitate laterally

Scaphoid

- Boat-shaped, with a body, waist and tuberosity
- Blood supply is from distal to proximal
- Fractures through the waist of the scaphoid can disrupt the blood supply, resulting in avascular necrosis of the proximal part

Carpal tunnel

- Fibro-osseous tunnel bound by the carpals dorsally and the flexor retinaculum on the volar aspect
- Contents
  - Median nerve
  - Tendons of the flexor digitorum

superficialis and profundus (in a
common sheath)
- Flexor pollicis longus
- Palmaris longus, flexor carpi radialis
and flexor carpi ulnaris are the three
tendons that are outside the carpal
tunnel

Joints of the lower limb

Pelvis and hip

- Synovial ball-and–socket joint between the
head of femur and the acetabulum
- The width of the symphysis pubis should
not exceed 7 mm on anteroposterior views
- A fibrocartilagenous rim (the labrum)
deepens the acetabulum
- The symphysis pubis is a secondary
cartilaginous joint
- Ligaments
  - Ischiofemoral ligament
  - Pubofemoral ligament, which is
triangular in shape
  - Iliofemoral, which is an inverted 'V'
shape
  - Ligament of the head of the femur
- Important relations
  - Anterior: the femoral vessels and the
femoral nerve
  - Posterior: the sciatic nerve
  - Shenton's line: seen on anteroposterior
radiograph of pelvis, it joins the inferior
edge of inferior ischiopubic ramus
to the inferior edge of the shadow of
neck of femur; discontinuity denotes a
fracture of the neck of femur

Imaging of the hip joint

- Von Rosen's view: 45° abduction and
internal rotation of the hip, used to
assess instability of the hip joint in
children

- The blood supply of the femoral head
comes from three sources
  - Along the capsule of hip joint, derived
from the trochanteric anastomosis

- From the shaft (the nutrient artery)
- Through the ligament of the head of the
femur
- The most important source is the capsular
artery, which can get disrupted in fractures
of the neck of the femur

The linea aspera

- A ridge of roughened surface on the
posterior aspect of the femur
- Attachments
  - Gluteus maximus
  - Short head of the biceps femoris
  - Pectineus and iliacus
  - Adductor magnus
  - Vastus medialis and vastus lateralis
  - Adductor brevis and adductor longus

Sacroiliac joint

- Synovial joint at its inferior two thirds
and a fibrocartilaginous articulation at its
superior one third (similar to the pubic
symphysis)
- Ligaments
  - Ventral and dorsal sacroiliac ligaments
  - Interosseous sacroiliac ligament
(strongest ligament in the body)

Knee joint

- Modified synovial hinge joint
- Consists of two joints between the femoral
and tibial condyles and the patellofemoral
joint

Bursas

- Important bursas are the suprapatellar,
pre-patellar, infrapatellar and popliteal
bursas

Ligaments

- Important ligaments
  - Medial collateral ligament: between
the medial femoral epicondyle and the
medial tibial condyle
  - Lateral collateral ligament: between
the lateral femoral epicondyle and the
fibular head
  - Anterior cruciate ligament: between the
anterior tibial intercondylar area and
the posterior part of the medial surface
of the lateral femoral condyle

– Posterior cruciate ligament: between the posterior tibial intercondylar area and the anterior part of the lateral surface of the medial femoral condyle; prevents the femur from sliding forwards on tibia

Menisci

- The menisci are semicircular, fibrocartilaginous bands
- They appear triangular on coronal and sagittal imaging as they taper from a height of 3–5 mm at the periphery to a sharp, thin, central free margin
- Medial meniscus is larger and more 'C'-shaped than its lateral counterpart
- Its posterior horn is larger than its anterior horn
- It is more closely attached to the joint capsule, and being less mobile has a greater risk of tearing
- The body of medial and lateral menisci show a 'bowtie' configuration on two contiguous sagittal 4 mm MRI scans
- Discoid meniscus (with predilection for the lateral meniscus) represents a thickened meniscus with a bowtie configuration seen on three or more sagittal MRI scans
- Meniscofemoral ligaments course from the posterior horn of the lateral meniscus to the medial femoral condyle
- If present anterior to the posterior cruciate ligament, it is called the ligament of Humphry; if posterior to the posterior cruciate ligament, it is called the ligament of Wrisberg

Patella

- Sesamoid bone
- Appears at the age of 3 years
- Can be bipartite in 10% of people
- Prone to lateral dislocation
- Fabella is found in 25% of adults and lies in the lateral head of the gastrocnemius
- The patellar tendon is a continuation of the quadriceps tendon and is attached to the tibial tuberosity

Popliteus muscle

- Origin is the lateral surface of the lateral femoral condyle
- Insertion is at the posterior tibia, deep to the lateral collateral ligament
- Action: 'Key' muscle that helps unlocking the knee at beginning of flexion by facilitating the slight inward rotation of the tibia
- Also attached to the lateral meniscus by ligaments

Ankle joint and foot

Articulation of the tarsals

- Navicular articulates with the talus proximally, the three cuneiform bones distally, and occasionally with the cuboid laterally
- Cuboid articulates with the fourth and fifth metatarsal bases distally the calcaneus proximally (forming the calcaneocuboid joint), and the lateral cuneiform bone and the navicular bone medially; the inferior surface has a groove at its distal third for the tendon of the peroneus longus muscles

- The fifth metatarsal
  - Articulates with cuboid and the fourth metatarsal
  - Peroneus tertius and peroneus brevis insert on it
  - Its normal apophysis is longitudinal to it, at the base of bone
  - Jones's fracture involves the metaphyseal–diaphyseal junction and should not be confused with the commoner distal, transversely oriented fracture that occurs at the base of the fifth metatarsal

Osteoarthritis

- Degenerative joint disease affecting males and females equally
- Due to intrinsic degeneration of articular cartilage or excessive wear and tear
- Affects the hips and knees more commonly than shoulders and elbows
- Note there is a rare erosive variant of OA that is seen in middle-aged women
- Small joint involvement
  - Primary osteoarthritis frequently involves the hand, wrist, acromioclavicular joint, hip, knee (medial compartment), foot and spine
  - Involvement of hands is 10 times more common in women than in men
  - In the hand, the distal interphalangeal (DIP) joints are the most commonly involved
  - Loss of cartilage in the first carpometacarpal (CMC) and metacarpophalangeal (MCP) joints is typical

Imaging features
- Cartilage destruction in the weight-bearing portions of the joint
- Absence of erosions
- Bone density preserved
- Narrowing of joint space is an early feature
- Osteophytosis
- Subchondral sclerosis
- Subchondral cysts, due to microfractures in the subchondral bone

Rheumatoid arthritis

- Erosive arthropathy affecting females more than males
- Rheumatoid factor may be negative early in the disease, but becomes positive in 90–95% of cases subsequently
- Rheumatoid factor may be falsely positive in older people

Imaging features
- Polyarticular synovitis with osteoporosis
- Uniform cartilage destruction
- No productive changes, i.e. absent osteophytes/periostitis
- Typically bilaterally symmetric involvement of the following joints
  - Wrist: the radiocarpal joints and the distal radio-ulnar joints
  - Hand: the MCP joints and the PIP joints
  - Foot: the metatarsal phalangeal (MTP) joints and the retrocalcaneal bursa
- Rotator cuff tears at the shoulder, valgus deformity of knee and protrusio deformity of the hips are associated features
- Upper cervical spine may display facet erosions and atlantoaxial subluxation

Juvenile rheumatoid arthritis/ juvenile chronic arthritis

- Still's disease is a type of juvenile rheumatoid arthritis, presenting as an acute illness with pyrexia, anaemia, leukocytosis, hepatosplenomegaly, lymphadenopathy and polyarthritis
- Only 10% of cases are positive for rheumatoid factor
- Radiographic features are generally mild and only about 25% of patients develop chronic and destructive arthritis
- Commonly affected joints: knees, elbows and hips
- Metaphyseal and epiphyseal ballooning (due to hyperaemia)
- The growth plate closes early as a result of hyperemia and there is asymmetric maturation of ossification centres
- Can cause ankylosis in the carpus, tarsus and spine
- Atlantoaxial subluxation is not a common finding and occurs in seropositive cases

Ankylosing spondylitis

- An autoimmune spondyloarthropathy

associated with ulcerative colitis, enteritis, iritis and aortic valve disease
- Commoner in males
- Median age 15–35 years

Imaging features
- Sacroiliitis is the hallmark feature. Involvement of the axial skeleton is more common than peripheral skeleton. Unilateral early on, then becomes bilateral
- Changes in the spine include: vertical syndesmophytes (bamboo spine), squaring, marginal syndesmophytes
- Spine fractures easily at cervicothoracic and thoracolumbar junctions
- Peripheral large joint erosive arthritis is also a feature

Psoriatic arthropathy

- Seronegative spondyloarthropathy involving synovial and cartilaginous joints
- Occurs in 5% of patients with psoriasis and may occur before the onset of skin changes
- Five clinical and radiological types
  - Polyarthritis with predominant involvement of the DIP joints
  - Seronegative rheumatoid-like polyarthritis
  - Oligoarticular arthritis
  - Spondyloarthritis mimicking ankylosing spondylitis
  - Arthritis mutilans

Imaging features
- DIP joints more severely affected than PIP joints
- Bone density preserved
- Periostitis and 'sausage digit' (soft tissue swelling of the entire digit) may help distinguish psoriatic arthropathy from rheumatoid arthritis
- 'Pencil-in-cup' deformity may be seen, secondary to erosions that are initially periarticular and progress to involve the entire articular surface
- Tuft resorption or reactive sclerosis in distal phalanx ('ivory phalanx')
- Asymmetric sacroiliitis and spondylitis with paravertebral ossification
- Bulky asymmetric osteophytoses

Reiter's syndrome

- Clinical triad of arthritis, uveitis and urethritis
- Males are more frequently affected than females
- May be sexually transmitted or occur following dysentery
- HLA-B27 positive in 80% of cases

Imaging features
- Identical to psoriasis, but usually involves lower extremity instead
- Osteoporosis is a feature of acute disease, but not of recurrent or chronic disease
- Calcaneal erosions with spur formation are typical
- Bulky asymmetric paravertebral ossification are seen in the thoracolumbar spine

Systemic lupus erythematosus

- Over 80% have symmetric, non-erosive, non-deforming polyarthritis affecting the small joints of the hands, wrists, knees, shoulders
- Bilateral and symmetrical
- Reducible deformities:
  - ulnar subluxation of the MCP joints and the first CMC joint
  - flexion or extension deformities of the interphalangeal joints
- Associated with avascular necrosis in unusual sites such as the talus
- Soft tissue calcification (usually in the lower extremities) in 10% of cases

Jaccoud's arthropathy

- Irreversible deformities
- Ulnar drift at the MCP joints as well as swan-neck and boutonière deformities
- Seen in rheumatic fever

Scleroderma

- 50% of patients have articular involvement

- The fingers, wrists and ankles are commonly affected
- Erosions may be seen at the DIP joints, the first MCP joints, the CMC joints and the MTP joints
- Acro-osteolysis with soft tissue atrophy is a feature
- Soft tissue calcification may be associated

Amyloidosis

- Primary or secondary
- Bulky nodular synovitis
- Well-marginated erosions
- Wrists, elbows and shoulders can be affected
- The cervical spine is classically involved in dialysis-related spondyloarthropathy

Charcot's joints (neuropathic arthropathy)

- Severely destructive, rapidly progressive arthropathy
- Usually monostotic
- Common causes include diabetes mellitus, syphilis, syringomyelia and spinal cord injury
- Rarer causes are multiple sclerosis, hereditary sensorimotor neuropathy (Charcot–Marie–Tooth disease), alcoholism, amyloidosis, intra-articular corticosteroids, congenital insensitivity to pain, scleroderma and dysautonomia (Riley–Day syndrome)
- Three forms are described: hypertrophic (accounting for 20% of cases), atrophic (40%) and mixed (40%)

Imaging features

- Classic description of the hypertrophic form is of 'five Ds': normal Density, joint Distension, bony Debris, joint Disorganisation, Dislocation
- The atrophic form shows severe bone resorption, with little or no debris
- All forms are invariably associated with large effusions

- No juxta-articular osteoporosis is seen unless the joint is infected

Gout

- Sodium urate crystal arthropathy
- Middle-aged and elderly men are usually affected
- Long latent period between onset of symptoms and bony changes

Imaging features

- Normal bone density, and cartilage is often intact
- No joint space narrowing till late, since this is primarily a non-inflammatory process with recurrent acute, intermittent episodes rather than chronic progression
- Olecranon bursitis is commonly associated
- Often asymmetric and monoarticular
- The first MTP joints, the DIP joints and the patellofemoral joints are the most frequently involved joints
- Erosions are sharply marginated and may be intra-articular or para-articular
- An overhanging edge of a para-articular erosion is pathognomonic
- Gouty tophus may rarely show amorphous calcification
- Gouty tophus is seen on MRI as low on T1-weighted images (T1WI) and variably high or low on T2-weighted images (T2WI), depending on calcium content and status of calcium hydration

Pyrophosphate arthropathy

- May be idiopathic or associated with hyperparathyroidism or hemochromatosis
- Chondrocalcinosis is usually present
- Symmetric involvement of the knees, wrists and MCP joints
- Presents clinically with a sudden onset of pain and fever, with a tender, swollen, red joint that has a reduced range of movements

Findings in calcium pyrophosphate dihydrate deposition disease

- Knee: patellofemoral disease predominates
- Wrist: radiocarpal disease, progress to scapholunate advanced collapse (SLAC)
- Hand: involves the second and third MCP joints
- Large subchondral cysts may be seen

Bone sarcoid

- Bony involvement is rare (occurs in up to 15% of known cases)
- The most frequently noted abnormality is lytic lesions with lacy trabeculae, usually in the middle or distal phalanges
- Generalised osteopenia, sclerosis of phalangeal tufts, and focal or generalised sclerosis are other known manifestations

Marfan's syndrome

- Connective tissue disorder of unknown cause
- Autosomal dominant
- One in 10,000
- Commonest locations are the lumbar spine and sacrum
- Skeletal manifestations
  - Kyphoscoliosis
  - Posterior scalloping, due to dural ectasia
  - Increased interpedicular distance
  - Increased anterior translation and subluxation at the C1–C2 level
  - Increased height of the odontoid process
  - Basilar invagination
  - Biconcave vertebrae
  - Early osteoarthritis
  - Protrusio acetabuli
  - Pectus excavatum
  - Pes planus, club foot, hallux valgus and hammer toes

Primary hyperparathyroidism

- Increased levels of parathyroid hormone
- Increased serum calcium and decreased serum phosphate
- Parathyroid adenomas account for over 90% of cases
- Middle-aged women most commonly affected
- Common clinical manifestations include nephrolithiasis, hypertension, peptic ulcer, pancreatitis, bone pain and psychiatric disorders
- Incidence of bone lesions is 25–40%
- Associations
  - Multiple endocrine neoplasia type 1 (Wermer's syndrome), with pituitary adenoma and pancreatic islet cell tumour
  - Multiple endocrine neoplasia type 2 (Sipple's syndrome), with medullary thyroid carcinoma and phaeochromocytoma

Imaging features

Plain X-ray
- Subperiosteal bone resorption (seen in only 10% of cases), commonly along the radial aspect of the middle phalanges of the second and third digits (other sites include the tufts, the medial metaphysis of the proximal humerus, the femur and the tibia)
- Resorption at other sites, which can be intracortical, endosteal, subchondral, subligamentous (in the calcaneus or clavicle) or trabecular
- Osteopenia in the majority of cases
- Cortical thinning
- Soft tissue calcifications
- Rarely, brown tumours
- Erosions in the sacroiliac joints, symphysis pubis, ligamentous insertions
- Resorption of the distal or medial end of the clavicle and the vertebral endplates (aggressive Schmorl's nodes)

- 'Pepper-pot' skull
- Diffuse osteosclerosis (rare)
- Chondrocalcinosis in 10–20% of cases, characteristically in the knee, symphysis pubis and wrist

Bone scan
- Normal in 80% of cases
- 24-hour study shows increased retention of phosphate tracers, focal uptake in affected areas, and brown tumours

Primary hyperparathyroidism versus secondary hyperparathyroidism

- Adenomas commonly in primary
- Brown tumours are seen in primary more than in secondary
- Soft tissue calcification is seen in secondary more than in primary
- Bone sclerosis is seen in secondary more than in primary
- Periostitis is seen in secondary more than in primary

Osteoporosis

- Characterised by diminished bone mass, with a normal ratio of non-mineralised to mineralised bone
- Multiple causes
  - Diminished oestrogen levels
  - Family history
  - Low levels of weight-bearing exercise
  - Smoking
  - Alcohol abuse
  - Drugs, e.g. corticosteroids, heparin, phenytoin, phenobarbital
  - Poor nutrition

Imaging features

Plain X-ray
- Insensitive for the detection of osteoporosis: 50% bone loss is required before the loss can be seen

- Cortical thinning
- Fractures with delayed healing and poor callus formation

Dual energy X-ray absorptiometry (DEXA) scan
- The most precise way of estimating disease burden
- It works by comparing a patient's bone density with normal ranges in age-matched populations (giving the Z score) and young populations (giving the T score)
- The T score is more useful as they give an indication of fracture risk
- T scores 1–2 standard deviations below the mean density are defined as being osteopenic
- T scores < 2 standard deviations below the mean density are defined as indicating osteoporosis

Renal osteodystrophy

- Bone changes in chronic kidney disease
- Secondary hyperparathyroidism, osteomalacia, bone sclerosis and aluminium toxicity all contribute to the findings in renal osteodystrophy

Imaging features
- Osteopenia and/or osteosclerosis
- Changes due to osteomalacia and rickets: coarsened, blurred trabeculae and metaphyseal fraying or cupping
- Secondary hyperparathyroidism, with typical changes of bone resorption, brown tumours, periosteal new bone formation and chondrocalcinosis

- 'Rugger jersey' spine: bands of hazy sclerosis in parallel with the end-plates
- Profuse soft tissue calcifications and tumoural calcinosis

Acromegaly

- Excess of growth hormone
- Leads to gigantism in skeletally immature people
- Leads to bone widening and acral growth in adults

Imaging features
- Soft tissue thickening over the phalanges and heel pad
- Enlarged sella turcica
- Prominence of facial bones, increased vertebral body and disc height with posterior vertebral scalloping
- Exaggerated thoracic kyphosis is associated
- Enlarged paranasal sinuses with increased pneumatisation
- Spade-like phalanges

Hypothyroidism

- Mild osteoporosis
- Soft tissue swelling
- Delayed skeletal maturity
- Delayed dental development
- Wormian bones
- Bullet-shaped vertebrae at the thoracolumbar junction
- Stippled epiphyses

Infections

Osteomyelitis

Aetiology

- Haematogenous spread is the commonest mode
  - Neonates: *Staphylococcus aureus*, group B streptococci, *Escherichia coli*
  - Children: *Staphylococcus aureus*
  - Sickle cell anaemia: staphylococci still predominate, but with a higher incidence of *Salmonella*
  - Adults: *Staphylococcus aureus*
  - IVDU: Gram-negative bacteria (*Pseudomonas*, *Klebsiella*)
- Contiguous spread from soft tissue ulcers
- Spread along fascial planes from soft tissue infections of the hand

Imaging features of acute osteomyelitis

- Obliteration of soft tissue fat planes is often the first sign
- Osseous changes may not be evident for 1–2 weeks

- This is followed by signs of intramedullary destruction: a subtle permeative pattern within the bone or indistinctiveness of the cortex
- Cortical destruction follows, with accompanying endosteal cortical scalloping and periosteal reaction
- A sequestrum and involucrum eventually develop if left untreated
- Cloaca: a cortical and periosteal defect through which pus drains from infected medullary cavity

Imaging features of chronic osteomyelitis

- Brodie's abscess
- Thickened cortex (host reaction) with mixed bone density

Tuberculous osteomyelitis

- Slower course and less host reaction than in pyogenic osteomyelitis
- In children tuberculosis may first manifest itself in the small bones of the hands and feet, where it causes dactylitis (spina ventosa)

MRI findings in osteomyelitis			
Situation	T1WI	T2WI	T1WI plus gadolinium
Marrow inflammation	Low signal	High signal	High signal
Intraosseous abscess	Low signal	High signal	High signal in rim
Sequestrum	Low signal	Low signal	High signal around sequestrum
Cortical breech	Intermediate signal	Intermediate or high signal	Intermediate signal
Cloaca	Hard to see in low-signal periosteum	High signal	Not seen
Sinus tract	Not seen	High signal	High signal

Infection versus neuropathy in diabetes: diabetic dilemma

	Osteomyelitis	Neuroarthropathy
Location	Adjacent to ulcers Metatarsal heads Calcaneal tuberosity Distal phalanges Malleoli	Joints Tarsometatarsal (Lis franc) Talonavicular and Calcaneocuboid Ankle and subtalar joint
Other features	Cortical destruction Sequestrum Abscess	Bone fragmentation Malalignment
Non-discriminatory	Effusion Soft tissue oedema Bone marrow oedema Periosteal reaction	

Causes of rickets

< 6 months of age	> 6 months of age
• Hypophosphatasia • Prematurity • Primary hyperparathyroidism • Maternal deficiency of vitamin D	• Dietary deficiency of vitamin D • Liver dysfunction • Malabsorption • Chronic renal disease

Diabetic dilemma

- The dilemma is: infection versus neuropathy? (See table above)

Septic arthritis

- Early joint effusion
- Osteoporosis and cartilage destruction follow secondary to local hyperaemia
- Erosion and destruction make way to osteomyelitis
- Ankylosis may eventually occur
- Tuberculous and fungal septic arthritides are more chronic processes than bacterial arthritis; cartilage destruction is slow and the joint space remains relatively well preserved till late

Nutritional, metabolic and haematological diseases

Rickets

- Osteomalacia in the skeletally immature
- Caused by vitamin D deficiency (e.g. inadequate dietary intake or reduced exposure to sunlight); see table above

Imaging features

- Calcification of cartilage and osteoid does not occur, leading to widening of the zone of provisional calcification, which is perceived as metaphyseal widening on plain X-rays
- Widened and irregularly shaped metaphyses with flaring is caused by stress at sites of ligamentous attachments

- Microfractures of the primary spongiosa are caused by protrusion of physeal cartilage
- Physeal width is 2.5–3 mm in rickets (normal range is 0.9–1.9 mm)
- Cupping and fraying of the metaphyses is typical
- Metaphyseal spurs are also a feature
- Poorly mineralised epiphyseal centres with delayed appearance
- Periosteal reaction may be present
- Coarse trabeculation is noted (but ground-glass appearance is not a feature)
- Soft bones with deformities such as bowing
- Risk of Salter–Harris type I fractures in weight-bearing areas
- Skull: frontal bossing, premature fusion of the sagittal suture, delayed dentition and hypoplasia of enamel
- Ribs: cupping of the ends of the ribs, with widening of rib epiphyseal cartilage, giving a 'rachitic rosary' appearance
- Spine: scoliosis and biconcave vertebral bodies
- Pelvis: coxa vara, and triradiate pelvis caused by inwardly migrating sacrum and acetabula
- Knees: genu varum or valgum

Osteomalacia

- Vitamin D deficient state in adults
- Osteoid formation is normal, but mineralisation does not occur

Associations include neurofibromatosis type 1 and haemangiopericytoma

Imaging features

- Generalised bone demineralisation: lucent bones with indistinct trabecular detail and thinned cortex
- Soft bones with various deformities such as protrusio acetabuli
- A specific feature is the appearance of looser zones, or pseudofractures; these are characteristically located in the medial aspects of the proximal femurs, the pubic bones, the dorsal aspect of the proximal ulnas and the distal aspect of the scapula bones and ribs

Scurvy

- Caused by a long-term deficiency of vitamin C

Imaging features

- Ground-glass osteoporosis
- Increased density and widening of the zone of provisional calcification (white line of Frankl)
- Metaphyseal spurs or marginal fractures (Pelkan's sign)
- Transverse radiolucent band at the metaphysis subjacent to the zone of provisional calcification (scurvy line or Trummerfield's zone, which is a site of fractures and infarction)
- Parke corner sign: subepiphyseal infarction leading to cupping of the epiphysis
- Ring of increased density surrounding the epiphysis (Wimberger's sign)
- Periosteal elevation
- Sites of abnormalities include the distal end of femur, the proximal and distal ends of the tibia and fibula, the distal end of the radius and ulna, the proximal humerus, and the distal ends of the ribs

Haemophilia

- Bleeding disorder
- X-linked-recessive inheritance, hence found only in males

Imaging features

- Multiple episodes of haemarthroses, commonest in the knee, elbow and ankle joints (large joints)
- Dense effusions
- Hypertrophied synovium with haemosiderin deposits (low signal on T1WI and T2WI)
- Resulting hyperaemia causes osteoporosis of adjacent bones and epiphyseal overgrowth (enlargement and ballooning) with early closure
- Hence there is widening of the intercondylar notch on the femur
- Cartilage destruction, erosions and subarticular cysts are typical
- Secondary degenerative joint disease invariably ensues

- A pseudotumour of haemophilia may be seen: a non-neoplastic mass lesion appearing secondary to a bleed; pressure erosion occurs at the cortical region, with extrinsic or intrinsic scalloping and extensive periosteal reaction. A soft tissue mass may be associated with this

Sickle cell anaemia and thalassaemia

- Haemoglobinopathy (glutamic acid in position 6 is substituted by valine)
- Autosomal-recessive inheritance

Imaging features

- Patchy bone density secondary to chronic bone infarcts
- Avascular necrosis
- Chest radiograph should be evaluated for cardiomegaly and pulmonary infarcts
- Gallstones and autosplenectomy may be seen
- Three characteristic features
  - Marrow hyperplasia; in thalassaemia, marrow hyperplasia is florid with widening of the diploic space, with a 'hair-on-end' appearance; the paranasal sinuses are often obliterated. AVN is uncommon in thalassaemia
  - Marrow infarction (dactylitis is a common manifestation in the young; it is a periosteal reaction with soft tissue swelling and avascular necrosis of the hip and humeral head)
  - Osteomyelitis; while *Salmonella* osteomyelitis is known to occur in this patient group, staphylococci remain the commonest pathogens overall

Paget's disease

- Chronic skeletal disease characterised by abnormal osteoblastic and osteoclastic activity resulting in abnormal bone remodelling
- Rare before the age of 40 years; 3% occur in those > 40 years of age, 10% in those > 80 years of age
- Males are more commonly affected than females
- Most commonly affects the skull, followed by the spine, the pelvis and then long bones such as the femur
- Normal calcium and phosphate levels; raised alkaline phosphatase levels
- Three stages of disease: lytic, mixed and sclerotic
- Complications
  - Osteoarthritis (in 50–96% of cases)
  - Basilar skull invagination (in 30% of cases)
  - Insufficiency fractures, protrusions and proximal femoral varus deformity may be seen
  - Deafness (both types), due to spinal stenosis
  - Sarcomatous transformation (in < 1% of cases)
  - Osteomyelitis and metastases are more common in Paget's bones, owing to hypervascularity

Imaging features

- Pathognomic triad
  - Bone expansion
  - Cortical thickening
  - Trabecular bone thickening
- Disease starts at one end of the bone and progresses along the shaft
- Osteoporosis circumscripta of skull in the active stage, cotton-wool appearance with mixed lytic and blastic pattern of the thickened calvarium in late stages
- Paget's disease of the spine
  - Upper cervical spine, low thoracic spine and the mid-lumbar spine are the sites most commonly affected
  - Enlarged vertebral body, with a 'bone-within-bone' appearance
  - Ivory vertebrae
  - Ossification of spinal ligaments, paravertebral soft tissue and disc spaces

Osteopetrosis

- Increased bone density due to impaired osteoclastic function
- Bone marrow failure ensues in severe forms, contributing to mortality
- Pathological fractures (usually heal well)
- Associated with rickets (secondary to sequestration of calcium within bones)

Imaging features

Skull imaging

- Narrowed foramina
- Underdeveloped paranasal sinuses
- Retention of deciduous teeth
- Hypertelorism

Vertebral imaging

- 'Bone-within-bone' appearance
- 'Picture-frame' vertebrae with sclerotic borders
- Tendency to infection

Cervical spine

- The normal basion–axial distance and the normal basion–dental distance is 12 mm

Injury mechanisms

Hyperflexion

- Hyperflexion sprain
- Hyperflexion dislocation (without facet lock or with unilateral or bilateral facet lock)
- Comminuted ('tear-drop')
- Burst: two-column injury, with the fracture extending to involve the posterior cortex of the vertebral body
- Hyperflexion fracture–dislocation
- Occipito-atlantal dislocation or subluxation
- Atlantoaxial dislocation
- Anterior or lateral fracture–dislocation of the dens
- Clay shoveler's fracture: a fracture through the spinous process at the C6–T1 levels

Hyperextension

- Hangman's fracture: hyperextension and traction injury of the second cervical vertebra
- Hyperextension sprain
- Posterior fracture: dislocation of the dens
- Posterior atlantoaxial dislocation

Axial compression

- Jefferson's fracture, from a compression force to the first cervical vertebra; typical in diving injuries
- Occipital condyle fracture type 3

Unstable injury patterns

- Bilateral locked or jumped facets
- Flexion tear-drop fractures
- Hangman's fracture
- Hyperextension dislocation–fracture
- Jefferson's facture
- Odontoid fracture (particularly type 2)

Thoracic and lumbar spine injuries

- Injury patterns
  - Compression and wedge fractures
  - Burst fractures
  - Chance fractures: 'lap-belt' injury caused by sudden, severe flexion that is usually centred on the thoracolumbar region; injury can be purely bony, purely ligamentous or a combination of the two

Spondylosis

- Defect in the pars interarticularis
- A form of chronic stress fracture, with non-union, typically seen in adolescents who engage in sport
- Commonly seen at the L4–L5 and L5–S1 levels

Spondylolisthesis

- Bilateral pars defects lead to ventral subluxation of the vertebral body
- Aetiologies include dysplastic, isthmic (commonest type secondary to spondylolysis), degenerative, traumatic and pathological changes
- Four grades are described, based on the degree of anterior displacement

Upper limb trauma

Thumb fractures

- Bennett's fracture
  - Unstable fracture
  - Intra-articular fracture involving the base of the first metacarpal
  - The distal metacarpal fragment is pulled dorsally and laterally by the abductor pollicis longus muscle
- Rolando's fracture
  - Unstable fracture
  - Intra-articular, comminuted fracture of the base of the first metacarpal

- Extra-articular fracture
  - Stable injury
  - The CMC joint is not involved
  - Treated by closed reduction
- Gamekeeper's or skier's thumb
  - Injury to the ulnar (medial) collateral ligament at the MCP joint, occasionally accompanied by an avulsion fracture of the proximal phalangeal base
  - Steners lesion represents an abnormally interposed adductor aponeurosis between the torn ulnar collateral ligament and its distal attachment to the proximal phalangeal base

Carpal injuries

- Fractures of the scaphoid account for 60–70% of all carpal injuries, fractures of the triquetrum for 7–20%, while trapezoid fractures are the rarest type
- Scaphoid fracture
  - Peak age is 15–40 years
  - The arterial supply enters the waist of the scaphoid on the anterolateral surface
  - 70% in waist, 10% proximal pole, 20% distal pole
  - Healing without periosteal callus
  - Delayed or non-union is encountered in practically every proximal pole fracture and 30% of waist fractures

Imaging features

- Views in a scaphoid series: posteroanterior, lateral, 45° pronation oblique, and posteroanterior view with ulnar deviation

MRI

- Fracture line appears as low signal on T1WI, high signal on T2WI
- Sagittal images show scaphoid flexion (humpback deformity)
- Avascular necrosis is seen as loss of marrow signal, low signal on T1WI and T2WI; the risk of avascular necrosis is highest with proximal pole fractures, while there is no such risk with fractures of the distal pole

Bone scan

- May be negative in the first 48 hours (unlike MRI, which will be positive)

Dorsal intercalated segment instability (DISI) or dorsiflexion instability

- The lunate is angulated dorsally
- The scapholunate angle is increased (30–60° is normal, 60–80° is questionably abnormal, > 80° is abnormal)
- The capitolunate angle is increased (< 30° is normal)

Volar intercalated segmental instability (VISI), volarflexion instability or palmar flexion instability

- The lunate is tilted in a palmar direction
- The scapholunate angle is decreased (to < 30°)
- VISI may be a normal variant, especially if the wrist is very lax

---

- Lunate dislocation
  - Most severe carpal injury, and associated with a trans-scaphoid fracture
  - The lunate dislocates anteriorly (in a volar direction); the radius and capitate remain in a straight line
  - Triangular appearance of lunate on frontal projection
- Perilunate dislocation
  - Results from fall on the outstretched, hyperextended hand
  - Less common than lunate dislocation
  - Associated with scaphoid waist fractures
  - Whole of the carpus, except the lunate is displaced posteriorly; the radius and lunate remain in a straight line, and the capitate lies posteriorly and out of line
  - Triangular appearance of lunate on frontal view
- Triangular fibrocartilage tears
  - The triangular fibrocartilage is composed of the dorsal and volar radioulnar ligaments, as well as the articular disc

- It is a biconcave disc of hypointense signal on MRI
- Triangular fibrocartilage tears are a cause of ulnar-sided wrist pain and are associated with positive ulnar variance, while negative ulnar variance is associated with Kienböck's disease (avascular necrosis of the lunate)
- On MRI, the presence of fluid extending across the articular disc or discontinuity in the contour of the triangular fibrocartilage is pathognomonic
- Chondromalacia of the lunate, triquetrum or ulna are related findings, particularly when there is positive ulnar variance
- Likely to need surgical intervention in patients < 40 years of age, in whom trauma is often the aetiology
- Degenerative tears are common in patients > 40 years of age, and treatment is usually conservative

Fractures of the distal radius

- Colles' fracture
  - Dorsally angulated, impacted distal radial fracture with dorsal and radial displacement of the distal fracture segment
  - More frequent in osteoporotic women
- Smith's fracture
  - Reverse Colles' fracture, with volar angulation and volar displacement of distal fracture segment
- Barton's fracture
  - Unstable intra-articular fracture of the distal radius
  - The fracture extends through the dorsal margin of the radius, with associated dorsal dislocation of the carpus
- Reverse Barton's fracture
  - The anterior (volar) cortex of the distal radius is involved
  - A highly unstable injury

Fractures of the radius and ulna

- Monteggia fracture
  - Fracture of the shaft of the ulna associated with dislocation of the head of the radius

- Galeazzi fracture
  - Fracture of the shaft of the radius associated with dislocation at the distal radio-ulnar joint
- Fractures of the olecranon
  - Account for 20% of all elbow injuries
  - Apophysis fuses by the age of 14–16 years
  - Inability to extend the elbow is characteristic of olecranon injuries and is caused by triceps tendon dysfunction or injury
  - Soft tissue swelling in the olecranon bursa indicates injury
  - A posterior fat pad is a typical imaging feature

Elbow dislocation

- Commonest site of dislocation in children
- Posterior or posterolateral (displacement of radius and ulna in relation to the humerus) in 80–85% of cases
- Other forms are lateral, anterior and medial
- Associated with fractures in 20–60% of cases, most commonly of the medial condyle or epicondyle, followed by the head or neck of the radius
- Myositis ossificans appears in 3% of all elbow injuries, but in 89% of fractures and dislocations about the elbow in adults with associated head injury
- Usually appears within 3–4 weeks of injury
- Usually anterior to the joint
- Incidence increased by too early return to activity following an injury

Supracondylar injuries

- These fractures account for > 60% of all elbow fractures in children
- Hyperextension type of injury caused by a fall on the outstretched hand in > 95% of cases
- The elbow becomes locked in hyperextension
  The olecranon is displaced superiorly into the olecranon fossa, causing the anterior humeral cortex to bend and eventually break
- If the force continues, both the anterior and posterior humeral cortices can fracture

- If there is only minimal or no displacement, these fractures can be occult on X-ray, and the only sign will be a positive fat pad sign
- Usually there is some displacement, and the anterior humeral line will not usually pass through the centre of the capitellum; rather it will traverse the anterior third of the capitellum or even pass further anterior to the capitellum

Shoulder dislocation

- The most commonly dislocated joint
- Anterior dislocation: arm held in abduction and external rotation; account for 95–98% of emergency/casualty admissions for shoulder dislocation
- Posterior dislocation: common during seizure or electrocution, arm held in adduction and internal rotation
- Inferior dislocation: arm fully abducted with elbow commonly flexed; account for 0.5% of emergency/casualty admissions for shoulder dislocation

Imaging features

Plain X-ray

- Anteroposterior view
  - Anterior dislocation characterised by subcoracoid position of the humeral head
  - Posterior dislocation characterised by 'light-bulb' appearance of the humeral head, although this is not always seen; it can be diagnosed radiographically by identifying subtle asymmetry of the glenohumeral joint space in a post-trauma setting
- Injuries associated with anterior dislocation
  - Labral lesions, e.g. anteroinferior Bankart's tear, which is the most common lesion in anterior glenohumeral instability and is associated with a torn scapular periosteum
  - Bony glenoid lesions, e.g. osseous anterior glenoid rim fractures in 44% of cases
  - Ligamentous lesions (particularly of the anterior band of the inferior

glenohumeral ligament), leading to joint laxity
  - Hill–Sachs lesions in 77% of cases
  - Rotator cuff tears
  - Anterior labroligamentous periosteal sleeve avulsion (ALPSA), which represents a cartilaginous variant of Bankart's tear in which the torn labroligamentous complex is displaced medically and inferiorly and the scapular periosteum is preserved at the site of the labral tear
  - Perthes' lesion, another Bankart variant, in which the scapular periosteum remains intact but is stripped medially, and the anterior labrum is avulsed from the glenoid but remains partially attached to the scapula by the intact periosteum
  - Glenoid labral articular disruption (GLAD), a tear of the anteroinferior labrum with avulsion of the adjacent glenoid hyaline cartilage; the lesion is clinically stable because the labrum is not detached; the mechanism of injury is glenohumeral impaction in the ABER (ABduction and External Rotation) position
- Injuries associated with posterior dislocation
  - Posterior labral tear or detachment (reverse Bankart's tear)
  - Tear of the posterior band of the inferior glenohumeral ligament
  - Reverse Hill–Sachs lesion (impacted fracture of the anterior aspect of the humeral head), giving a 'trough' sign
  - Teres minor injury

Subacromial subdeltoid bursal impingement

- Compression of the supraspinatus muscle between humeral head and the coracoacromial arch
- Common in occupations and sports that involve overhead activities
- Anatomical variants that predispose to the impingement
  - Curved acromial arch
  - Anteroinferiorly hooked acromion

- Enthesophyte underneath the acromion
- Lateral acromial downsloping
- Os acromiale

Imaging features

Ultrasound
- Bunching of the subacromial subdeltoid bursa during abduction

MRI
- Thickened heterogeneous or torn tendon, with fluid in the subacromial bursa,
- Increased signal in the distal supraspinatus tendon on T1WI and T2WI

Lower limb trauma

Pelvic injury
- Pelvic fractures can be stable or unstable
- Stable pelvic fractures
  - Consist of single breaks in the pelvic ring or fractures of the peripheral margins that do not disrupt the ring
  - Account for two thirds of all pelvic injuries
  - Unilateral fracture of the pubic ramus (commonest pelvic fracture)
  - Iliac wing fracture (Duverney's fracture) involves the lateral margin of the ala and is caused by direct lateral compression; associated with paralytic ileus and abdominal rigidity (due visceral injury or irritation of the peritoneum by the underlying haematoma)
  - Sacral fractures are usually transverse and in the S3–S4 region
- Unstable fractures are those that disrupt the pelvic ring
  - Typical examples include Malgaigne's fracture, straddle fracture, pelvic dislocation and bucket-handle fracture
- Posterior arch fractures have a higher morbidity than anterior arch fractures
- Overall mortality in pelvic fractures is between 9-19%

Malgaigne's fracture
- Commonest unstable pelvic fracture (accounting for 14% of all types)
- Vertical shearing force involves both the anterior arch and the posterior arch on the ipsilateral side
- Results in double vertical fractures, most commonly through superior and inferior pubic rami and sacrum/ilium
- Usually results in superior displacement of the affected hemipelvis and hip

Straddle fracture
- Injury resulting from landing on a hard object in the straddle position, as seen in bicycle accidents
- Bilateral fractures of pubic and ischial rami
- Medial fracture fragments are usually elevated
- Associated with urethral and bladder injuries in 20% of cases

Pelvic dislocation
- Sprung pelvis ('open-book' injury) is usually associated with genitourinary injury with disruption of the pubic symphysis and bilateral sacroiliac joints
- Occurs secondary to an anteroposterior compression force
- Normal sacroiliac joint space is 1–4 mm
- Normal width of the pubic symphysis is 5 mm

Bucket-handle fracture
- Fracture of the anterior arch and the contralateral posterior arch
- Rare

Incidences of types of pelvic injury

- Vertical shearing: 10%
- Anterior compression: 15%
- Lateral compression: 65%
- Mixed: 10%

Acetabular fracture
- 20% of all pelvic fractures involve the acetabulum
- CT is the best modality of evaluating acetabular fractures
- Acetabular fractures are classified into four types: posterior rim fractures, transverse acetabular fractures, anterior column fractures and posterior column fractures

- Posterior rim fracture
  - Most common acetabular fracture, seen in 33% of cases
  - Occurs with posterior hip dislocation, the commonest type of hip dislocation
- Transverse acetabular fracture
  - Separates the bone into the halves
  - Disrupts along the iliopubic and ilioischial lines
  - May be associated with central dislocation of femoral head
- Anterior column fracture
  - Fracture through the iliopubic line
  - May be associated with central dislocation of femoral head
- Posterior column fracture
  - Fracture through the ilioischial line
  - May be associated with central dislocation of femoral head

Avulsion fractures of the pelvis: patterns and affected attachments

- Ischial tuberosity (hamstrings)
- Anterior inferior iliac spine (rectus femoris-straight head)
- Anterior superior iliac spine (sartorius)
- Iliac crest (abdominal muscles)

Complications and associated injuries

- Haemorrhage
  - Occurs 75% of cases of pelvic fracture
  - Usually arises from laceration of one or more branches of the internal iliac artery, particularly the superior gluteal branch
- Urinary tract injury
  - All patients who have sustained a pelvic fracture must be assumed to have a urinary tract injury until proven otherwise
  - Urethra is injured in 4–17% of cases, almost exclusively in males
  - The urethra at or above the level of the urogenital diaphragm (posterior or membranous urethra) is the most susceptible to injury
  - The bladder is injured in 4% of cases, and in 60–80% of these cases the injury is extraperitoneal
- Visceral injury
  - Occurs in 20% of cases

  - Most commonly involves the liver, spleen and the left side of the diaphragm
- Neural injury
  - The sciatic nerve is susceptible to injury in posterior fracture–dislocation injuries
  - Reported incidence of neurological deficits in conjunction with pelvic fractures is approximately 12%; they are more likely to occur in sacral fractures
- Bowel injury
  - Rare but carries a high mortality
  - Small bowel is more susceptible than the large bowel
  - Paralytic ileus is a common occurrence in pelvic injuries
- Infections
  - Retroperitoneal abscesses may form, even 3 months after injury if there has been an open fracture

Knee injuries

Meniscal tears

- Meniscal tears occur in two primary planes, vertical and horizontal
- Three basic shapes of meniscal tears: longitudinal, horizontal and radial; complex tears are a combination of these basic shapes
- Two most important criteria for detecting meniscal tears
  - Abnormal shape
  - High signal intensity unequivocally reaching the meniscal articular surface (superior or inferior, or both) on sagittal or coronal proton-density images

Displaced tears

- Bucket-handle tear is a displaced longitudinal tear, which is best recognised on coronal images
- Flap tear is a displaced horizontal tear
- Parrot-beak tear is displaced radial tear; it is an unstable tear
- Normally there are only two structures in the intercondylar fossa: the anterior and posterior cruciate ligament; any other structure in the intercondylar fossa is abnormal and should raise suspicion for a displaced meniscal fragment

Meniscal cyst

- Horizontal tears divide the meniscus into top and bottom parts
- If a horizontal tear extends all the way from the apex to the outer margin of the meniscus, it may result in the formation of a meniscal cyst
- Synovial fluid runs through the horizontal tear and accumulates peripherally, resulting in a meniscal cyst
- A meniscal cyst can lose its communication with the joint space and hence may not fill with contrast on MR arthrography

The three criteria for the diagnosis of a meniscal cyst

1 Horizontal tear
2 Focal area of fluid accumulation (bright on T2WI)
3 Adjacent to the peripheral margin of meniscus

Discoid meniscus

- Large dysplastic meniscus with loss of the normal semilunar shape
- Commonly affects the lateral meniscus and may be bilateral
- Patients usually present with pain, clicking and snapping of the knee
- Continuous appearance of the meniscus on three consecutive, 4–5 mm thick sagittal slices is characteristic

Ligamentous injury

Anterior cruciate ligament

- Normally an intracapsular extrasynovial structure
- Primary stabiliser against anterior tibial subluxation
- Composed of between three and five layers of fibres
- Between the fibres there can be fat or synovium or sometimes a small amount of fluid. This explains the fact that the anterior cruciate ligament is not entirely of low signal on proton-density images
- Oriented at a 55° incline to the tibial plateau

- There is non-visualisation of 5–10% of normal anterior cruciate ligaments on sagittal-plane views
- Injury mechanisms and patterns
  - Valgus and anterolateral rotatory subluxation of the knee typically causes injury to the anterior cruciate ligament
  - Commoner in females and young, active people
  - Location of rupture is mostly near femoral origin of the ligament
  - MRI does not accurately differentiate between partial and complete tears
  - On X-rays an important indirect sign of an anterior cruciate ligament tear is a Segond fracture, which is a bony avulsion injury of the iliotibial band or the lateral collateral ligament (anterior oblique band)

Indirect signs of an anterior cruciate ligament tear

High specificity
- Deep lateral femoral notch sign
- Abnormal orientation of the posterior cruciate ligament

Low sensitivity
- Bone contusions of the posterior aspect of the lateral tibial plateau and the mid-portion of the lateral femoral condyle
- Anterior tibial translocation
- Uncovering of the posterior horn of the lateral meniscus
- Visualising the lateral collateral ligament in just one coronal image (rather than two or three images)
- Fracture with high association of anterior cruciate ligament tears, including a Segond fracture

Posterolateral corner injury

- Infrequent injury
- Usually associated with anterior cruciate ligament and/or posterior cruciate ligament injuries
- Severe disability ensues from unrecognised injury, owing to instability and articular degeneration

- Missed injury can result in failure of reconstructed anterior cruciate ligament or posterior cruciate ligament
- If a bone bruise is seen anteromedially, ligamentous injury on the contralateral side (the posterolateral corner) ought to be suspected

Posterolateral corner of the knee

The posterolateral corner (or posterolateral complex) is a complex anatomical system that contains seven or eight structures. The orthopaedic surgeon is interested particularly in three of these structures, which are easily visualised on MRI:

1 Lateral collateral ligament (fibular collateral ligament)
2 Biceps femoris muscle and tendon
3 Popliteus tendon

Contusion patterns in knee trauma

- Pivot shift injury: contusion in the posterolateral tibial plateau and the mid-portion of the lateral femoral condyle
- Dashboard injury: contusion in the anterior aspect of the proximal tibia
- Hyperextension injury: kissing contusion between the anterior aspect of the proximal tibia and distal femur; an anteromedial bone bruise is seen
- Clip injury: contusion in the lateral and medial femoral condyles
- Lateral patellar dislocation: oedema in the inferomedial patella and the anterior aspect of the lateral femoral condyle

The 'unhappy' triad (O'Donoghue's triad)

Commonly occurs in contact sports such as football when the knee is hit from the outside, which causes an injury to three knee structures:

1 Anterior cruciate ligament
2 Medial cruciate ligament
3 Medial meniscus

Posterior cruciate ligament

- Prevents posterior subluxation of the tibia
- Isolated injuries to the posterior cruciate ligament are rare
- A typical scenario would be a dashboard injury, which is a hyperflexion mechanism of injury

Medial cruciate ligament

- Extends from the medial epicondyle to insert along the medial tibia, usually 7 cm below the joint space
- A long ligament, which firmly adheres to the joint capsule and the medial meniscal body

Lateral collateral ligament (fibular collateral ligament)

- Part of the posterolateral complex of the knee
- Originates in a sulcus along the lateral femoral condyle to insert as a conjoint tendon with the biceps femoris tendon on to the fibular head

Sites of post-traumatic avascular necrosis

- Hip involvement of one hip increases the risk to the contralateral hip (in such cases, avascular necrusosi is seen in up to 70%)
- Blount's disease (also called tibia vara) is avascular necrosis of the medial tibial condyle
- Kienböck's disease is avascular necrosis of the lunate bone
- Köhler's disease is avascular necrosis of the tarsal bone

Perthes' disease

- Avascular necrosis of the femoral head in children
- Peak age is 4–8 years
- Bilateral in up to 10% of cases
- Males are five times more commonly affected than females

- Usually idiopathic, but may be secondary to trauma

Imaging features

Plain X-ray
- Smaller femoral epiphysis on the affected side, typically with sclerosis
- Widened joint space (secondary to thickened intra-articular cartilage, joint fluid or joint laxity)
- Later, a lucent subchondral fracture line appears, followed by fragmentation of the femoral head

CT
- Loss of asterisk in the centre of the femoral head ('asterisk' refers to the stellate pattern of crossing trabeculae in the centre of a normal femoral head)

MR
- Marrow signal from femoral epiphysis is low on T1WI and high on T2WI
- Double-line sign: sclerotic rim between viable and non-viable bone is edged by a high-signal rim of granulation tissue

Slipped femoral epiphysis

- Atraumatic fracture through the physeal plate
- Usually one-sided
- Associations
  - Trauma (Salter-Harris type I injury)
  - Growth spurt (commonly seen in boys aged 8–17 years)
  - Renal osteodystrophy and rickets
  - Childhood irradiation
  - Growth hormone or steroid treatment
  - Developmental dysplasia of the hip
  - Perthes' disease
  - Endocrine problems, e.g. hypothyroidism, hypoestrogenism, acromegaly, cryptorchidism, pituitary adenoma, parathyroid adenoma
- Complications
  - Avascular necrosis (seen in 10–15% of cases)
  - Coxa vara
  - Osteoarthritis (in 90% of cases)
  - Discrepancy in limb length

Imaging features

- Widened growth plate (prior to the slip)
- Posteromedial displacement of head during the slip
- Decrease in the neck–shaft angle
- If long-standing, then one sees sclerosis and irregularity with a widened physis

Stress fractures

- May be an insufficiency fracture or a fatigue fracture
- Insufficiency fracture
  - Normal stresses but abnormal bone
  - Causes include osteoporosis, osteomalacia, steroids, Paget's disease, hyperparathyroidism, rheumatoid arthritis and radiation
- Fatigue fracture
  - Abnormal stress on normal bone
  - Causes include new activity, poor equipment and abnormal biomechanics

Osteochondritis dissecans

- Subchondral fracture
- Often seen in athletes
- Typically affects the lateral aspect of the medial femoral condylar articular surface
- Other sites include the weight-bearing surfaces of the lateral femoral condyle, tibia, talus, patella and capitellum

Imaging features

- Subchondral fracture line paralleling the joint surface in a concave fashion

MRI
- The focus is seen as low signal on T1WI and T2WI, with variable amounts of oedema
- Loose osteochondral fragment are demonstrated on all MR sequences
- An osteochondral fragment is unstable when a T2 high-signal line (representing fluid) separates an undisplaced osteochondral fragment from native bone
- Other signs of instability are a displaced fragment and adjacent cyst formation

Tendon injuries in the lower limb

Achilles tendon tear

- Typically seen in middle-aged men who participate in athletic sports
- Usually ruptures 2–6 cm superior to the os calcis
- The tendon tears at its myotendinous junction in cases of direct trauma

Imaging features

MRI

- Normal tendon is uniformly hypointense on all sequences
- Disruption in continuity with or without a wavy retracted tendon is diagnostic
- Haemorrhage, fluid and interposed fat can appear hyperintense

Tibialis posterior tendon tear

- May be spontaneous or associated with synovitis, corticosteroid injections or trauma
- Chronic degeneration occurs in women in their fifth and sixth decades
- Clinically presents with medial foot pain and flat foot
- Unilateral in 90% OF CASES
- Usually ruptures within 6 cm proximal to the navicular insertion

Anterior talofibular ligament tear

- The anterior talofibular ligament is the lateral ankle ligament that tears most commonly
- Caused by inversion and internal rotation combined with plantar flexion
- Associated with anterior displacement of the talus and contusion of the medial part of the talus

Myositis ossificans

- Formation of mature bone within soft tissues

- Occurs after trauma and burns and in the neurological impairment
- The thigh and the elbow are common locations, but it can occur anywhere
- Related to the time since the trauma
  - < 2 weeks after the trauma: soft tissue mass that is painful, warm and doughy to the touch
  - 3–4 weeks after the trauma: amorphous density within the mass, with associated underlying bony periosteal reaction
  - 6–8 weeks after the trauma: amorphous bone matures into compact bone that surrounds a lacy pattern of less mature bone
  - Maturation proceeds centripetally, and it takes 5–6 months to form mature bone

Imaging features

MRI

- Early: isointense to muscle on T1WI, high signal on T2WI, with prominent surrounding oedema; periosteal reaction and bone marrow oedema may be present
- After 8 weeks: inhomogeneous centre and a rim that is low intensity on all sequences
- Parosteal osteosarcoma is the closest differential diagnosis to myositis ossificans; it shows as reverse-zoning organised bone centrally and as less mature bone peripherally

Progressive myositis ossificans (fibrodysplasia ossificans progressiva)

- Hereditary mesodermal disorder
- Autosomal-dominant inheritance
- Progressive ossification of striated muscle, tendons and ligaments
- Muscle involvement secondary to pressure atrophy from interstitial tissues
- Acute torticollis is the most frequent presentation
- Bridging heterotopic bone seen in severe cases
- Death may result from respiratory failure caused by chest wall restriction

Benign tumours of bone

- Mnemonic from Helms (2005):
  'FEGNOMASHIC' (Fibrous dysplasia,
  Enchondroma, Giant cell tumour, Non-
  ossifying fibroma, Osteoblastoma,
  Metastatic disease, Aneurysmal bone cyst,
  Simple bone cyst, Hyperparathyroidism,
  Infection (osteomyelitis),
  Chondroblastoma).

Fibrous dysplasia

- Monostotic (most commonly) or
  polyostotic (in 30% of cases)
- Predilection for the pelvis, femur, ribs and
  skull
- Polyostotic type occasionally occurs
  in association with McCune–Albright
  syndrome
- When seen in the tibia and jaw, consider
  adamantinoma (a rare malignant tumour
  that radiologically and histologically
  resembles fibrous dysplasia

Imaging features

- Expansile, with ground-glass matrix and a
  sclerotic rind
- Often purely lytic, but may progress to
  matrix calcification and appear sclerotic
  (lesions in skull may be densely sclerotic)
- No periosteal reaction unless fractured

Enchondroma

- Metaphyseal cartilage tumour
- Can be central or eccentric, expansile or
  non-expansile
- 50% of cases occur in tubular bones
  (phalanges) of hands and feet, where the
  tumour appears lucent
- Calcified chondroid matrix is invariably
  present except when located in the
  phalanges
- Sclerotic margin is absent or thin
- No periosteal reaction

Imaging features

MRI
- Lobulated, bright signal on T2WI with
  low-signal calcification, arcs (chondroid
  matrix) and ring-enhancement pattern

Multiple enchondromas (Ollier's disease)

- Not premalignant on its own
- Not hereditary
- Called Maffucci's syndrome when
  associated with soft tissue haemangiomas,
  and predisposes to malignancy

Eosinophilic granuloma

- Peak age is 5–10 years
- Usually monostotic, but progresses to
  polyostotic disease within 6 months in
  10–20% of cases

Imaging features

- Variable appearances: lytic or sclerotic,
  well defined or ill defined, periosteal
  reaction present or absent
- Periosteal reaction, when present, is thick,
  wavy and uniform
- May appear aggressive with a permeative
  pattern and a soft tissue component
- May occasionally have a bony sequestrum

Giant cell tumour

Four important criteria, according to Helms:
- Occurs only in patients with a closed
  epiphysis
- Lesion is epiphyseal and abuts the
  articular surface
- Eccentric location
- Sharp non-sclerotic zone of transition

Non-ossifying fibroma and fibrous cortical defect

- Metaphyseal defect
- Common in children (30% of cases occur
  in children; rarely seen after the age of 30
  years)
- Males are twice as commonly affected as
  females
- Involutes after 2–4 years
- Known as a non-ossifying fibroma when
  large (> 2 cm in length)

Imaging features

Plain X-ray
- Most commonly around the knee, but can
  occur in any long bone

- Sclerotic border with mild endosteal scalloping
- Slightly expansile
- No periosteal reaction

Bone scan and MRI
- Minimal or mild uptake, hot during 'healing' phase
- MRI shows that 80% of cases are hypointense on both T1WI and T2WI; others are hypointense on T1WI and hyperintense on T2WI
- Intense contrast enhancement in 80% of cases
- Hypophosphatemic rickets a known complication

Jaffe–Campanacci syndrome
- Non-ossifying fibroma with extraskeletal manifestations in children
- Associations include mental retardation, hypogonadism, ocular defect, congenital heart defect and café-au-lait spots

Osteoblastoma
- Most commonly occurs in the posterior elements of the vertebral bodies
- Speckled calcification or ossification seen in half of all cases
- Expansile, lytic lesion

Metastatic disease
- Commonest malignant tumours affecting the skeleton
- Good evidence suggests that distant metastases spread from venous tumour emboli, rather than via arterial or lymphatic routes
- Common organs for the primary malignancy are the breast, bronchus, prostate, kidney and thyroid
- The site of the primary carcinoma may remain unknown in as many as 17.6% of patients even after full investigation
- Skeletal biopsy is confirmatory
- Bones containing red marrow are the most commonly involved (85–90% of cases), and the axial skeleton is more commonly involved than the appendicular skeleton
- Common sites are the vertebrae, pelvis, proximal femur (the lesser trochanter in particular), the skull, the ribs and the proximal humerus
- Breast primary tumour
  - Bone involvement in 24% of early cases and 84% of advanced cases
  - Osteolytic (most commonly) or osteoblastic (in 10% of cases) or mixed (in 10% of cases)
  - Common sites are the vertebrae, pelvis and ribs
- Prostate primary tumour
  - Predominantly blastic or mixed
  - Florid periosteal 'sunburst' appearance is known to occur
- Lung primary tumour
  - Usually primaries are small cell carcinoma and oat cell carcinoma: majority of bone secondaries are osteolytic
  - Adenocarcinoma and bronchial carcinoid normally produce focal or diffuse densely blastic lesions
- Kidney or thyroid primary tumour
  - Almost all bone secondaries are lytic
- Gastrointestinal primary tumour
  - Bone secondaries are usually lytic, but sclerotic metastases are seen with adenocarcinoma
- Bladder primary tumour
  - Bone secondaries usually lytic, but exuberant periosteal new bone may be seen occasionally
  - Predilection for the bones of the legs

Imaging features
- Features favouring a diagnosis of metastases rather than primary malignancy include a diaphyseal location and involvement of the vertebral body and pedicles
- Consider an alternate diagnosis in the absence of bone expansion, florid periosteal reaction, new bone formation and a large soft tissue mass
- Kidney, lung, thyroid and breast primaries commonly give lytic bony metastases
- Prostate and breast primaries commonly give sclerotic bony metastases; bladder and carcinoid primaries uncommonly give sclerotic bony metastases

Bone scan

- Most cost-effective modality
- 5% of metastases have a normal scan
- Abnormal uptake relies on intact local blood flow and increased osteoblastic activity
- Superscan may be seen with diffuse osteoblastic metastases from the prostate or breast: presence of generalised increase in skeletal activity with reduced or absent renal activity seen on scanning
- Baseline scan has a high sensitivity for breast, prostate and lung metastases, but a poor sensitivity for infiltrative lesions like multiple myeloma, neuroblastoma and histiocytosis
- Follow-up scan: a stable scan suggests a relatively good prognosis
- However, increased activity in a follow-up scan may be seen
  - Enlargement of lesions
  - New lesions
  - Healing flare with treatment (this does not signify tumour is responding favourably to treatment)
  - Avascular necrosis
  - Radiation-induced changes
- Decreased activity implies osteolytic lesions, or it may occur following radiotherapy

MRI

- Most metastases are located in the medulla and show reduced signal intensity on T1WI and increased signal intensity on T2WI and short inversion time inversion recovery (STIR) sequences
- Osteoblastic metastases may appear hypointense on all sequences
- Identification of a halo of high signal around a lesion is a suggestive feature of metastasis on T2WI

Multiple myeloma

- Solitary or multiple punched-out, lytic lesions
- Diffuse osteopenia
- Plasmacytoma shows as a focal lytic expansile lesion
- Bone scan and skeletal survey are complementary
- MRI may be used as a survey tool

Imaging features

MRI

- Low tumour burden: normal scan
- Focal involvement: identical picture to that seen with metastases
- Pre-treatment:
  - T1 signal equal to or lower than that of muscle
  - Diffuse enhancement with contrast
- Post-treatment
  - Complete response: resolution with no enhancement or persistent lesions with no (or rim) enhancement (plain X-rays may show sclerotic rim around the lytic lesions)
  - Incomplete response: persistent enhancement

Osteoid osteoma

- A hamartoma composed of osteoid and woven bone, < 1.5 cm in diameter
- Peak ages is the second and third decades
- Males are 2.5 times more commonly affected than females
- Pain responsive to aspirin
- Commoner in the appendicular skeleton
- Painful scoliosis: concave towards lesion
- No site in the body is exempt
- Can involve the medulla or cortex or be subperiosteal; can involve the metaphyses or diaphyses

Imaging features

- Nidus may be lucent or sclerotic, is 10 mm or less in diameter and is surrounded by reactive sclerosis

Bone scan

- Double-density sign (focal increased activity surrounded by area of slightly lesser intensity, caused by reactive sclerosis

CT

- Cortical tumors often show a lucent nidus with surrounding reactive sclerosis and periosteal reaction
- Brodie's abscess can have a similar appearance
- CT guidance is necessary for radiofrequency ablation, the current

commonly practised method for treatment of osteoid osteomas

MRI
- Complements CT and bone scan
- Shows intense oedema on STIR sequences around the nidus

> ### Intra-articular osteoid osteoma
>
> - A rare form of the disease
> - Usually presents as a rounded soft-tissue mass
> - May result in joint effusions or synovial inflammation
> - Difficult to visualise on CT or MRI

Aneurysmal bone cyst

- Primary or secondary to benign or malignant conditions, e.g. trauma, giant cell tumour, osteosarcoma
- Occurs in patients < 30 years of age
- Males and females are equally affected
- Presents with local pain and swelling, and with neurological signs if the spine is involved
- Can occur at any site, but predominantly in the vertebrae (usually in the appendage) and long bones (metaphyseal or diaphyseal)

Imaging features

Plain X-ray
- Classically an expansile, eccentric lesion in the metaphysis of a child
- Matrix entirely lytic
- Thin 'egg-shell' cortex
- Rapid growth
- No periosteal reaction, unless a fracture is seen

CT
- Complex cystic lesion within the periosteal membrane
- Absence of matrix calcification

MRI
- Heterogeneous lesion, with blood products

- Fluid–fluid levels (a non-specific feature since this can be seen in several other bone tumours)

Solitary bone cyst

- Most commonly occurs in the first and second decades of life
- Commonest sites are the proximal humerus (in 50% of cases) and the proximal femur (in 20% of cases)
- Central, metaphyseal location
- Mildly expansile with cortical thinning, narrow zone of transition and a fine sclerotic rim
- 'Fallen fragment' sign: a fractured fragment that settles in the dependent portion of the fluid-filled cyst

Chondroblastoma

- Eccentrically located epiphyseal lesion
- Occurs in patients < 30 years of age
- Commonest site is the proximal humerus
- Calcification occurs in 40–60% of cases
- Can show surrounding oedema on MRI

Chondromyxoid fibroma

- Rare, benign cartilaginous tumour
- Most frequently seen in the second and third decades
- Usually located eccentrically within the metaphysis, commonly in the proximal third of the tibia
- Thick sclerotic margin with mild cortical expansion is typical
- Malignant transformation is rare
- High recurrence rate following curettage

Imaging features

- Eccentric, lobulated, lucent lesion involving the cortex and medulla
- Characteristic sclerotic endosteal border with scalloped margins
- No periosteal reaction
- Soft tissue extension os uncommon
- Calcification of the matrix is very rarely seen on imaging
- MRI is non-specific, with high signal on T2WI

Malignant tumours of bone

Osteosarcoma

- Commonest malignant primary bone tumour
- Occurs in patients < 30 years of age, although some present in older patients with malignant degeneration of Paget's disease
- Originates in the metaphysis and extends across the physeal plate to the epiphysis
- Central and parosteal are the two common forms
- Telangiectatic osteosarcoma is a rare type, which appears similar to an aneurismal bone cyst on imaging
- Parosteal osteosarcoma
  - Median age is older than for the commoner central type
  - Posterior aspect of the distal femur is a common location
  - Wraps around underlying bone as it grows, and therefore prognosis is better than for the central type because it can be relatively easily resected

Ewing's sarcoma

- Commonest primary malignant bone tumour in the first decade of life
- 95% occur in patients aged 4–25 years
- Bone and lung metastases are common at the time of presentation (and give a 5-year survival rate of 50%)

Imaging features

Plain X-ray
- Typically, permeative lesion in the diaphysis of long bones; however, lesions may be metaphyseal or diametaphyseal with a wide zone of transition
- 75% of cases involve the pelvis or long tubular bones; other sites include the shoulder girdle, rib and vertebral body
- 'Onion-skin' periosteal reaction is typical, but 'sunburst' and amorphous forms can be present atypically

MRI
- Low signal on T1WI, high signal on T2WI, with a particularly large soft tissue component, often with central necrosis

Chondrosarcoma

- Cartilage-producing sarcoma, often appearing radiologically non-aggressive
- A lytic, destructive lesion with amorphous 'snow-flake' calcification in a patient > 40 years should prompt the diagnosis
- Endosteal cortical scalloping of > 70% of the cortex in a minimally aggressive lesion should also suggest the diagnosis, as should increasing pain and size of an exostosis in an adult

Chondrosarcoma versus enchondroma

Points that favour chondrosarcoma:
- Lesional pain
- Larger size
- Axial location
- Epiphyseal (particularly clear cell type)
- Oedema in adjacent marrow or soft tissues
- Any destructive change
- Significant depth and length of cortical scalloping (involving more than two thirds of the cortex)

Malignant fibrous histiocytoma (fibrosarcoma)

- Peak age range is 30–60 years
- Most commonly arises as a primary lesion, but may be secondary to another lesion, e.g. Paget's disease, radiation-induced changes
- High-grade lesions carry a 5-year survival rate of 25%

Imaging features

MRI
- Usually detected on MRI
- Isointense to muscle on T1WI, high signal on T2WI
- Occasionally shows dystrophic calcification

Bone lymphoma

- Primary lymphoma of the bone is almost exclusively non-Hodgkin's lymphoma

- Accounts for 1% of all cases of non-Hodgkin's lymphoma
- Average age at presentation is 24 years
- Males are more commonly affected than females
- Affects the appendicular skeleton (most commonly the femur, followed by the tibia and then the humerus)
- Bone involvement in non-Hodgkin's lymphoma is usually permeative osteolytic (in 77% of cases); it is sclerotic in 4% of cases

Diagnostic criteria for primary lymphoma of the bone

- Only a single bone involved
- Unequivocal histological evidence of lymphoma
- Other disease is limited to regional areas at the time of presentation
- Primary tumour precedes metastasis by at least 6 months

Secondary lymphoma

- More frequently seen in children
- The axial skeleton is involved more commonly than the appendicular skeleton
- Secondary bony involvement is seen in 20% of patients with Hodgkin's disease; primary Hodgkin's disease of the bone is extremely rare
- Bone involvement in Hodgkin's disease is sclerotic or mixed; Hodgkin's disease can cause ivory vertebral body

Imaging features

MRI
- Modality of choice for staging and follow-up; MRI can upstage by nearly 30%
- Tumour infiltration of low signal on T1WI; high signal on STIR sequences

Hodgkin's disease

- Soft tissue disease may involve adjacent bones
- Classic finding is the sclerotic 'ivory' vertebra
- Direct invasion of the bone by local lymph node disease is denoted by the suffix 'E', added to the appropriate stage
- Involvement of the bone marrow indicates stage 4 disease: worse prognosis than involvement of other viscera and osseous bone

Osteochondroma

- Cartilage-capped exostosis
- Generally accepted to be a developmental anomaly
- Childhood radiotherapy is an association
- Presents from 2–60 years (median age is 20 years)
- Males are 1.4 times more commonly affected than females
- Occurs in long bones
- Metaphyseal in origin but migrates to the diaphysis as growth occurs (away from joint, causing a 'coat-hanger appearance')
- Typically occurs around the knee
- Pedunculated and sessile forms are known
- Diaphyseal aclasis: multiple cartilaginous exostoses constituting an autosomal-dominant disorder
- Malignant change in occurs in < 1% of cases of osteochondroma
- Malignant change in diaphyseal aclasis occurs in up to 5% of cases

Imaging features

MRI
- Cortical and medullary continuity between the osteochondroma and parent bone
- Evaluates the hyaline cap (normally < 1 cm in thickness)

Malignant transformation in osteochondroma

- Cartilage cap thickness is > 2 cm
- Dispersed calcification in the cap
- Increased uptake on bone scan
- Clinical criteria: growth after maturation, pain, enlargement

Synovial lesions

Bursitis

- Benign uni- or multilocular soft tissue masses
- Fluid-filled and lined by synovium
- Commonest sites are the subacromial or subdeltoid, olecranon, iliopsoas, prepatellar and semimembranosus–gastrocnemius bursas
- Baker's cyst involves the semimembranosus bursa
- Note that ganglia, unlike bursas, are not lined by synovium

Imaging features

Ultrasound
- Anechoic or hypoechoic

CT
- Hypodense relative to muscle

MRI
- Hyperintense on T2WI and STIR sequences (rim can enhance minimally post-contrast); variable signal intensity on T1WI depending on protein content

Pigmented villonodular synovitis

- Monoarticular synovial proliferative disorder
- Presents as a painless soft tissue mass
- Males and females are equally affected
- Diffuse and focal nodular forms are known

Imaging features

Plain X-ray
- Effusion is typical
- Variably sized erosions with sclerotic margins may be seen

CT
- Irregular and thickened synovium on arthrography
- Absence of calcification is typical

MRI
- Diffusely thickened synovium with low-signal intensity on all sequences, owing to the hemosiderin deposits, resulting in a characteristic blooming artefact on gradient-echo MRI
- Focal mass typically adjacent to the patella in Hoffa's fat pad (focal nodular synovitis or focal pigmented villonodular synovitis)

Synovial chondromatosis

- Synovial metaplasia of unknown aetiology with development of cartilaginous and osteocartilaginous nodules within the metaplastic synovium
- Males are more commonly affected than females
- Typically occurs in the third, fourth of fifth, but it is seen in all age groups
- Most commonly occurs in the knee, followed by the hip, shoulder and elbow

Imaging features

Plain X-ray
- Multiple round bodies of similar size and variable mineralisation within an effusion
- Mechanical erosions may be formed by the bodies, and changes of secondary osteoarthritis may be seen in the long term

MRI
- Round bodies that conform to the signal characteristics of bone or cartilage, depending on their constitution

Synovial sarcoma

- Synovial sarcoma is a misnomer that arose because the tumour appears histologically similar to synovium; however, this tumour does not arise from the joint synovium
- Indolent expansile malignancy
- Exact origin of the tumour is unknown but it arises from soft tissues in proximity to a joint

- Despite the misnomer, only 10% are intra-articular
- Peak age range is 30–50 years
- Females are more commonly affected than males
- Commonly seen in the lower extremity (especially the knee and foot)
- Usually occurs within 5 cm of a joint
- Calcification is seen in 30% of cases, in more peripheral part of lesion
- Involves the adjacent bone in around 20% of cases, with periosteal reaction

Imaging features

MRI
- Poorly defined lesion
- Low on T1WI, but high if haemorrhage is present; heterogeneous on T2WI (cystic, solid or fibrous)
- Fluid–fluid levels can be seen

The prosthetic joint

- The initial films serve as baseline study and are used as reference films for follow-up imaging

Dislocation

- Most commonly occurs in the immediate postoperative period (occurs in 3% of patients)
- Can also occur as a late complication in prostheses that are not well positioned

Loosening

- Radiographic manifestations
  - A lucent zone > 2 mm at the interface (indicative of loosening)
  - Component migration (diagnostic of loosening): seen for example in the hip joint as interval tilting or cranial migration of the acetabular cup or as subsidence (> 10 mm) and varus tilting of the femoral stem

Particle disease (cement disease)

- Mostly seen in non-cemented hips as a reaction to small polyethylene particles in the prosthesis
- Granulomatous lesions seen as focal radiolucencies of varying size around the prosthesis
- Tends to occur 1–5 years after surgery and is associated with smooth endosteal cortical scalloping
- The key feature is that it produces no secondary bone response (unlike infection)

Infection

- Ill-defined bone resorption
- Absence of a sclerotic margin
- Ill-defined endosteal surface

Fracture

Frequency of fractures postoperatively
  - Cemented total hip arthroplasty: 0.4%
  - Revision hip arthroplasty: 7.2%

Achondroplasia

- Autosomal-dominant, rhizomelic, short-limb dwarfism
- Normal intelligence and life span

Imaging features

Plain X-ray
- Lumbar kyphosis in infancy progressing to exaggerated lordosis in adulthood
- Bullet-shaped vertebral bodies in infancy, vertebra plana in adulthood
- Posterior vertebral scalloping
- Interpedicular distance progressively decreases caudally
- Spinal and cranial stenoses are the major causes of morbidity
- Spinal stenosis occurs secondary to degenerative disease superimposed on congenitally short pedicles
- Squared iliac wings in pelvis
- 'Champagne glass' inlet in the pelvis
- Long bones are short and wide
- Enlarged skull with narrowed foramina
- Bone mineral density preserved

Osteogenesis imperfecta

- Collagen disorder of the bone
- Blue sclerae (in 90% of cases), osteoporosis, scoliosis, grey teeth, hearing loss (due to otic bone fractures)
- Wormian bones are frequently associated
- Severe osteopenia and multiple fractures with excessive callus
- Non-accidental trauma is the main differential diagnosis

Types of osteogenesis imperfecta

Type I: commonest form
Type II: most severe form, lethal in the neonatal period
Type III: severely deforming, but compatible with life
Type IV: mild form, no blue sclera

Transient osteoporosis of the hip

- A form of regional osteoporosis
- Commonly seen in middle-aged men (bilaterally) and pregnant women (usually in the left hip)
- Presents clinically with a sudden onset of severe hip pain
- Self-limiting, and warrants no treatment; however, it however recur in other joints
- Pathological fracture may occur through the affected bone
- In comparison, regional migratory osteoporosis (another form of regional osteoporosis) affects multiple consecutive joints

Imaging features

Plain X-ray
- Severe osteopenia of the acetabulum and femoral head with loss of subchondral cortex. The joint space is preserved

MRI
- Striking oedema in the proximal femur, usually associated with a joint effusion
- Low signal on T1WI, high signal on T2WI and STIR sequences with contrast enhancement throughout the femoral head and neck
- No subchondral sclerosis
- MRI abnormalities subside in 6–10 months

Musculoskeletal effects of phenytoin

- Gum hypertrophy
- Osteomalacia
- Thickening of the skull vault

Avascular necrosis of the femoral head

- Causes
  - Trauma
  - Steroids
  - Alcoholism
  - Sickle cell disease
  - Gaucher's syndrome

  - Caisson's disease
  - Radiation
  - Systemic lupus erythematosus (which can cause avascular necrosis in unusual sites, such as the talus or humerus)

Imaging features

Plain X-ray
- Sclerosis, followed by subchondral fracture and flattening ('snow cap' sign)
- Cartilage remains intact until the onset of secondary degenerative arthritis

Radionuclide study
- Initially shows a photopenic region, followed by increased activity with revascularisation and repair

MRI
- Initial oedema
- Subsequently the 'double-rim' sign develops: distinct abnormality of the marrow signal in the subchondral region, with peripheral low-intensity rim on both T1WI and T2WI sequences and an adjacent inner rim of increased intensity on T2WI

Avascular necrosis of the spine

- Air within the vertebral body is characteristic (MR signal void)
- 'H'-shaped vertebra, due to collapse of superior and inferior endplates (typically seen in sickle cell disease)

Baker's cyst

- Synovium-lined bursa that lies between the medial head of the gastrocnemius muscle and semimembranosus muscle
- A contralateral, subclinical Baker's cysts is a common finding
- Affects 15% of the population
- Commoner in males
- Associated with osteoarthritis of the knee joint

Imaging features

MRI

- Low signal on T1WI unless haemorrhagic, high signal on T2WI
- May be septated, with complex features
- Intra-articular bony or cartilaginous bodies can lie within the cyst as a result of underlying knee joint pathology

Ultrasound

- Anechoic with posterior enhancement
- Extension through the knee capsule is not seen with an intact cyst

2.8 Lists to remember

Widening of the femoral intercondylar notch

- Mnemonic: 'BAIT'
  - Blood disorder, e.g. hemophilia
  - Arthritis, e.g. gout, rheumatoid arthritis and juvenile rheumatoid arthritis, psoriasis
  - Infection, e.g. tuberculosis
  - Tumour, e.g. pigmented villonodular synovitis

Raised alkaline phosphatase

- Causes
  - Paget's disease
  - Osteomalacia and rickets
  - Renal osteodystrophy
  - Metastases
  - Primary bone tumour, e.g. sarcoma
  - Recent fracture
  - Puberty

Acro-osteolysis of the terminal phalanx

- Causes
  - Hyperparathyroidism
  - Psoriasis, rheumatoid arthritis, Reiter's syndrome
  - Raynaud's disease, scleroderma
  - Dermatomyositis
  - Diabetes mellitus
  - Sarcoidosis
  - Pyknodysostosis
  - Lesch–Nyhan syndrome
  - Leprosy
  - Polyvinyl chloride workers

Accelerated bone maturation

- Causes
  - Hyperthyroidism
  - Pseudohypoparathyroidism
  - Hypothalamic hamartoma
  - McCune–Albright syndrome
  - Idiopathic precocity
  - Adrenal and gonadal tumours
  - Acrodysostosis

Juxta-articular osteoporosis

- Causes
  - Rheumatoid arthritis, juvenile rheumatoid arthritis
  - Tuberculosis or pyogenic infection
  - Reiter's syndrome
  - Scleroderma
  - Haemophilia

Fusion of the cervical spine

- Mnemonic: 'PIKRAD'
  - Post-trauma
  - Infection, e.g. tuberculosis
  - Klippel–Feil syndrome
  - Reiter's syndrome, rheumatoid arthritis, psoriasis
  - Ankylosing spondylitis
  - Diffuse idiopathic skeletal hyperostosis (DISH)

Protrusio acetabuli

- Abnormal medial position of the femoral head compared with the pelvis
- Primary (otto pelvis) form is bilateral, familial and more common in women
- Causes
  - Rheumatoid arthritis, osteoarthritis
  - Turner's syndrome
  - Pelvic trauma
  - Bone-softening conditions, e.g. Paget's disease, fibrous dysplasia, osteomalacia, renal osteodystrophy
  - Marfan's syndrome

Sclerotic pedicle

- Contralateral pedicle congenitally absent
- Osteoid osteoma
- Unilateral spondylolysis
- Sclerotic metastases

Vertebra plana

- Flattening of the vertebral body
- Causes
  - Trauma
  - Tumour (myeloma, metastases, leukaemia)
  - Infection
  - Steroids
  - Haemangioma
  - Eosinophilic granuloma

Periarticular calcification

- Hypercalcaemic states
  - Sarcoidosis
  - Hypervitaminosis D
  - Renal failure with secondary hyperparathyroidism
  - Tumoral calcinosis
- Degenerative changes
  - Calcium pyrophosphate dihydrate deposition disease (CPPD)
  - Calcium hydroxyapatite deposition disease
- Inflammatory conditions
  - Dermatomyositis
  - Gout
  - Bursitis
  - Scleroderma
- Neoplasms
  - Synovial chondromatosis
  - Synovial sarcoma

Sacroiliitis

- Changes of sacroiliitis typically begin in the lower and middle thirds of the sacroiliac joint
- The iliac side of the joint is more severely affected than the sacral side
- Erosive changes initially lead to pseudo-widening of the joint space
- Bony ankylosis ensues from progressive subchondral sclerosis
- Eventually, the bones return to normal density
- Bilaterally symmetrical sacroiliitis
  - Ankylosing spondylitis
  - Inflammatory bowel disease
  - Late psoriatic arthropathy (in 50% of cases)
  - Late rheumatoid arthritis
  - Gout, pseudogout
  - Acromegaly, ochronosis
  - Osteitis condensans ilii (seen in young, multiparous women)
- Bilaterally asymmetric sacroiliitis
  - Early ankylosing spondylitis
  - Early psoriatic arthropathy (50%)
  - Reiter's syndrome
  - Juvenile rheumatoid arthritis
- Unilateral sacroiliitis
  - Infections
  - Osteoarthritis

Erlenmeyer's flask deformity

- Condition where the distal end of long bones is expanded
- Most common bone to get affected is the femur
- Results from a wide metaphysis secondary to failure of osteoclastic function
- Causes
  - Osteopetrosis
  - Haemolytic anaemias, e.g. thalassaemia, sickle cell anaemia
  - Storage disorders, e.g. Gaucher's disease, Niemann-Pick disease
  - Pyle's disease (metaphyseal dysplasia)
  - Lead poisoning
  - Rickets, hypophosphatasia
  - Fibrous dysplasia
  - Down's syndrome
  - Achondroplasia
  - Leukaemia

Acromioclavicular joint injury grades

- Grade I: acromioclavicular ligament sprain
- Grade II: acromioclavicular ligament rupture with coracoclavicular ligament intact; acromioclavicular joint space > 5mm, coracoclavicular < 11–13 mm
- Grade III: acromioclavicular and coracoclavicular rupture
- Grade IV: clavicle dislocated posteriorly: anteroposterior views may be normal; MRI can assess for soft tissue pathology

Diffusely increased bone density

- Causes
  - Myelofibrosis
  - Mastocytosis
  - Metastatic disease
  - Sickle cell disease
  - Paget's disease
  - Pyknodysostosis
  - Renal osteodystrophy
  - Osteopetrosis
  - Fluorosis

Dense metaphyseal bands

- Causes
  - Normal finding
  - Lead poisoning
  - Vitamin D excess
  - Stress lines
  - Post-treatment rickets
  - Scurvy

Bowed long bones in children

- Causes
  - Rickets
  - Osteogenesis imperfecta
  - Trauma
  - Madelung's deformity
  - Neurofibromatosis

Neurofibroma of bone

- Scoliosis: short segment
- Prone to rapid progression
- Enlarged neural foramina
- Posterior vertebral body scalloping
- Dural ectasia
- Hypoplastic cranial bones
- Anterior distal tibial bowing
- Pseudoarthroses
- Multiple non-ossifying fibromas
- Ribbon ribs

Pseudoarthrosis

- Causes
  - Non-union of a fracture

- Fibrous dysplasia
- Neurofibromatosis
- Osteogenesis imperfecta
- Congenital

Excessive callus

- Causes
  - Steroids
  - Neuropathic
  - Congenital insensitivity to pain
  - Paralysis
  - Osteogenesis imperfecta
  - Renal osteodystrophy
  - Burns
  - Scurvy

Common sites of mandibular fractures

Fracture type	Prevalence
Body	30–40%
Angle	25–31%
Condyle	15–17%
Symphysis	7–15%
Ramus	3–9%
Alveolar	2–4%
Coronoid process	1–2%

Superscan

- Metabolic disorders
  - Renal osteodystrophy
  - Osteomalacia
  - Hyperparathyroidism
  - Hyperthyroidism
- Lesional causes
  - Diffuse metastases
  - Myelofibrosis
  - Aplastic anaemia
  - Leukaemia
  - Waldenström's macroglobulinaemia
  - Systemic mastocytosis
  - Widespread Paget's disease

No uptake of technetium-99m-methylene diphosphonate

- Causes
- Bone island
- Osteopoikilosis
- Non-ossifying fibroma, fibrous cortical defect
- Osteopathia striata
- Calcified gall stones

Associations of slipped femoral epiphysis

- Growth spur
- Perthes' disease
- Renal osteodystrophy
- Rickets
- Childhood irradiation
- Growth hormone therapy
- Trauma
- Malnutrition
- Developmental dysplasia of the hip
- Endocrine disorders, e.g. hypothyroidism, hypo-oestrogenic conditions, acromegaly, gigantism, cryptorchidism, pituitary adenoma, parathyroid adenoma

Stippled epiphysis

- Causes
  - Normal finding
  - Avascular necrosis
  - Hypothyroidism
  - Chondrodysplasia punctata
  - Multiple epiphysial dysplasia
  - Down's syndrome
  - Hypoparathyroidism
  - Homocystinuria
  - Zellweger's syndrome

'Bone-within-bone' appearance

- Causes
  - Endosteal new bone formation
  - Normal finding in the thoracic and lumbar vertebra in infants
  - Growth lines
  - Caffey's disease
  - Sickle cell and thalassemia
  - Congenital syphilis
  - Osteopetrosis
  - Radiation
  - Acromegaly
  - Paget's disease
  - Gaucher's disease

Wormian bones

- Sutural bones
- Causes
  - Cleidocranial dysostosis
  - Pyknodysostosis
  - Osteogenesis imperfecta
  - Hypothyroidism
  - Down syndrome

Permeative pattern in bone

- Causes
  - Lymphoma, leukaemia
  - Multiple myeloma
  - Ewing's sarcoma
  - Neuroblastoma
  - Osteomyelitis

Lytic bone lesions in children

- Causes
  - Infection
  - Eosinophilic granuloma
  - Leukaemia
  - Neuroblastoma metastases
  - Ewing's sarcoma

Ivory vertebra

- Causes
  - Paget's disease
  - Lymphoma
  - Haemangioma
  - Metastases

MRI findings

Entities that shorten T1 (high signal intensity on T1WI)

- Lipoma
- Haematoma

- Intralesional haemorrhage
- Gadolinium
- Fatty stroma of haemangioma, lipoma
- Protein
- Melanin
- Calcium in some cases

Low signal on T2WI

- Scar
- Dense mineralisation
- Melanin
- Subacute hematoma
- Gas

MRI findings		
Structure	T1 signal	T2 signal
Haematoma (acute)	Intermediate to high	High
Haematoma (subacute)	Intermediate to high	High
Haematoma (chronic)	Low	Low
Haemangioma	Intermediate (higher than muscle)	High
Lipoma	High	Intermediate
Protein	High	High
Fluid	Low	High
Air	Low	Low
Red marrow	Low	Intermediate
Hyaline cartilage	Intermediate	Intermediate
Cortical bone	Low	Low
Tendons	Low	Low
Ligaments	Low	Low
Fibrocartilage	Low	Low
Scar	Low	Low
Fat, fatty marrow	High	Intermediate
Muscle, nerves	Low to intermediate	Intermediate

Haematoma signal on MRI			
Hyperacute	Oxyhaemoglobin	T1: iso	T2: iso/bright
Acute	Deoxyhaemoglobin	T1: intermediate/low	T2: dark
Subacute, early	Intracell methaemoglobin	T1: bright	T2: dark
Subacute, late	Intracell methaemoglobin	T1: bright	T2: bright
Chronic	Haemosiderin	T1: dark	T2: dark

- Vascular flow void
- Foreign body
- Hemosiderin
- Pigmented villonodular synovitis
- Giant cell tumor of the tendon sheath (a form of pigmented villonodular synovitis)
- Synovial pannus tissue
- Gouty tophus
- Amyloid

Signal and resolution on MRI

- Good signal but poorer resolution
  - • Increased slice thickness
  - • Increased field of view
  - • Decreased imaging matrix
- Better resolution but worse signal
  - • Decreased slice thickness
  - • Decreased field of view
  - • Increased imaging matrix

Gadolinium

- Paramagnetic at room temperature
- Atomic number 64
- Electrons per shell: 2, 8, 18, 25, 9, 2; however, paramagnetic gadolinium-3+ has seven unpaired electrons in its outer shell
- Shows increased signal on T1WI
- Adverse effects include nephrogenic systemic fibrosis and nephrogenic dermopathy

STIR sequence

- Repetition time (TR) > 2000 milliseconds; echo time (TE) > 30 milliseconds
- Fat-suppression technique
- Should not be used with gadolinium
- Good for imaging bone, cartilage and muscle
- Useful when there is significant artefact from metal prosthesis
- Tissues with short T1 are bright
- Tissues with long T2 are bright

Low marrow signal

- Diffusely low signal
  - Bone marrow infiltration, e.g. leukaemia, myeloma

- Haemopoitic marrow
- Mastocytosis
- Haemosiderosis
- Myelofibrosis
- Osteopetrosis
- Focal low signal
  - Bone island
  - Sclerotic metastasis
  - Vacuum phenomenon

Haematoma signal on MRI

- Remember that imaging features of soft tissue haematomas can be quite variable (unlike those of intracranial haemorrhages)
- See table

MRI appearances of denervation

- Normal nerves appear slightly hyperintense to muscle on T2WI
- Acute (< 2 weeks since denervation): normal signal
- 1–12 months since denervation: high on T2WI, owing to extracellular intramuscular oedema
- > 12 months since denervation: high on T1WI, owing to fatty infiltration

Osseous lesions containing high signal on T1WI

- Intraosseous lipoma
- Bone infarct
- Hemangioma
- Paget's disease

Osseous lesion containing low signal on T2WI

- Sclerosis, calcification or matrix
- Fibrous lesions
- Primary bone lymphoma

Chapter 3

Gastrointestinal system

Liver anatomy

- The liver is a large gland situated in the right upper quadrant of the abdomen
- The gland anatomy can be studied under the three parts
  - Bile duct anatomy
  - Functional segmental anatomy
  - Vascular anatomy

Bile duct anatomy

- The intrahepatic ducts follow the portal venous and the hepatic arterial branches
- The intrahepatic ducts join to form the right hepatic duct and the left hepatic duct, which then form the main intrahepatic duct or common hepatic duct (CHD)
- The main intrahepatic duct is joined by the cystic duct to form the common bile duct (CBD)
- The CBD then joins the pancreatic duct at the ampulla of Vater (the major duodenal papilla) and drains into the duodenum
- Normal diameter of the bile ducts
  - CBD: 6–7 mm; > 8 mm is dilated
  - CHD at the porta hepatis: 5 mm

Bile duct variants

- Variants found in 1–3% of all autopsies
- Variants of important for postoperative bile leaks and obstruction
  - Aberrant intrahepatic dusts
  - Cystic duct entering hepatic duct
  - Duplication of cystic ducts
  - Ducts of Luschka (numerous ducts draining directly into the cystic duct)
  - Congenital tracheobiliary fistula

Cystic duct variants

- Account for 15–25% of bile duct variants
- Commonest is the cystic duct inserting into the middle third of the extrahepatic duct (75% of cases)
- < 1% of cases show insertion into the right hepatic duct

Functional segmental anatomy

- Based on hepatic and portal venous anatomy

- Middle hepatic vein divides the liver into the right and left lobes
- The portal vein divides the liver into an upper and lower portion
- The segments are then numbered around the inferior vena cava (IVC) from 1 to 8
- The caudate lobe is segment 1
- Segments 4a and 4b are found between the middle hepatic vein and the left hepatic vein, above and below the portal vein

Vascular anatomy

- The liver gets its blood supply from the hepatic artery and the portal vein
- 80% of its supply is from the portal vein, with 20% from the hepatic artery

Hepatic artery

- In 50–60% of people, the hepatic artery originates from the common hepatic artery, which is a branch of the celiac axis
- The common hepatic artery further divides into the gastroduodenal artery and the hepatic artery proper
- Commonest variants
  - The common hepatic artery divides into the gastroduodenal artery and the right hepatic artery (in 10% of people)
  - The common hepatic artery divides into the gastroduodenal artery and the left hepatic artery (in 10% of people)
- The hepatic artery waveform is pulsatile and low-resistance and shows a rapid systolic upstroke with a continuous diastolic flow
- The normal velocity measures 30–60 cm/second with a resistive index of 0.6 ± 0.06

Portal vein

- Formed by the confluence of the splenic vein and the superior mesenteric vein
- Cross-sectional diameter is approximately 12–14 mm
- Flow is non-pulsatile, in a hepatopetal direction with mild respiratory variation and a flow velocity of 20–30 cm/second

Hepatic veins

- Waveform is triphasic, with both respiratory and cardiac variation
- Hepatic vein sampling should occur at its confluence

Hepatitis

- Inflammation of the liver resulting in deranged liver functions followed by imageable changes
- Two main types: acute and chronic

Acute hepatitis

- Markedly raised AST and ALT with increased serum conjugated bilirubin
- Clinically causes abdominal pain and jaundice with either a normal or palpable liver
- Common causes
  - Viral (hepatitis A)
  - Drug-induced
  - Alcoholic use
  - Alcoholic liver disease
  - Fatty liver disease
  - Alcoholic hepatitis
  - Alcoholic cirrhosis

Imaging features

Ultrasound
- Appearance depends on the severity and stage of disease
- Typically shows as a diffuse decrease in liver echogenicity

Chronic hepatitis

- Defined as hepatitis lasting at least 6 months
- Common causes
  - Primary biliary cirrhosis
  - Hepatitis B, C and D
  - Primary sclerosing cholangitis
  - Wilson's disease
  - Alpha-1 antitrypsin deficiency

Imaging features

Ultrasound
- Increased liver echogenicity
- Coarse echotexture
- Loss of definition of portal vessels

Cirrhosis

- Chronic diffuse liver disease
- Aetiology is vast but most cases (75%) are due to alcoholic liver disease
- Causes
  - Toxins: alcohol, drugs such as methotrexate, nitrofurantoin, isoniazid
  - Inflammatory: from hepatitis of various causes, most commonly hepatitis B or C
  - Biliary disease: inflammatory bowel disease, cystic fibrosis
  - Nutritional: severe steatosis, malnutrition
  - Hereditary disorders: haemochromatosis, Wilson's disease, alpha-1 antitrypsin deficiency
  - Auto-immune disorders: primary biliary cirrhosis, primary sclerosing cholangitis
  - Idiopathic
- Three morphological types
  - Micronodular cirrhosis
  - Macronodular cirrhosis
  - Mixed cirrhosis
- Nodular lesions are of four main types
  - Regenerative nodules, consisting of hepatocytes and stroma
  - Cirrhotic nodules, which are regenerative nodules with surrounding fibrosis
  - Dysplastic nodules, which are hepatic adenomas with areas of dysplasia within then (a tissue diagnosis and not seen on imaging); they are seen in cirrhosis from hepatitis B and hepatitis C
  - Hepatocellular carcinoma
- Clinical presentation is usually with anorexia, nausea and vomiting; with symptoms and signs of portal hypertension such as variceal bleeding, ascites; or with symptoms and signs of hepatic encephalopathy such as confusion

Imaging features

Ultrasound
- Usually non-specific
- Hepatomegaly and an irregular outline to the liver edge seen in early disease

- A shrunken liver is seen in late stage
- Diffuse increase in echogenicity with a coarse echotexture
- Spares the caudate lobe, which may become hypertrophic
- Regenerative nodules are not seen unless they are large
- Decrease in definition of the portal vein wall
- Ancillary signs of liver failure include ascites and portal hypertension with splenomegaly and varices

CT
- Similar findings to ultrasound
- Characteristically there is a decrease in size of the right lobe and the medial segment of the left lobe, with compensatory hypertrophy of the caudate lobe
- The regenerative nodules are seen if they are siderotic, in which case they show as high-attenuation nodules without enhancement during the arterial phase but as similar to surrounding liver in portal venous phase
- Main use is to identify complications including bacterial peritonitis
- May also help in characterising focal lesions
- Nodular outline with hypertrophy of the caudate lobe and relative atrophy of the quadrate lobe
- Low-attenuation focal nodules are more suspicious of malignancy

MRI
- Problem-solving tool to characterise focal lesions
- Benign regenerative nodules show an increased signal on T1-weighted images (T1WI) and a decreased signal on T2-weighted images (T2WI) as a result of siderosis
- Dysplastic nodules show a homogeneously increased signal on T1WI and a very much decreased signal on T2WI, with enhancement with gadolinium (similar to findings with hepatocellular carcinoma)
- Neoplastic nodules in cirrhosis show variable appearances, but

characteristically there is enhancement in the arterial phase with wash-out during the portal venous phase. A 'nodule-in-nodule' appearance is characteristic on T2WI, with a neoplastic nodule that shows an increased T2 signal being seen within a dysplastic nodule that shows a decreased T2 signal

Haemochromatosis

- Abnormal deposition of iron in the liver
- Causes
  - Primary, due to an autosomal-recessive disorder that causes an increased uptake of transferrin
  - Secondary to iron deposition, which may be erythrogenic, due to Bantu siderosis or transfusional (after > 30 units of blood)
- Clinical findings
  - Hyperpigmentation
  - Arthralgias
  - Diabetes mellitus in 30–40% of cases
  - Liver failure in long-standing cases

Imaging features

CT
- Generalised increase in liver attenuation
- Portal vein branches seen as prominent, low-attenuation structures

MRI
- Reference tissue is skeletal muscle
- Liver is low signal on both T1WI and T2WI, and is best seen on gradient-echo T2WI, which shows magnetic susceptibility artefacts
- Pancreas also shows low signal late in the disease
- Spleen is normal in primary disease but low signal in secondary disease

Liver abscess

- Localised collections of pus within the liver
- Most commonly bacterial in aetiology (in 80–90% of cases)
- Fungal abscesses account for < 10% of cases, amoebic abscesses for 5% of cases

Pyogenic liver abscess

- Commonly polymicrobial, although *Escherichia coli* and streptococci account for the majority of organisms grown
- Aetiology varies: biliary spread is the commonest (20–30%); others include contiguous spread, trauma, portal venous
- Most commonly seen in those aged 60–70 years
- Right lobe is the commonest location (in > 50% of cases)
- Multiple abscesses are more common that a single abscess
- Central lesions are common

Amoebic liver abscess

- *Entamoeba histolytica* is the causative organism
- Most commonly seen in those aged 30–50 years
- Usually located in the right lobe of the liver and in the periphery
- Typically a single lesion
- Size varies; often the abscess is > 5 cm in diameter

Imaging features

Plain X-ray
- Raised right dome of the diaphragm
- Right basal atelectasis
- Right pleural effusions

Ultrasound
- In early stages the abscess appears as a hypo-echoic, ill-defined area
- Later it becomes better defined, with posterior enhancement and a thick reflective wall
- Simple or multi-loculated
- Single or multiple
- Central (pyogenic) or peripheral (amoebic)
- Depending on the type, the abscess contents may be homogeneous (in amoebic and pyogenic abscesses) or more heterogeneous, with low level foci of echogenicity (in pyogenic or fungal abscesses)

CT
- Low-attenuation lesion causing mass effect

- Peripheral wall enhancement on contrast studies
- Simple or multiloculated with nodularity of the wall
- Pyogenic abscesses contain gas whereas amoebic abscesses do not
- Two signs specific to pyogenic abscesses
  - Double target sign: wall enhances, with a surrounding hypodense zone caused by oedematous liver tissue
  - Cluster sign: several abscesses cluster together, looking as if they might coalesce

MRI
- Low signal on T1WI, high signal on T2WI
- Enhancement of wall on gadolinium
- Target sign on T2WI: cavity shows a high T2 signal with the wall showing a low T2 wall and peri-lesional oedema producing a high T2 signal

Nuclear medicine imaging
- Uptake of the sulphur colloid of technetium-99m and of labelled white blood cells
- The sulphur colloid is taken up by abscesses, giving rise to a focal area on imaging
- Gallium is taken up by pyogenic abscesses but not by amoebic abscesses

Hepatic haemangioma

- Commonest benign liver lesions, accounting for 70–80% of liver lesions
- Usually single (in 90% of cases) and peripheral
- Associated with focal nodular hyperplasia and Osler–Weber–Rendu syndrome
- May present with spontaneous haemorrhage or with Kasabach–Merritt syndrome (haemangioma plus thrombocytopenia)
- Usually < 4 cm in diameter; produces a giant cavernous haemangioma when > 4 cm
- Blood supply comes from the hepatic artery
- May rupture spontaneously

Imaging features

Plain X-ray
- Calcifications within the liver

Ultrasound
- Variable features
- Majority are hyperechoic although can be hypoechoic
- May show acoustic enhancement
- No flow on colour Doppler

CT
- Well-circumscribed, predominantly low-attenuation lesion
- On contrast enhancement there is a peripheral nodular enhancement that fills in over time as seen on delayed images
- Small lesions, though they enhance immediately

MRI
- Sharply defined lesion
- Low signal on T1WI and markedly hyperintense on T2WI
- Central fibrous scar present
- Similar enhancement pattern to that seen on CT, with peripheral nodular enhancement that progresses centripetally with central uniform enhancement taking approximately 15 minutes

Focal nodular hyperplasia

- Second commonest benign liver lesion
- Peak age is 30–50 years, with a female predominance
- Associated with hepatic haemangiomas
- More commonly located in the right lobe
- Solitary lesion < 5 cm in diameter
- Tumour-like lesion that is seen on the surface of the liver
- Non-encapsulated, sometimes pedunculated
- Central scar that contains an arteriovenous malformation
- Very vascular and contains Kupffer cells
- No calcification within the lesion

Imaging features

Ultrasound
- Hyperechoic lesion showing as a homogeneous mass

- Hypoechoic central scar seen in 15–20% of cases
- Lesion displaces vessels around it
- Colour Doppler imaging shows enlarged vessels within the lesion, with a central artery and large peripheral draining veins

CT
- Ill-defined, low-attenuation mass
- Transient hyperintensity in the portal venous phase of contrast injection that then leaches away to isointensity to the surrounding tissue in the equilibrium phase
- 'Spoke-wheel' pattern with a central scar is seen in 20–30% of cases
- Central scar is seen in delayed images

MRI
- On T1WI the lesion is isointense, with a well-defined hypointense central scar
- On T2WI the lesion is usually isointense, with a hyperintense central scar in 75% of cases
- On gadolinium-enhanced dynamic imaging, there is intense enhancement in the arterial phase that progressively becomes less intense
- The central scar enhances early and is a characteristic finding
- Kupffer cell-specific agents, such as superoxides, cause enhancement of the lesion

Differential diagnoses

- Fibrolamellar hepatocellular carcinoma (HCC)
- Hepatic adenoma
- Well-differentiated HCC
- Giant cavernous haemangioma
- Hypervascular metastasis
- Intrahepatic cholangiocarcinoma

Hepatocellular adenoma

- Seen in women on oral contraceptives
- Peak age is 20–40 years
- Men on anabolic steroids may develop it

- Most commonly seen in the right lobe in a subcapsular location
- Typically 5–10 cm in diameter
- Adenomas consist of hepatocytes and Kupffer cells with fat but no portal tracts within it. The lesion has areas of haemorrhage and necrosis within it

Imaging features

Ultrasound
- Heterogeneous solid lesion
- Variable echotexture depending on constituent elements
- Hypoechoic rim due to compression of liver tissue around the tumour

CT
- Well-defined rounded lesion
- May have hyperdense areas if there has been haemorrhage within the tumour

MRI
- The appearances cannot be reliably distinguished from those of HCC
- Areas of haemorrhage of differing ages results in a lesion that is heterogenous in appearance on various sequences
- Predominantly hyperintense on T1WI
- Isointense on T2WI

Nuclear medicine imaging
- Photopenic lesion on sulphur colloid scintigraphy, surrounded by a rim of increased uptake
- No uptake on gallium scan

Hepatocellular carcinoma (HCC)

- Also known as a hepatoma
- Commonest visceral malignancy
- Peak age is 60–70 years; when seen in children it is usually in those > 10 years old

Aetiology of HCC	
W	Wilson's disease
H	Haemochromatosis
A	Alpha 1 antitrypsin deficiency
T	Tyrosinosis
H	Hepatitis
C	Cirrhosis
C	Carcinogens

- Causes
  - Cirrhosis from hepatitis B or C (40–50% of cases)
  - Alcohol cirrhosis (< 10% of cases)
  - Vascular neoplasm
- Solitary in 30% of cases, multifocal in 60–70% and diffuse in 5%
- Invades the portal vein in 50–60% of cases; invades the hepatic vein or the IVC in < 20%
- Also invades the bile ducts
- Metastasis are seen in 70% of cases
- Commonest lymphatic site for metastases is the hepatoduodenal nodes
- Commonest sites for haematogenous spread are the lungs, adrenal glands and bone
- Pathogenesis follows a stepwise process: regenerative nodules progress to an adenomatous nodule, which becomes a dysplastic nodule, then a small HCC (< 2 cm in diameter) and then a large HCC

Imaging features

Ultrasound
- Variable echogenicity
- Background of cirrhosis
- Invasion to hepatic or portal veins seen by colour flow

CT
- Best seen with dynamic CT
- Heterogenous enhancing mass with focal necrosis
- Calcification is seen in 10% of cases
- Invasion is best demonstrated with CT
- Features of portal venous invasion are arterial–portal fistulae, periportal streaks of high attenuation, and dilatation of portal vein and branches
- No enhancement of the segment of the liver that is blocked
- Intrinsic portal vein obstruction is specific to HCC
- Portal vein thrombosis is differentiated from HCC by the lack of enhancement of the thrombus

MRI
- Focal liver lesions with high signal on T2WI and variable intensity on T1WI
  - Low T1 signal in 30–40% of cases

- High T1 signal in 40–50% of cases
- Isointense T1 signal in 10–20% of cases
- High-grade dysplasia and small HCCs show a "nodule-in-nodule appearance especially within siderotic nodules
- At dynamic gadolinium imaging intense enhancement is seen
- Characteristic features of large HCC
  - Mosaic pattern: confluent small nodules separated by thin septae, best seen on T2WI and giving a heterogenous appearance on gadolinium-enhanced images
  - Tumour capsule is present in 60–80% of cases and is hypointense on both T1WI and T2WI
  - Extracapsular extension with satellite nodules is seen in 50–70% of cases
  - Vascular invasion (as seen on CT), seen on MRI as the presence of high signal on T1WI and T1 gradient-echo images within the portal vein, and enhancement of the tumour thrombus in the arterial phase and a filling defect in later phases on gadolinium-enhanced imaging

Nuclear medicine imaging
- Sulphur colloid scan shows a cold spot
- Avid uptake on gallium scan

Fibrolamellar HCC

- Special type of HCC
- Peak age is 30–40 years
- No underlying cirrhosis or other risk factors for HCC
- Solitary lobulated lesion with a central scar
- Encapsulated with a pseudocapsule of compressed hepatic tissue
- Central amorphous calcification seen in 30–40% of cases
- Regional lymphadenopathy seen in 50–60%; commonest site is the porta hepatis
- Distant metastases are uncommon
- Good prognosis

Imaging features

Ultrasound
- Heterogenous, predominantly hyperechoic central scar

CT
- Lobulated mass
- Enhancing mass with central scar that does not enhance
- Pseudocapsule

MRI
- Hypointense on T1WI
- Hyperintense on T2WI
- Scar is typically hypointense on both T1WI and T2WI
- Heterogenous gadolinium enhancement of the lesion but no enhancement of the scar
- Not typically known to cause vascular invasion

Fatty liver disease

- Complication of many toxic, ischaemic and metabolic insults to the liver
- May be diffuse or focal
- May be lobar, segmental or nodular

Imaging features

Ultrasound
- Hyperechoic
- Impaired visualisation of hepatic vessels
- If focal then the margins are poorly visualised

CT
- Areas of low attenuation with average of 10 Hounsfield units
- Liver spleen density is reversed
- Hyperdense intrahepatic vessels
- Focal fatty infiltration has no mass effect and the vessels course normally through the area of infiltration

MRI
- High signal on T1WI
- Low signal on T2WI
- Conventional imaging insensitive for fatty infiltration
- Opposed-phase imaging turns the fat-infiltrated areas dark on out-of-phase imaging

Metastases to the liver

- One of the commonest organs for metastases

- Commonest malignant lesion of the liver, usually arising from primary in the colon, breast, lung or pancreas
- Both lobes are involved in 75% of cases
- Lesions are solitary in 10% of cases

Imaging features

Ultrasound
- Focal metastases are space-occupying lesions that distort the liver anatomy
- Variable echogenicity
- Echogenic liver lesions are usually from the gastrointestinal tract or the urogenital tract
- No Doppler signal is generated, the exception being carcinoid tumours

CT
- Attenuation is variable but most are predominantly low-attenuation lesions
- Peripheral ring enhancement occurs frequently
- Cystic metastases can be differentiated from benign cysts by mural nodule, fluid–fluid levels or septations
- Most sensitive imaging modality is CT angiography, which is used to assess potentially resectable metastases

Exclusion criteria for metastatectomy

- Advanced stage of primary tumour
- More than four metastases
- Extrahepatic metastases
- < 30% of liver tissue left after resection

- Causes of calcified liver metastases
  - Gastric carcinoma
  - Malignant melanoma
  - Renal cell carcinoma
  - Colon carcinoma
  - Ovarian carcinoma
- Causes of hypervascular metastases
  - Thyroid carcinoma
  - Renal cell carcinoma
  - Carcinoid
  - Melanoma
  - Pancreatic islet cell tumours

- Causes of haemorrhagic metastases
  - Colon carcinoma
  - Thyroid carcinoma
  - Breast carcinoma
  - Choriocarcinoma
  - Melanoma

Budd–Chiari syndrome

- Occlusion of the venous outflow of the liver: occlusion of the hepatic vein or the IVC
- Presents clinically with hepatomegaly and ascites
- Aetiology is diverse, but most often idiopathic (in 60–70% of cases)

Thrombotic obstruction (Virchow's triad)
- The three features of Virchow's triad
  - Blood flow problems
  - Problems of the constituents
  - Problems with the walls
- Causes are the 'five Ps'
  - Pregnancy
  - Pill
  - Polycythemia rubra vera
  - Platelets – abnormal/excess
  - Paroxysmal nocturnal haemoglobinuria

Non-thrombotic obstruction
- Causes
  - Right heart failure
  - Constrictive pericarditis
  - Right atrial tumour
  - IVC membranes

Imaging features
Ultrasound
- Hepatomegaly
- Caudate lobe hypertrophy
- Gallbladder wall thickening
- Obliteration of the hepatic veins and/or the IVC
- Portal vein enlargement and change in flow dynamics
- Hepatopetal or hepatofugal flow may be seen in the portal vein
- Portosystemic anastomosis and the azygos and hemiazygos systems become prominent

- Doppler studies show absence of flow or reversal of flow within the hepatic veins, with dampening of the IVC waveform
- Hepatic artery resistance index > 0.7

CT
- Hepatomegaly and ascites
- Non-homogeneous liver enhancement with a predominantly central area of enhancement and delayed enhancement of the periphery
- The periphery may show low attenuation
- The caudate lobe is enlarged and enhances floridly
- Poor identification of the hepatic veins
- Identification of the cause of obstruction may be possible
- Thrombosis in the IVC and hepatic veins may be difficult to see

MRI
- Peripheral liver gives low signal on T1WI and high signal on T2WI
- Liver parenchyma is not homogeneous
- Gadolinium enhancement is variable
- Comma-shaped intrahepatic varices, caused by intrahepatic collateral vessels, are characteristically seen on coronal images
- Reduction in calibre or absence of the hepatic veins and IVC

Major differential diagnoses

- Cirrhosis
- Hepatic veno-occlusive disease
- Right heart failure

Hepatic veno-occlusive disease

- Commonly caused by radiation or chemotherapy in transplant patients
- Demonstrated on MRI by occlusion of the small centrilobular venules without major hepatic vein thrombosis
- Ultrasound shows bidirectional flow in the portal veins without evidence of hepatic vein or IVC obstruction, with gallbladder wall thickening

Portal vein thrombosis

- Thrombosis of the portal vein is a a causative factor for the development of portal hypertension in children

- Occurs in 30% of cases of HCC and in 5–10% of cases of cirrhosis
- Can be acute or chronic
- Clinical manifestations include haematemesis, hepatic encephalopathy and abdominal pain

Causes of portal vein thrombosis

- Idiopathic in neonates
- Malignancy (HCC, cholangiocarcinoma, pancreatic carcinoma, liver metastases)
- Hypercoagulable states
- Trauma, especially iatrogenic by introduction of umbilical vein catheter
- Intraperitoneal inflammation
- Umbilical sepsis
- Pancreatitis
- Peritonitis
- Ascending cholangitis

Imaging features

Ultrasound
- Echogenic material within the portal vein in the acute phase that becomes less well visualised with age
- Increased portal vein diameter
- Thickened lesser omentum in the acute phase

CT
- There is low attenuation thrombus within the portal vein on portal venous phase
- Decrease in attenuation of the liver
- In chronic stages multiple peripheral collaterals are seen

MRI
- Gradient-echo imaging shows flow voids in the portal vein
- Depending on the age of the thrombus, signal changes differ, with high T1 and T2 signal within the first 5 weeks and high T2 signal after that

Peliosis hepatis

- Rare benign disorder characterised by dilatation of sinusoidal blood-filled spaces and of blood-filled spaces within the organs of the reticuloendothelial system

- Affects the liver, spleen, bone marrow, lymph nodes and lungs
- Causes
  - AIDS
  - Chronic infections, e.g. tuberculosis
  - Anabolic steroids
  - Chronic renal failure
  - Tamoxifen

Imaging features

Ultrasound
- Multiple echogenic or hypoechoic areas

CT
- Enhancing, round lesions within the organs
- The lesions are initially hypoattenuating; they become isoattenuating with time

Anatomy

- The biliary tree transports bile from the liver to the second part of the duodenum
- Bile duct variants are common, the most important being the aberrant cystic duct
- Variations of the cystic duct occur in < 25% of cases
- 75% of cystic ducts insert into the middle third of the extrahepatic CHD
- 10% insert into the distal CHD
- < 1% have a gallbladder draining directly into the CBD

Choledochal cysts

- One of a spectrum of cystic dilatations of the biliary system, characterised by cystic dilatation of the extrahepatic bile ducts
- Classification is based on the extent and morphology of the choledochal cysts
- Usually presents before the age of 10 years, with 30–40% presenting before the age of 1 year
- Associated with anomalies of the biliary and pancreatic ductal systems and with liver cysts
- Clinical manifestations (triad seen in 25% of cases)
  - Intermittent obstructive jaundice
  - Recurrent right upper quadrant pain
  - Right upper quadrant mass

Imaging features

Ultrasound
- Cyst adjacent to gallbladder
- Intrahepatic bile duct dilatation, caused by pressure on the CHD
- May be seen in antenatal scans

MRI
- MR cholangiopancreatography (MRCP) confirms the presence of the cyst and identifies the anomalous anatomy

Nuclear medicine imaging
- Delayed filling of the choledochal cyst on hepatobiliary imino-diacetic acid (HIDA) scans
- Differential diagnoses include hepatic cysts, pancreatic pseudocysts and enteric duplication cysts

Cholelithiasis and cholangiolithiasis

- Prevalence increases with age
- Causes
  - Haemolytic disease
  - Cholestasis
  - Metabolic disorders
  - Malabsorption
  - Increased incidence in diabetics
- Cholangiolithiasis is the commonest cause of bile duct obstruction

Main types

- Cholesterol stones
  - Account for 70–80% of stones
  - Radiolucent
  - 70% are mixed and 20% are radiopaque
  - Strong association with cirrhosis
- Pigment stones
  - Account for 30% of stones
  - 2–5 mm in diameter and faceted
  - Predominantly contain calcium bilirubinate
  - 50% are radiopaque

Imaging features

Ultrasound
- Specific and sensitive for gallstones
- Echogenic
- Mobility needs to be assessed on ultrasound
- Wall–echo shadow complex is seen when the gallbladder is contracted over the gallstones

CT
- Hyperdense stones can be seen on CT
- Inverse relationship between the cholesterol in the stones and degree of attenuation

MRI
- Less sensitive for visualising stones than CT
- However, MRCP is often done to provide a further assessment of the anatomy and to visualise the stones better
- Stones are seen as signal voids or filling defects within the biliary tree

Acute calculous cholecystitis

- Inflammation of the gallbladder
- Peak age is 50–70 years
- Complications
  - Gangrene
  - Abscess
  - Emphysematous cholecystitis
  - Bouveret syndrome (erosion of gallstones into the duodenum)
  - Empyema
  - Gallstone ileus

Imaging features

Ultrasound
- Echogenic
- May be mobile
- Gallstones may be impacted in the neck
- Sludge within the gallbladder
- Gallbladder wall thickening > 3 mm
- Pericholecystic fluid
- Positive sonographic Murphy's sign

CT
- Distended gallbladder
- Multiple gallstones
- Pericholecystic fat stranding
- Increased attenuation of bile

MRI
- MRCP shows gallstones within the biliary tree
- Dilatation of the CBD
- Intrahepatic duct dilatation if there is proximal stone or if Mirizzi's syndrome is present

Chronic cholecystitis

- Commonest gallbladder disease

- Gallbladder is contracted and may be calcified ('porcelain' gallbladder)
- Hepatobiliary imino-diacetic acid (HIDA) scanning is useful for looking at biliary obstruction

Acalculous cholecystitis

- Caused by gallbladder dysmotility and super-added bacterial infection
- Seen in burns, serious injury and extrinsic inflammation
- Similar ultrasound appearances to those of calculous cholecystitis, but without the gallstones
- Reduced motility with cholecystokinin
- Complications include gangrene of the gallbladder and perforation

Emphysematous cholecystitis

- Ischaemia of gallbladder wall secondary to inflammation and vasculitis
- Typically seen in diabetes
- Plain radiographs show gas around the gallbladder
- Pneumobilia

Imaging features

Plain X-ray
- Gas around the gallbladder
- Pneumobilia

Ultrasound
- Gas obscures the wall of the gallbladder
- Pericholecystic fluid
- Pneumobilia

Xanthogranulomatous cholecystitis

- Inflammation of the gallbladder with intramural nodules
- Peak age is 70–80 years
- Thick gallbladder wall and intramural hypoechoic nodules
- Focal fatty inflammation
- Biliary obstruction

Cholangiocarcinoma

- Associated with primary sclerosing cholangitis
- Most commonly located in the hilum or in the distal CBD (in 30–40% of cases)

- Predisposing factors
  - Inflammatory bowel disease
  - Primary sclerosing cholangitis
  - Cholelithiasis
  - Choledochal cysts
  - Caroli's disease
  - Biliary atresia
  - Adult polycystic kidney disease
  - Congenital hepatic fibrosis
  - Papillomatosis of the gallbladder

Intrahepatic cholangiocarcinoma

- Peak age is 50-60 years
- Mass with satellite nodules
- Dilated biliary tree with a predominantly hyperechoic mass (in 75% of cases)
- Shows homogeneous delayed enhancement on CT, with dilated intrahepatic ducts
- A Klatskin's tumour is located at the confluence of the right and left hepatic ducts; indirect signs are segmental dilatation of the main ducts, portal vein obstruction and lobar atrophy

Extrahepatic cholangiocarcinoma

- Peak age is 60–70 years
- 10% present with cholangitis
- Pure intrahepatic duct dilatation
- Mass seen in the extrahepatic biliary tree
- Usually an infiltrating lesion of low attenuation that shows delayed enhancement

Mirizzi's syndrome

- Impaction of the gallstone in the neck of the gallbladder
- Obstructs the cystic duct
- Gives rise to cholecystitis

Cholangitis

- Inflammation of the bile ducts
- Most commonly due to obstruction

Obstructive cholangitis

- Caused by benign obstruction by surgery or calculi in 60% of cases
- Malignant obstruction may be due to an ampullary tumour
- Acutely non-suppurative in 10–20% of cases; suppurative in 80–90% cases
- *Escherichia coli* is the commonest causative organism

Imaging features

Ultrasound
- Shows the cause of the obstruction
- May show pneumobilia

CT
- Peri-biliary enhancement on arterial phase imaging

Primary sclerosing cholangitis

- Chronic obliterative fibrotic inflammation of the biliary tree
- Intrahepatic bile ducts are more often involved than extrahepatic bile ducts
- Associations
  - IBD
  - Pancreatitis
  - Sjögren's
  - Retroperitoneal fibrosis
  - Peyronie's disease
- CBD is always involved

Imaging features

Ultrasound
- Echogenic portal triads

CT
- Pruning of the biliary tree and beading of the ducts, with wall nodularity

Cholangiogram
- Characteristic beading of the ducts with pruned appearance

MRI
- MRCP shows pruning of the biliary tree and similar pruning appearance

Anatomy

- Retroperitoneal structure within the anterior pararenal space at the T12–L1 level
- Four parts are described: the head, the body, the tail and the uncinate process
- Central pancreatic duct feeds into the ampulla of Vater, together with the CBD
- They enter via the major duodenal papilla into the second part of the duodenum
- Accessory pancreatic duct entering into the minor duodenal papilla
- Relations
  - Retroperitoneal, lying in the pararenal space along with the retroperitoneal colon and duodenum
  - Lies anterior to the IVC, the aorta and the first part of the duodenum at the level of the superior mesenteric artery
  - Lies anterior to the confluence of the superior mesenteric vein and the splenic vein
  - Lies posterior to the lesser sac and the mesentery of the transverse colon
  - To the left the tail is related to the hilum of the spleen
  - To the right the tail is related to the second part of the duodenum
  - Blood supply is via the superior pancreaticoduodenal artery (a branch of the gastroepiploic artery) and the inferior pancreaticoduodenal artery (a branch of the superior mesenteric artery)

Embryology

- Formed by the fusion of the dorsal and ventral buds of the foregut in the fourth week of gestation
- The dorsal duct (Santorini's duct) drains the body and tail of the pancreas through the minor papilla
- The ventral duct (Wirsung's duct) drains the uncinate process through the major papilla
- The dorsal and ventral ducts fuse so that the main duct of Wirsung consists of the ventral duct and proximal segment of the dorsal duct; it drains into the major papilla
- The distal dorsal duct regresses and drains as Santorini's duct through the minor papilla

Pancreatic anomalies

Frequency of anomalies
• Dual drainage (accessory papillae) (30% of cases)
• Pancreas divisum (< 10% of cases)
• Ectopic pancreatic tissue (< 10% of cases)
• Annular pancreas (one in 7000 cases)

Pancreas divisum

- Formed by failure of the dorsal and ventral buds to fuse
- The dorsal and ventral ducts drain separately
- The dorsal duct drains the body, tail and superior part of the head of the pancreas through the minor duodenal papilla
- The ventral duct drains the uncinate process and the inferior part of the head through the major papilla
- Presents with non-alcoholic recurrent pancreatitis in the dorsal segment, caused by stenosis of the minor papilla

Imaging features

ERCP
- Difficult cannulation of the minor papilla
- Obvious absence of connection between the dorsal and ventral ducts

CT
- May show increase in the craniocaudal length and a fat plane between the dorsal and ventral elements

MRCP
- Similar findings to those of ERCP

Annular pancreas

- A rotational anomaly
- Located in the second part of the duodenum
- May cause obstruction in neonates or be asymptomatic

Imaging features

Plain X-ray
- 'Double bubble' sign in neonates, caused by duodenal obstruction
- Upper gastrointestinal (GI) series shows eccentric or concentric narrowing of the duodenum with delayed gastric emptying; the duodenal mucosa is flattened, with no ulceration

CT
- Mass around the duodenum

Endoscopic retrograde cholangiopancreatogram (ERCP)
- Ventral duct wrapped around the second part of the duodenum

Pancreatitis

- Commonest pathology in the pancreas
- Causes
  - Idiopathic
  - Alcohol (15% of cases)
  - Cholelithiasis (75% of cases), mainly acute
  - Metabolic disorders
  - Hypercalcaemia in hyperparathyroidism
  - Hereditary pancreatitis

- Hyperlipidaemia types I and V
- Kwashiorkor
- Infection or infestation
- Trauma (iatrogenic in a Billroth II gastrectomy, a splenectomy or choledochal surgery)
- Structural abnormalities
- Diuretics (thiazides and frusemide)
- Anticancer drugs (azidothymidine, asparaginase)
- Antibiotics (sulphonamides, tetracycline)
- Antidiabetic drugs (phenformin)
- Malignancy (metastasis and lymphoma)

Acute pancreatitis

- May be diffuse (50% of cases) or focal (50% of cases)
- Commonly caused by gallstones
- Two main pathological forms: oedematous and necrotising
- Haemorrhagic pancreatitis is characterised by fat necrosis and haemorrhage
- Suppurative pancreatitis is caused by super-added bacterial infection
- Presents with abdominal pain radiating to the back and raised levels of serum amylase, lipase and calcium
- Signs of haemorrhagic pancreatitis
  - Cullen's sign: periumbilical ecchymoses
  - Grey–Turner sign: ecchymoses on the flanks
  - Fox sign: infrainguinal ecchymoses

Imaging features

AXR
- Generalised or focal ileus (sentinel loop)
- Renal halo, caused by perirenal oedema
- Gas in the pancreatic region
- Ascites

CXR
- Basal subsegmental atelectasis
- Pleural effusions
- Elevation of the left hemidiaphragm
- Adult respiratory distress syndrome
- Pulmonary oedema
- Pulmonary infarction or infiltrates

Imaging features

Upper GI contrast study
- Non-specific findings
- Widening of duodenal sweep
- Thickened duodenal folds
- 'Reverse three' sign (tethering of folds)
- Enlarged major papilla
- Anterior displacement of the stomach
- Jejunal or ileal fold thickening

Ultrasound
- Enlarged pancreas
- Diffuse or focal hypoechoic areas
- Frequently difficult because overlying bowel obscures the area

CT
- Modality of choice
- Interstitial oedematous pancreatitis
  - Pancreatic and peripancreatic oedema
  - Contour changes
  - Duct dilatation
  - Altered pancreatic attenuation
  - Differentiated from acute necrotising pancreatitis by the presence of contrast enhancement of the whole pancreas, whereas in necrotising pancreatitis there is patchy enhancement

- Necrotising pancreatitis
  - Focal or diffuse areas of necrosis of pancreatic parenchyma
  - Associated peripancreatic fat necrosis
  - Contrast-enhanced CT shows patchy enhancement of the pancreas
  - Morbidity and mortality is high, and it carries a poor prognosis and is an indication for surgery
  - Complications include pancreatic abscess, pseudocyst, fistulae, pseudo-aneurysms and exocrine or endocrine deficiency
  - Pancreatic abscess needs to be differentiated from necrosis: a well-marginated fluid collection is seen in an abscess but not in necrosis
  - Rate of infection with necrosis is high, and infection cannot be detected accurately on CT
- Acute fluid collections
  - Caused by the mesentery originating from the pancreas, with spread of fluid and subsequent ileus in the hepatic flexure, transverse colon and splenic flexure
  - Fluid is seen to accumulate in the lesser sac first followed by anterior perirenal space
  - The fluid then may spread cephalad to the bare area or caudad to the pelvis via the psoas muscle
  - 'Halo' sign around the kidneys as a result of fluid in the anterior perirenal space

Pancreatic pseudocyst

- Cyst formation within the pancreas, usually secondary to inflammation (mostly chronic pancreatitis); acute collections in the pancreas or lesser sac are not pseudocysts
- Requires > 4 weeks to form and matures in 6–8 weeks
- Two-thirds are seen within the pancreatic tissue, with the omental bursa the second commonest site for a pseudocyst
- Complications
  - Rupture into peritoneum (generalised peritonitis) or into a loop of bowel (decompression/fistulation)

    – Haemorrhage from vessels in wall or pseudoaneurysm
    – Air in pseudocyst must raise the possibility of a fistula. The site can usually be determined by a contrast study

Imaging features

Upper GI contrast study

- Depending on where the pseudocyst lies and on its size, it can cause smooth extrinsic indentations of either the stomach and duodenal sweep or the splenic flexure
- Gastric outlet obstruction is a known complication

Ultrasound

- Usually a single, unilocular cyst
- May show debris within it
- May increase in size with time
- Rarely obstructs the CBD or the pancreatic duct, leading to a clinical presentation of jaundice

CT

- Starts as a subtle area of low density and then walls off
- Contrast enhancement of the walls
- Fluid in pseudocyst 0–30 Hounsfield units, but depends on the protein concentration of the fluid

Pancreatitis abscess

- Collection of pus close to the pancreas
- Usually occurs 2–4 weeks after severe acute pancreatitis
- Most commonly caused by *Escherichia coli* or polymicrobial
- *Candida* abscesses may occur in immunocompromised patients
- May gas with some Gram-positive infections

Vascular complications

- Can cause vascular occlusion, haemorrhage or pseudo-aneurysm
- Occlusion of the splenic artery and vein is common
- Pseudoaneurysm formation occurs in 10% of causes, and 30–40% of these have associated haemorrhage
- Usually affects the splenic artery followed by the gastroduodenal and pancreaticoduodenal artery branches, and it can be confused with a pseudocyst
- Haemorrhage occurs in up to 5% of cases of pancreatitis as well as in relation to pseudocysts and pseudoaneuryms

Emphysematous pancreatitis

- Pancreatitis with super-added infection with gas forming bacteria
- Commonest causative organism is *Escherichia coli*
- High mortality and morbidity
- Majority of cases resolve with conservative treatment
- Differential diagnoses include duodenal diverticulum, penetrating ulcer of the stomach or duodenum, GI fistulae from surrounding structures and iatrogenic aetiologies, e.g. following an ERCP or roux-en-Y surgery

Chronic pancreatitis

- Recurrent or continued inflammation of the pancreas leading to irreversible changes to the anatomy and function of the pancreas
- Clinical features include recurrent abdominal pain and steatorrhea
- Often results in diabetes mellitus

Causes of chronic pancreatitis

Calcifying type
- Juvenile tropical pancreatitis
- Hereditary pancreatitis
- Hyperlipidaemia
- Hypercalcaemia

Obstructive type
- Trauma
- Renal failure
- Cystic fibrosis
- Sclerosing cholangitis
- Ampullary tumour
- Ampullary stenosis

Imaging features

Abdominal radiographs

- Irregular calcification in the region of the pancreas

CT and ultrasound

- Gland size depends on fibrosis and inflammation, which may be diffuse or focal
- Hence there may be no change in size of the pancreas, or atrophy or enlargement
- Associated loss of fat plane can be seen, appearing like a tumour encasement
- Calcification is irregular and most commonly first occurs in the head
- Duct involvement is important because duct obstruction may cause symptoms and can be relieved surgically
- Decalcification of the gland is a known entity
- Beading ('chain of pearls' appearance) is seen in the pancreatic duct in 68% of cases

MRI

- Loss of signal on fat-saturation T1WI
- Poor contrast enhancement of the pancreas
- MRCP shows duct dilatation and beading

Pancreatic duct adenocarcinoma

- Accounts for 80% of all pancreatic malignancies
- Peak age is 50–80 years
- Causes
  - Smoking
  - Diabetes mellitus
  - Alcohol
  - Hereditary pancreatitis
- Commonest site is the head of the pancreas (in 60–70% of cases)
- Presents clinically with weight loss, abdominal pain and obstructive jaundice

Imaging features

Ultrasound

- Heterogeneous hypoechoic mass in the pancreas
- Contour deformity
- Pancreatic duct dilatation if the lesion is an obstructing one

Barium meal

- 'Inverted three' sign
- Antral padding

- Mass or filling defect in the ampullary region of duodenum

CT

- Adenocarcinoma can be seen on CT in 95% of cases
- Tumours of the head and body of the pancreas produce a diffuse enlargement of the gland
- Usually heterogeneous with central low attenuation
- Biliary tree and pancreatic dilatation may be seen
- Biliary tree dilatation occurs with tumours of the head of pancreas tumours; this is abrupt compared with pancreatitis, in which the dilatation is concentric and gradual
- Invasion of contiguous organs, including the duodenum, stomach and mesenteric root
- Adenocarcinomas rarely calcify (commonly non-functioning islet cell tumours)
- Local extension to vessels is suggested when there is a loss of the fat plane between the mass and vessel
- Local extension may also cause dilatation of the pancreaticoduodenal vein
- Lymph node spread is to the peripancreatic and porta hepatis nodes, which can be seen in the hepatoduodenal area and the root of the mesentery
- Liver metastases occur commonly

Intraductal papillary mucinous tumour of the pancreas

- Low-grade pancreatic malignancy arising from the epithelial cells of the ducts
- Contains mucin
- Presents with abdominal pain and pancreatitis
- Two main types
  - Main duct intraductal papillary mucinous tumour of the pancreas
  - Branch duct intraductal papillary mucinous tumour of the pancreas
- Branch type has good prognosis with partial pancreatectomy

Imaging features

CT

- Dilatation of the main pancreatic duct
- Papillary projections into the main duct seen on thin-section CT
- Multilobulated cystic lesions in the uncinate process
- Main duct dilatation of > 10 mm has a higher risk of being malignant
- Main duct dilatation may be segmental or focal, and the appearance may be of that of a pseudocyst
- The branch duct type is seen usually in the uncinate process
- Two patterns are seen, microcystic and macrocystic

Cystic carcinomas of the pancreas

- Group of cystic tumours within the pancreas
- May affect the main duct or branch ducts
- Usually presents clinically with abdominal pain or weight loss
- May be completely asymptomatic and discovered incidentally
- Two main types
  - Mucinous cystadenoma or cystadenocarcinoma (macrocystic type), which is thought to be malignant
  - Serous cystadenoma or cystadenocarcinoma (microcystic type), which is thought to be benign

Mucinous (macrocystic) type

- Includes both cystadenoma and cystadenocarcinoma
- Accounts for 5–10% of all cystic pancreatic neoplasms
- Peak age is 40–50 years
- Female predominance (19 times commoner in females)
- Commonly seen in the body and tail of the pancreas
- Usually fewer than six cysts of varying diameters but > 2 cm
- Calcification is present and non-specific
- There may be solid papillary projections into the cyst
- Invasion of other organs is known

Imaging features

Ultrasound

- Cystic lesions with low-level internal echoes

CT

- Single cyst or multiple cysts
- Cysts are large and septate, with fluid attenuation within them; attenuation value varies depending on the presence of protein or haemorrhage
- Papillary or nodular excrescence is known

MRI

- Similar findings to those of CT
- Hyperintense or hypointense lesions within cysts on T1WI, depending upon protein content
- On T2WI the cysts are hyperintense with hypointense septae
- Intracystic excrescences are seen
- Enhancement of the septae and solid components of the cyst

Serous (microcystic) type

- Usually benign
- Accounts for 40–50% of all cystic pancreatic neoplasms
- Peak age is 60–70 years
- Female predominance
- Predominantly located in the head of the pancreas, although any part can be affected
- Associated with von Hippel–Lindau disease
- Multiple cysts (usually more than six), measuring < 2 cm in diameter, although a few large cysts may be seen
- Calcification is present and is non-specific
- Good prognosis; can be surgically resected

Imaging features

Ultrasound

- Multiple echogenic, predominantly solid areas

CT

- Low-attenuation cystic areas
- Good enhancement on contrast, with numerous small and medium-sized cysts that may be difficult to separate
- A stellate late-enhancing scar is seen in 30% of cases

MRI
- High-signal cystic lesions on T2WI, with well-defined septae
- Hypointense on T1WI
- Central scar not well seen
- Delayed contrast enhancement

> ### Cystic lesions of the pancreas
>
> - Pancreatic collections or pseudocysts
> - Serous cystadenoma (second commonest cause)
> - Pancreatic abscess
> - Benign pancreatic cysts
> - Parasitic cysts
> - Pancreatic dermoid cysts
> - Pancreatic haematoma and traumatic pancreatitis

Pancreatic islet cell tumours

- Derivatives of the amine precursor uptake decarboxylase (APUD) cells or the islet cells of Langerhans
- Associated with multiple endocrine neoplasia type 1
- Functional in 80–90% of cases

Imaging features

Ultrasound
- Mass in the head of the pancreas
- Hypoechoic

CT
- Mass in the head of the pancreas, with or without necrosis
- Coarse calcification
- Enhances with contrast

Insulinoma
- Commonest islet cell tumour
- Peak age is 40–60 years
- Usually < 2 cm in diameter
- May be multiple
- No specific predilection for any location
- Presents with Whipple's triad
  - Spontaneous hypoglycaemia
  - Blood glucose below 50 mg/ml
  - Relief by administration of glucose

- Benign in 90% of cases, malignant in 10%
- Single in 90% of cases, multiple in 10%
- Sporadic in 90% of cases
- < 5 cm in 90% of cases
- Intrapancreatic in 90% of cases

Gastrinoma
- Second commonest islet cell tumour
- Peak age < 20 years
- Sporadic in 70% of patients
- Mostly benign and multiple
- Associated with multiple endocrine neoplasia type 1, in which case they are malignant
- Usually in the head of the pancreas
- Gastrinoma triangle: porta hepatis at the apex with the second and third parts of the duodenum as the base
- Up to 30% are ectopic
- Presentation is with Zollinger–Ellison syndrome
- Increased risk peptic ulcer disease

Non-functioning islet cell tumours
- Third commonest islet cell tumour
- May be benign or malignant
- The benign type are usually asymptomatic and do not grow large enough to be diagnosed
- Malignant tumours needs to be differentiated from each other because the treatment differs
- 80–100% of all benign non-functioning islet cell tumours eventually turn malignant
- May cause a mass effect and compression or invasion of structures
- Associated with multiple endocrine neoplasia type 1
- Peak age is from the third decade onwards
- Nodular calcification seen in 20–30% of cases
- Usual location is the pancreatic head

Glucagonoma
- Uncommon
- 75% are malignant
- Almost all are symptomatic
- Associated with multiple endocrine neoplasia type 1

- Peak age is 50–79 years
- Female predominance
- Commonest location is in the body or tail of the pancreas, although ectopic sites seen
- Clinical presentation
  - Necrolytic erythema migrans
  - Diarrhoea
  - Diabetes mellitus
  - Glossitis
  - Weight loss
  - Unexplained thromboembolic complications (deep venous thrombosis, pulmonary embolism) in 25% of cases
- Large masses seen in the pancreas on imaging
- Liver metastases occur in 50% of cases

VIPoma

- Secretes vasoactive intestinal peptide (VIP)
- Two thirds occur in women
- Location
  - Pancreas: in the body and tail
  - Extra-pancreatic: in the retroperitoneum and mediastinum in children, usually from a neurogenic tumour, e.g. ganglioblastoma, neuroblastoma
- Clinical presentation
  - Watery diarrhoea, hypokalaemia, hypochlorhydria (Verner–Morrison's syndrome)
  - Gallbladder dilatation, caused by paralysis of smooth muscle secondary to the VIP secretion
  - Commonly malignant, with metastasis to the liver in approximately 59% of cases at presentation

Somatostatinoma

- Predominantly located in head of the pancreas
- Peak age is 50 years

- Presents clinically with diabetes mellitus or steatorrhea
- Usually < 3 cm in diameter
- Malignant tumour that metastasises to the liver

Metastases to the pancreas

- Renal cell carcinoma
- Bronchogenic carcinoma
- Breast carcinoma
- GI stromal tumours
- Melanoma
- Carcinoid
- Adrenal carcinoma
- Thyroid carcinoma
- Angiosarcoma
- Can affect any part of the pancreas, although the head is the commonest area
- Usually associated with metastases to other areas
- Differential diagnosis includes ductal carcinoma

Multiple endocrine neoplasia

- Group of syndromes associated with endocrine hyperplasia
- Autosomal-dominant condition
- Hyperplasia of glands
- Type 1 is also known as Wermer's syndrome
- Type 2 is also known as Sipple's syndrome
- Type 3 is also known as mucosal neuroma syndrome

Type 1

- The glands involved have multiple tumours
- May be malignant

- Commonest sites are parathyroid glands, the pancreas (mostly islet cell tumours) and the anterior pituitary gland
- Peak age is 30–50 years
- An all-or-none phenomenon, i.e. all the above sites are affected in this syndrome
- Multiple lipomas and angiofibromas may lead to the diagnosis before the endocrine manifestations are found

Type 2A

- Accounts for most cases of multiple endocrine neoplasia
- Usually RET oncogene-positive
- Commonest sites are the thyroid (medullary C cell carcinoma), the adrenal glands (phaeochromocytomas, which are bilateral in 70% of cases) and the parathyroid gland (hyperplasia)
- Associated with carcinoid and Cushing's syndrome

Type 2B

- Accounts for 5% of all cases of multiple endocrine neoplasia type 2
- Marfanoid features with mucosal neuromas
- Aggressive form that frequently manifests itself in childhood
- Commonly causes medullary thyroid carcinoma, phaeochromocytomas, and oral, intestinal mucosal neuromas
- May cause intussusception as a result of neuromas in the bowel

Carney's complex

- Rare type of multiple endocrine neoplasia
- Causes primary pigmented adrenocortical disease, pituitary adenomas, Sertoli cell tumours, thyroid nodules and non-endocrine features including cardiac myxomas and schwannomas

Congenital oesophageal atresia and tracheo-oesophageal fistula (TOF)

- Oesophageal atresia refers to a congenitally interrupted oesophagus
- One or more fistulae may be present between the malformed oesophagus and the trachea or the TOF
- Presents clinically with an inability to swallow or with aspiration
- Variants
  - Type A: oesophageal atresia without fistula or so-called pure oesophageal atresia (10% of cases)
  - Type B: oesophageal atresia with proximal TOF (<1% of cases)
  - Type C: oesophageal atresia with distal TOF (85% of cases)
  - Type D: oesophageal atresia with proximal and distal TOF (< 1% of cases)
  - Type E: TOF without oesophageal atresia or so-called H-type fistula (4% of cases)
  - Type F: congenital oesophageal stenosis (< 1% of cases)

Imaging features

Antenatal ultrasound
- Polyhydramnios, which occurs in 33% of fetuses with oesophageal atresia and distal TOF and in almost 100% of fetuses with oesophageal atresia without fistula

CXR
- May show tracheal compression and deviation
- Absence of gastric air bubble indicates type A or type B oesophageal atresia
- Aspiration pneumonia into the posterior segment of the upper lobes
- Nasogastric tube 'coils' following insertion
- Contrast swallow may be necessary to identify the position of the fistula but

---

Associated anomalies (VACTERL)

- **Vertebral defects:** multiple or single hemivertebrae, scoliosis, rib deformities

- **Anorectal malformations:** imperforate anus of all varieties, cloacal deformities

- **Cardiovascular defects:** ventricular septal defect (the commonest cardiac defect), tetralogy of Fallot, patent ductus arteriosus, atrial septal defects, atrioventricular canal defects, aortic coarctation, right-sided aortic arch, single umbilical artery, others

- **Tracheo-oesophageal defects:** oesophageal atresia

- **Renal anomalies:** renal agenesis (including Potter's syndrome, bilateral renal agenesis, bilateral reanal dysplasia), horseshoe kidney, polycystic kidneys, urethral atresia, ureteral malformations

- **Limb deformities:** radial dysplasia, absent radius, radial ray deformities, syndactyly, polydactyly, lower-limb tibial deformities

VACTERL syndrome occurs when three or more of these associated anomalies are present

the examination carries a high risk of aspiration

- There is an association of right sided aortic arch, seen in 5% of patients with TOF, and this is important for surgical planning

Acquired TOF

Iatrogenic acquired TOF

- Traumatic TOF occurs secondary to either blunt trauma or open avulsion to the neck or thorax
- Usually located at the level of the carina and appears several days after initial injury
- An endotracheal tube cuff can increase the pressure posteriorly when there is a nasogastric tube in the oesophagus, giving rise to a TOF
- The risk is increased in patients with poor nutrition, as occurs in long-term intensive care unit patients
- Rarely occurs in relation to tracheostomy tubes

Malignant acquired TOF

- Malignant TOF is most commonly associated with oesophageal malignancies, although associations with lung carcinoma and with metastatic squamous cell laryngeal carcinoma are also recognized
- Most often occurs in the trachea (50% of cases) and bronchi (40% of cases)
- Prognosis is poor because there is a high risk of aspiration pneumonitis
- Imaging to demonstrate aspiration is by contrast swallows or CT
- Chest X-rays may imply the presence of aspiration by evidence of recurrent aspiration pneumonia

Achalasia

- Failure of peristalsis and relaxation of lower oesophageal sphincter

- Dysphagia for solids, exacerbated by stress and cold liquids
- May be idiopathic or caused by Chagas' disease (infiltration of Auerbach's plexus by *Trypanosoma cruzi*)
- Complications include oesophageal carcinoma (in 2–7% of cases) and aspiration pneumonia caused by regurgitation of pooled secretions and food particles
- Treatment is with balloon dilatation or surgical myotomy (Ramsted's operation)
- Main differential diagnosis is malignant pseudoachalasia secondary to gastric and oesophageal carcinoma; the main differentiator is timing of symptom onset (pseudoachalasia characteristically has a more rapid onset)

Imaging features

CXR
- Double right mediastinal stripe
- Convex opacity behind right heart border
- Air–fluid level in thoracic oesophagus (usually retrocardiac)
- Small gastric air bubble
- Aspiration pneumonia

Barium swallow
- Pooling of contrast with distal oesophageal dilatation (in 90% of cases)
- 'Birds beak' at the tip of the distal oesophagus (in 90% of cases)
- Failure of peristalsis to clear contrast
- Antegrade and retrograde motion of barium
- Associated epiphrenic diverticulae

Oesophageal cancer

- Accounts for 4–10% of all gastrointestinal cancers
- Males four times more commonly affected than females
- 20% occur in the upper third of the oesophagus, 30–40% in the middle third and 30–40% in the lower third

- Risk factors
  - Barrett's oesophagus
  - Alcohol abuse
  - Lye's stricture
  - Coeliac disease
  - Head and neck cancer
  - Smoking
  - Plummer–Vinson syndrome, achalasia, asbestosis or tylosis
- Prognosis is poor with a 5–20% 5-year survival rate
- Nodal involvement is a poor prognostic factor
- Staging
  - T1: invasion of lamina propria or submucosa
  - T2: invasion of the muscularis propria
  - T3: invasion of the adventitia
  - T4: invasion of adjacent structures
- Histology
  - Squamous cell carcinoma accounts for 50–70% of cases
  - Adenocarcinoma accounts for 30–50% of cases
  - Other types include spindle cell, mucoepidermoid, adenoid cystic, leiomyosarcoma, rhabdomyosarcoma, fibrosarcoma and metastases
- Criteria for unresectability
  - Pericardial effusion
  - Intraluminal mass in airway
  - Tumour extension between the trachea and the aortic arch or between the left main bronchus and the descending aorta
  - >90° contact with the aortic circumference
  - Pleural thickening or pleural effusion adjacent to tumour
  - Mediastinal or coeliac axis nodes

Imaging features

CXR
- Widened azygo-oesophageal recess
- Thick posterior or right tracheal stripe
- Wide mediastinum
- Tracheal deviation
- Retrocardiac mass
- Posterior tracheal indentation
- Aspiration pneumonia

Barium swallow
- Most accurate when done with a double-contrast technique
- Filling defect in the oesophagus or 'bird beaking' of the distal oesophagus
- Strictures are irregular and circumferential, with loss of superficial mucosa
- Ulceration may be seen

CT
- Useful in staging and surgical planning, as well as for reviewing postoperative features and recurrence
- Insensitive for identifying nodal disease because the major criteria currently used is node size

Endoscopic ultrasound
- More accurate than endoscopy in diagnosing recurrent disease and more accurate than CT in local disease staging
- Especially useful for disease that is confined to the mucosa and submucosa

Boerhaave's syndrome

- Oesophageal rupture caused by a sudden rise in intraluminal oesophageal pressure produced during vomiting
- Neuromuscular inco-ordination causes failure of the cricopharyngeus muscle to relax
- Commonest anatomical location of the tear is at the left posterolateral wall of the lower third of the oesophagus, 2–3 cm proximal to the gastro-oesophageal junction
- Second commonest site of rupture is in the subdiaphragmatic or upper thoracic area
- 80% of all patients are middle-aged men
- Overall mortality rate is 30%
- Mortality is usually due to subsequent infection, e.g. mediastinitis, pneumonitis, pericarditis, empyema
- Surgical intervention is required in most cases
- Patients who undergo surgical repair within 24 hours of injury have a 70–75% chance of survival
- This falls to 35–50% if surgery is delayed longer than 24 hours and to approximately 10% if delayed longer than 48 hours

Imaging features

CXR
- Useful in the initial diagnosis because in 90% of cases there is an abnormal finding after perforation
- Commonest finding is a unilateral effusion, usually on the left (as most perforations are left-sided)
- The V sign of Naclerio (seen in 20% of cases) is a specific but not a sensitive sign: air in the space between the heart and vertebral column, seen as a left paraspinal hyperlucency
- Continuous diaphragm sign
- Other findings may include pneumothorax, hydropneumothorax, pneumomediastinum, subcutaneous emphysema or mediastinal widening
- 10% of CXRs are normal
- Findings may take an hour or more to develop after perforation

Contrast swallow
- Non-ionic contrast is used
- Confirmatory test with up to 90% sensitivity
- Contrast is seen to enter the pleural cavity

CT
- Extraluminal air within the mediastinum in conjunction with the clinical picture gives up to a 90% correlation
- The air may be seen to track alongside the aorta
- Oesophageal wall haematoma
- Contrast extravasation
- Peri-oesophageal or mediastinal fluid
- If diagnosis has been delayed, there may be a mediastinal abscess or empyema

Oesophageal perforation

- Associated with a 20–60% mortality
- Causes
  - Iatrogenic (in 55% of cases)
  - Spontaneous (Boerhaave's syndrome)
  - Trauma
  - Oesophageal cancer
  - Retained foreign body
  - Barrett's ulcer

Upper and mid-oesophageal perforation

- Commonest site is the cricopharyngeus
- Iatrogenic condition

Imaging features

CXR
- Widening of the prevertebral fascia with air and fluid and a right-sided pleural effusion

Lower oesophageal perforation

Imaging features

CXR
- Pneumomediastinum
- Subcutaneous emphysema
- Widening of the mediastinum (secondary to mediastinitis)
- Hydrothorax (usually left-sided)
- Hydropneumothorax

Water-soluble swallow
- Single contrast swallow using a non-ionic contrast
- Entry of contrast into the mediastinum or pleural cavity proves the presence of rupture
- false-negative rate is approximately 10%

CT
- Similar findings to those seen in Boerhaave's syndrome
- Focal extraluminal collections of air adjacent to the site of rupture
- Obliteration of fat planes in the mediastinum
- Peri-oesophageal fluid collections
- Contrast extravasation into the mediastinum
- Delayed imaging may show the presence of mediastinal abscess formation, seen as an enhancing cavitating lesion with an air–fluid level

Mallory–Weiss tear

- Upper gastrointestinal bleeding secondary to longitudinal mucosal lacerations at the gastro-oesophageal junction or gastric cardia

- Bleeding stops spontaneously in 80–90% of patients
- With conservative therapy, most tears heal uneventfully within 48 hours
- Tears can easily be missed if endoscopy is delayed
- Clinical presentation is with haematemesis following a bout of retching or vomiting
- Associated with a hiatus hernia in 35–100% of cases
- Iatrogenic tears are uncommon
- Barium swallow and gastrografin studies should not be performed, owing to their low diagnostic sensitivity and interference with endoscopic assessment and therapy
- Endoscopy is the procedure of choice for both diagnosis and therapy
- Split is 2–3 cm in length and a few millimetres in width
- > 80% of cases present with a single tear
- The usual location of the tear is just below the gastro-oesophageal junction on the lesser curve of stomach
- Most patients have stopped bleeding at the time of endoscopy

Oesophageal rings and webs

- Commonest structural abnormalities of the oesophagus
- Most patients with oesophageal rings and webs are asymptomatic

Oesophageal ring

- Concentric, smooth, thin (3–5 mm) extension of the normal oesophageal tissue consisting of three anatomic layers of mucosa, submucosa and muscle
- Most oesophageal rings are found incidentally, are asymptomatic, and do not require treatment
- Those that are symptomatic may be treated with endoscopic dilatation or disruption and, rarely, with surgery
- Three main types of oesophageal rings, classified as A, B (Schatzki's ring) and C (indentation caused by the diaphragmatic crura); other rings may be seen that are either congenital or inflammatory in origin

A ring

- Seen 1.5 cm proximal to the squamocolumnar junction
- A muscular ring that may be seen intermittently on barium swallow studies

B ring (Schatzki's ring)

- Technically a web, since it consists of mucosa and submucosa
- Typically found at the squamocolumnar junction and forms the upper limit of a hiatus hernia
- A common complication is impaction of meat at this site

C ring

- A rare anatomical variant, which seen as an indentation of the lower oesophagus caused by the diaphragmatic crura

Oesophageal web

- A thin (2–3 mm), eccentric, smooth extension of normal oesophageal tissue consisting of mucosa and submucosa
- Can occur anywhere along the length of the oesophagus, but typically in the anterior postcricoid area of the proximal oesophagus
- Plummer–Vinson syndrome is characterised by a post-cricoid or upper oesophageal eccentric web and iron-deficiency anaemia
- A web can also be congenital or developmental in origin, or inflammatory or autoimmune in nature
- Barium swallow is the diagnostic test of choice; endoscopy is less sensitive

Oesophageal strictures

- Causes
  - Acid peptic disease
  - Autoimmune disease
  - Infection
  - Caustic injury
  - Congenital anomaly
  - Iatrogenic
  - Medication-induced
  - Radiation-induced
  - Malignancy
  - Idiopathic

- Peptic strictures account for 70–80% of cases, usually originate from the squamocolumnar junction and are typically 1–4 cm in length
- 10 times commoner in whites
- Symptoms include heartburn, dysphagia, odynophagia, food impaction, weight loss and chest pain
- Males are affected 2.5 times more commonly than females
- Medical management is with proton pump inhibitors
- Surgical management is by endoscopic dilatation, stricturoplasty, stenting or limited oesophagectomy

Classification

- Smooth oesophageal stricture
  - Inflammatory: acid peptic disease, scleroderma, corrosive injury, iatrogenic
  - Neoplastic: carcinoma, mediastinal tumour, leiomyoma
  - Achalasia
  - Skin disorders, e.g. epidermolysis bullosa, pemphigus
- Irregular oesophageal stricture
  - Neoplastic: carcinoma, leiomyosarcoma, carcinosarcoma, lymphoma
  - Inflammatory: acid reflux, Crohn's disease
  - Iatrogenic: radiotherapy, fundoplication

Diagnosis

- Barium swallow provides an objective baseline record of the oesophagus prior to medical therapy or endoscopic intervention
- Other tests include CT, endoscopic ultrasound, pH monitoring and manometry

Oesophageal varices

- Obstruction of the portal venous system leads to increased portal pressure
- Normal pressure in the portal vein is 5–10 mmHg; elevated portal venous pressure (> 10 mmHg) distends the veins proximal to the site of the blockage and increases capillary pressure in organs drained by the obstructed veins
- Gastroesophageal varices have two main in-flows: the left gastric or coronary vein and the splenic hilum via the short gastric veins
- Patients who have bled once from oesophageal varices have a 70% chance of rebleeding
- Approximately one third of further bleeding episodes are fatal
- Endoscopy is required at an early stage to formulate the management plan
- Obstruction and increased resistance can occur at three levels in relation to hepatic sinusoids
  - Pre-sinusoidal venous obstruction may be due to portal vein thrombosis, schistosomiasis or primary biliary cirrhosis
  - Elevated portal venous pressure (but with a normal wedged hepatic venous pressure) can occur with any cause of liver cirrhosis
  - Post-sinusoidal obstruction can occur in Budd–Chiari syndrome or veno-occlusive disease in which the central hepatic venules are the primary site of injury; the wedged hepatic venous pressure is characteristically elevated

Imaging features

Contrast studies

- Tortuous structures presenting as longitudinal filling defects projecting into the lumen of the oesophagus
- May also show as thickened oesophageal folds
- Scalloping of the borders on a single contrast examination

CT

- Imaging findings on non-contrast scans can appear similar to lymph nodes
- Post-contrast images show serpigenous tubular structures within the wall of the oesophagus that project into the lumen of the oesophagus
- Para-oesophageal varices are outside the oesophageal wall

Medical management

- Oesophageal varices with no history of bleeding are treated with non-selective beta-adrenergic blockers
- Bleeding varices
  - Endoscopic sclerotherapy is successful in controlling acute oesophageal variceal bleeding in up to 90% of cases
  - Endoscopic variceal ligation (banding) can also be used
  - Rebleeding occurs less frequently with ligation than with sclerotherapy (26% versus 45%)
  - Local complications are also less common with ligation than with sclerotherapy

Surgical management

- 5–10% of patients with oesophageal variceal haemorrhage have conditions that cannot be controlled by endoscopic or pharmacologic treatment
- Surgical options
  - Portosystemic shunt
  - Devascularisation of the lower 5 cm of the oesophagus and the upper two thirds of the stomach
  - Orthotopic liver transplantation

Radiological management

- Percutaneous transhepatic embolisation
- Transjugular intrahepatic portosystemic shunts (TIPS); complications include encephalopathy (in 20% of cases) and shunt occlusion (50% at 1 year)

Gastro-oesophageal reflux disease (GORD)

- Gastro-oesophageal disease is the commonest cause of oesophagitis
- Symptoms include dysphagia, odynophagia and heart burn
- Classification
  - Grade I: erythema
  - Grade II: linear, non-confluent erosions
  - Grade III: circular, confluent erosions
  - Grade IV: stricture or Barrett's oesophagus

- Complications
  - Strictures occur as a result of circumferential fibrosis secondary to chronic deep injury
  - Barrett's oesophagus

Barium swallow (to assess anatomy and complications)

- Oesophageal peristalsis: 50% of patients have ineffective swallow associated with GORD; this needs to be differentiated from achalasia and scleroderma, since they are the differential diagnoses
- Oesophagitis, stricturing and Barrett's oesophagus can also be looked for
- Hiatus hernias can be assessed and typed
  - Identification of the gastro-oesophageal junction and the diaphragmatic hiatus with more than 1.5 cm difference between them indicates a sliding hernia
  - Para-oesophageal hernias are those in which the gastro-oesophageal junction remains below the diaphragm and in which the fundus herniates
  - Type 3 hernias consist of hernias with both the above features
  - Type 4 hernias are herniation of all or part of the stomach with some element of organoaxial rotation
- Shortened oesophagus
- Reflux demonstrated on the swallow

Barrett's oesophagus

- Finding of specialized intestinal (columnar) metaplasia anywhere within the tubular oesophagus
- Commonest site is above the squamocolumnar junction
- Barrett's ulcers are deep penetrating ulcers and are usually associated with strictures; at times only a slowly tapering stricture without ulceration may be seen
- Risk factors
  - GORD
  - Hiatus hernia (in 75–90% of cases of Barrett's oesophagus)
  - Reduced lower oesophageal sphincter pressures

- Delayed oesophageal acid clearance time
- Duodenogastric reflux
- Risk of progression to adenocarcinoma of the oesophagus is estimated at approximately 0.5% per year in patients without dysplasia on initial surveillance biopsies
- Management
  - Antireflux surgeries, such as a Nissen fundoplication, have not been shown to reverse the outcome. Surgery seems to play no role in preventing the progression to cancer
  - Oesophagectomy when high-grade dysplasia is discovered and confirmed by a second pathologist

Imaging features

Barium swallow
- Reticular pattern (non-specific sign that is also seen in other forms of oesophagitis)
- There may be stricturing or ulceration
- Stricturing occurs at the squamocolumnar junction, is short and tight and typically eccentric in nature, whereas peptic strictures are more concentric and smooth
- An ascending stricture may be seen on serial barium swallows; this is caused by the proximal migration of the squamocolumnar junction and is specific to Barrett's oesophagus
- Sliding hiatus hernia is also associated with Barrett's oesophagus
- Needs confirmation with oesophagogastroduodenoscopy

Oesophagitis

- Causes include GORD (the commonest cause), infections, medications, radiation therapy, systemic disease and trauma
- Clinical features include dysphagia, pain, odynophagia and (in severe cases) malnutrition
- Diagnosis is by barium swallow or endoscopy
- Classification
  - Grade I: erythema
  - Grade II: linear, non-confluent erosions

- Grade III: circular, confluent erosions
- Grade IV: stricture or Barrett's oesophagus

Candida oesophagitis

- Predominantly occurs in immunosuppressed patients
- Oral thrush is a frequent finding and is often an indicator of oesophageal involvement
- However, oral thrush can be absent in 25% of cases of *Candida* oesophagitis
- *Candida* infection is frequently asymptomatic
- Predilection for the upper half of the oesophagus, with longitudinal orientation

Imaging features

Barium swallow
- Identified by double-contrast barium swallow in 90% of cases
- Initially starts as a plaque lesions
- Granular pattern of mucosal oedema, caused by confluence of the plaques
- In advanced cases, such as occur in AIDS patients, there may a shaggy appearance to the oesophagus, caused by pseudomembranes and confluent plaques
- Owing to the friable nature of the lesions, the barium sometimes dissects into the submucosa and gives a 'double-barrel' oesophagus

Grading scale

- Grade 1: A few raised, white plaques up to 2 mm in size; no ulceration
- Grade 2: multiple raised, white plaques > 2 mm in size; no ulceration
- Grade 3: confluent, linear, nodular, elevated plaques with ulceration
- Grade 4: grade 3 with narrowed lumen (stricturing)

Tuberculous oesophagitis

- Occurs with advanced mediastinal or pulmonary tuberculosis
- Mediastinal nodes are enlarged and erode into the oesophagus
- Oesophagogastroduodenoscopy reveals shallow ulcers, heaped-up lesions

that mimic neoplasia, and extrinsic compression of the oesophagus

- Primary tuberculous infection of the oesophagus is extremely rare but has been reported; it appears as mucosal plaques or serpiginous ulcers, strictures or fistulas

Cytomegalovirus (CMV) oesophagitis

- Almost always occurs in the immunocompromised patients and most commonly in patients with AIDS
- Presents with severe odynophagia and dysphagia, with evidence of dissemination
- One or more giant superficial erosions in the middle to distal oesophagus are observed
- The erosions are diamond-shaped, ovoid or serpiginous, with satellite ulcers and a halo of oedematous tissue, as in herpes simplex virus (HSV) oesophagitis
- With progression of the infection, shallow ulcerations may deepen and expand to up to 5–10 cm in diameter

HSV oesophagitis

- Second commonest type of oesophagitis
- Diagnosis is made at endoscopy
- Earliest oesophageal lesions are rounded vesicles 1–3 mm in diameter, located in the mid- to distal oesophagus
- The centres of the lesions slough to form discrete circumscribed ulcers with raised edges
- A halo of oedema is seen at the margins
- Advanced HSV oesophagitis may be indistinguishable from candidal oesophagitis: plaques, cobble stoning or a shaggy ulcerative appearance may be observed

Varicella–zoster virus oesophagitis

- The key to diagnosis is finding concurrent dermatological varicella–zoster virus lesions
- The appearance on endoscopy ranges from occasional vesicles to discrete ulcerative lesions to a confluence of ulcerations with necrosis

HIV oesophagitis

- Usually presents with acute-onset odynophagia plus a maculopapular rash
- Causes giant flat ulcers > 1 cm in diameter with satellite ulcers and a rim of oedematous tissue, similar in appearance to CMV oesophagitis, although no infectious aetiology is found
- Multiple, small, aphthoid lesions
- Later, giant deep ulcers extend up several centimetres
- Fistula formation, perforation, haemorrhage, or superinfection may complicate large ulcers

Behçet's disease

- Tunneling ulcers, fistulas and perforations seen

Scleroderma

- A more plastic deformity of the oesophagus with poor clearing and residual epithelial damage

Inflammatory bowel disease

- Oesophagitis is most commonly seen in Crohn's disease
- Ulcers are aphthoid
- Associated sinus, fistulous connections and polyps are seen
- Management is directed at the underlying cause

Duplication cyst

- Completely surrounded by muscularis propria
- Intramural masses
- Fluid density (high protein may cause high signal on T2WI)

Leiomyoma

- Commonest benign tumour of the oesophagus
- More common in the distal oesophagus (where there is smooth muscle)
- Arises from all layers of the wall of the oesophagus

- Multiple leiomyomas are associated with neural deafness and renal impairment (Alport's syndrome)
- Rarely associated with hypertrophic osteoarthropathy
- Predominantly an intramural lesion with potential exophytic components
- They may metastasise if they are malignant

Imaging features

CT

- Homogeneously enhancement or rim-like enhancement with intratumour calcification
- Well-defined mass with a smooth surface

Pharyngeal and oesophageal pouches and diverticula

Zenker's diverticulum

- Located in the posterior part of the oesophagus, usually to the left
- Forms between fibres of the inferior constrictor and cricopharyngeus muscles
- Symptoms include dysphagia, regurgitation, aspiration and hoarseness

Lateral pharyngeal pouch and diverticulum

- Located in the anterolateral wall of upper hypopharynx

- Appears through the thyrohyoid membrane
- Usually asymptomatic
- Commoner in patients with chronically elevated intrapharyngeal pressure, e.g. glass-blowers, trumpeters

Lateral cervical oesophageal pouch and diverticulum

- Appears through the Killian–Jamieson space, below the cricopharyngeus muscle
- Usually asymptomatic

Tertiary contractions in the oesophagus

- Unco-ordinated, non-propulsive contractions
- Occur in patients with impaired motor function due to muscle atrophy
- Commonest in elderly patients (seen in 25% of those > 60 years)
- Causes
  - Reflux oesophagitis
  - Obstruction at the gastric cardia
  - Presbyoesophagus
  - Neuropathy
  - Diabetes mellitus
  - Alcohol excess
  - Malignant infiltration of the oesophagus
  - Early achalasia

Gastritis

- Inflammation of the gastric mucosa
- The common mechanism of injury is an imbalance between the aggressive and the defensive factors that maintain the integrity of the gastric lining (the mucosa)
- Causes
  - Drugs, including non-steroidal anti-inflammatory drugs, which cause acute gastritis distally on or near the greater curvature of the stomach
  - Alcohol
  - Bile
  - Ischaemia
  - Bacterial (*Helicobacter pylori*), viral and fungal infection
  - Acute stress (shock)
  - Radiation
  - Allergy and food poisoning
  - Direct trauma

Helicobacter pylori gastritis

- *Helicobacter pylori* gastritis starts as acute gastritis in the antrum, causing intense inflammation, and over time, it may extend to involve the entire gastric mucosa resulting in chronic gastritis
- The acute gastritis encountered with *Helicobacter pylori* is usually asymptomatic
- The bacteria embed themselves in the mucous layer, a protective layer that coats the gastric mucosa
- The bacteria protect themselves from the acidity of the stomach through the production of large amounts of urease
- Infection produces inflammation via the production of a number of toxins and enzymes
- The intense inflammation can result in the loss of gastric glands responsible for the production of acid (atrophic gastritis)
- *Helicobacter pylori* is associated with 60% of gastric ulcers and 80% of duodenal ulcers
- It is also associated with gastric cancer

- *Symptoms:* Gnawing or burning epigastric distress, occasionally accompanied by nausea and/or vomiting. The pain may improve or worsen with eating
- Complications
  - Bleeding from an erosion or ulcer
  - Gastric outlet obstruction due to oedema limiting the adequate transfer of food from the stomach to the small intestine
  - Dehydration from vomiting
  - Renal insufficiency as a result of dehydration

Imaging features

Barium studies
- Thick folds, inflammatory nodules, coarse area gastrica, and erosions

Endoscopy
- May reveal a thickened, oedematous, non-pliable wall with erosions and reddened gastric folds
- Ulcers and frank bleeding are sometimes present

Phlegmonous gastritis

- Uncommon form of gastritis caused by numerous bacterial agents, including streptococci, staphylococci, *Proteus* species, *Clostridium* species and *Escherichia coli*
- Usually occurs in debilitated patients
- Associated with a recent large intake of alcohol, a concomitant upper respiratory tract infection and AIDS

Emphysematous gastritis

- Widespread phlegmonous gastritis caused by mucosal disruption
- Characterised by gas in the wall of the stomach
- Clinical features include bloody, foul-smelling emesis
- There may be vomiting of a necrotic cast of stomach, which is pathognomonic

Corrosive gastritis

- In acid-induced gastritis, the oesophagus is usually unharmed and gastric damage is severe
- In alkali-induced gastritis, the pylorus and antrum are frequently involved

Gastric cancer

- Third commonest GI malignancy
- Symptoms include GI bleeding, abdominal pain and weight loss
- Risk factors
  - Smoking
  - Nitrites and nitrates
  - Pickled vegetables
  - *Helicobacter pylori* gastritis
  - Chronic atrophic gastritis
  - Adenomatous and villous polyps
  - Gastrojejunostomy and partial gastrectomy
  - Pernicious anaemia
  - Ménétrier's disease
- Adenocarcinoma accounts for 95% of cases
- Overall 5-year survival rate is 5–18%
- Most are located in the distal third of stomach or in the cardia; 60% are on lesser curve, 10% on the greater curve and 30% at the gastro-oesophageal junction
- Staging
  - T1: limited to mucosa or submucosa
  - T2: involves muscle or serosa
  - T3: penetrates through serosa
  - T4a: invasion of adjacent contiguous tissues
  - T4b: invasion of adjacent organs, diaphragm or abdominal wall
- Metastases
  - Along peritoneal ligaments
  - To local lymph nodes
  - Haematogenous spread, including to the liver (25% of cases at presentation), the adrenal glands and bone
  - Peritoneal seeding, e.g. to the rectal wall (Blumer's shelf), ovaries (Krukenberg's tumour), the left supraclavicular node (Virchow's node)

Mucosa-associated lymphoid tissue (MALT) lymphoma

- Normal stomach does not contain lymphoid follicles but they can develop following infection with *Helicobacter pylori*
- Persistent antigenic stimulation by *Helicobacter pylori* is thought to lead to neoplastic transformation
- MALT lymphoma is usually locally contained at the time of diagnosis and has a better prognosis than non-Hodgkin's lymphoma
- Commonest site is the antrum
- Perforation is rare

Imaging features

Barium study
- Infiltrative focal lesion or a diffuse lesion
- Ulceration is rare

CT
- Thickening of the gastric wall with or without ulceration and enhancement
- Dissemination is commonly seen

Peptic ulcer disease

- Inflammatory injury in the gastric or duodenal mucosa, with extension beyond the submucosa into the muscularis mucosa
- Risk factors
  - *Helicobacter pylori* infection
  - Non-steroidal anti-inflammatory drugs
  - Cigarette smoking
  - Zollinger–Ellison syndrome (gastrinoma)
- Gastric and duodenal ulcers usually cannot be differentiated on the basis of clinical history alone
- Complications
  - Haemorrhage
  - Perforation
  - Gastric outlet obstruction
  - Gastric malignancy (the risk of malignant transformation is approximately 2% in the initial 3 years)

- Prognosis is excellent for benign ulcers, especially if *Helicobacter pylori* is completely eradicated and non-steroidal anti-inflammatory drugs are avoided

Gastric ulcer

- Classic gastric ulcer pain is described as occurring shortly after meals, for which antacids provide minimal relief
- Benign gastric ulcers are normally found on the lesser curvature
- These ulcers tend to project beyond the contour of the stomach, with radiating folds extending to the ulcer margin
- Malignant ulcers usually have irregular, heaped-up margins that protrude into the lumen of the stomach

Duodenal ulcer

- Duodenal ulcer pain often occurs hours after meals and at night. Pain is characteristically relieved with food or antacids
- More than 95% found in the first part of the duodenum
- Most < 1 cm in diameter

Diagnosis

- Double-contrast barium study performed by an expert GI radiologist has excellent accuracy in diagnosing a typical gastric ulcer
- Endoscopy is the modality of choice
- Provides the opportunity to perform multiple mucosal biopsies to check for *Helicobacter pylori* and to rule out malignancy
- A repeat endoscopy after 6 weeks of therapy is recommended to confirm healing of a gastric ulcer and to help to rule out gastric malignancy definitively

Treatment

- Medical therapy: mucosal protectants, histamine-2 blockers, proton pump inhibitors and *Helicobacter pylori* eradication (triple therapy has consistently been shown to eradicate the organism in > 90% of cases)
- Endoscopic therapy: injection therapy, coagulation therapy, haemostatic clips and argon plasma coagulation

- Surgery has a role in life-threatening haemorrhage, ulcer perforation, gastric outlet obstruction, giant gastric ulcer, and a transfusion requirement of more than 6 units in 24 hours

Gastric volvulus

- Abnormal degree of rotation of one part of stomach around another part
- > 180° rotation is required for complete obstruction)
- Associated with araoesophageal hiatus hernia and eventration of the diaphragm
- Two main types
  - Subdiaphragmatic gastric volvulus, which accounts for 30% of cases
  - Supradiaphragmatic gastric volvulus, which is seen in 60% of cases and is associated with para-oesophageal rolling hiatus hernias
- Axis of rotation can be organoaxial (in which the rotation is along a line from the cardia to the pylorus in 60% of cases) or mesenteroaxial (in which the rotation is around an axis extending from the lesser curve to the greater curve)
- Symptoms include violent retching (but no vomiting) and severe epigastric pain
- It may be impossible to pass a nasogastric tube
- In cases of recurrent volvulus, a hiatus hernia, eventration, diaphragmatic trauma and abdominal adhesions should be considered as possible predisposing factors

Imaging features

AXR
- Poor identifier but may show distended stomach and air–fluid levels with beaking at the gastro-oesophageal junction
- If a nasogastric tube has been passed it lies inferior to the gastro-oesophageal junction

CT
- Identifies the anatomy better than AXR, especially with the use of multiplanar reformats
- Can also evaluate for ischaemic complications

Hypertrophic pyloric stenosis

- Hypertrophy and hyperplasia of the circular muscle fibres of the pylorus, with proximal extension into gastric antrum
- Inherited as dominant polygenic trait
- Higher incidence in first-born boys
- Biochemistry shows hypokalaemic hypochloraemic metabolic alkalosis
- Adult type
  - Secondary to mild infantile form
  - Acute obstructive symptoms uncommon
  - Presents with nausea, vomiting and heartburn
- Infantile type
  - Presents at age 2–8 weeks
  - Clinical features include non-bilious projectile vomiting, a palpable olive-shaped mass and hypochloraemic metabolic acidosis

Imaging features

Ultrasound
- Target sign (hypoechoic ring of hypertrophied pyloric muscle around echogenic mucosa centrally)
- Elongated pylorus (17 mm or more)
- Pyloric muscle wall thickness (3 mm or more)
- Pyloric transverse diameter 13 mm or more with channel closed

Gastric gastrointestinal stromal tumour

- Commonest mesenchymal neoplasm of the GI tract
- Third commonest tumour of the GI tract (after adenocarcinoma and lymphoma)
- 50–70% originate in the stomach; the small intestine is the second-commonest site
- Can also originate in the mesentery and omentum
- Submucosal lesions, which most frequently grow endophytically in parallel with the lumen of the affected structure
- Clinical features include vague abdominal pain, obstruction and bleeding

- Associated with neurofibromatosis type 1 and Carney's triad (epithelioid gastric stromal tumours, pulmonary chondromas and extra-adrenal paragangliomas)
- Medical treatment is with imatinib mesylate (a selective tyrosine kinase inhibitor)
- Surgical treatment is resection, which is the definitive therapy

Imaging features

Barium study
- Double-contrast barium studies can usually detect tumours that have grown to a size sufficient to produce symptoms
- Submucosal lesions with a smooth overlying mucosa, thus preserving the are*ae* gastrica
- Larger lesions cause mucosal ulceration

CT
- Provides comprehensive information about the size and location of the tumour and its relationship to adjacent structures
- Lesions show rim enhancement or homogeneous enhancement
- Calcification may be present
- Larger masses undergo necrosis

PET-CT
- Useful for detecting metastases

Causes of thickened gastric mucosal folds (thickness > 1 cm)

- Inflammatory causes
  - Gastritis
  - Zollinger–Ellison syndrome
  - Acute pancreatitis
  - Crohn's disease
- Infiltrative and neoplastic causes
  - Lymphoma
  - Carcinoma
  - Pseudolymphoma
  - Eosinophilic gastroenteritis
- Other causes
  - Ménétrier's disease
  - Varices

Causes of linitis plastica

- Neoplasia
  - Gastric carcinoma
  - Lymphoma
  - Metastases
  - Local invasion from pancreatic carcinoma
- Inflammatory causes
  - Corrosives
  - Radiotherapy
  - Granulomas
  - Eosinophilic enteritis

Causes of target lesions in the stomach

- Submucosal metastases (from melanoma, lymphoma, carcinoma or carcinoid)
- Leiomyoma
- Ectopic pancreatic tissue (pancreatic rest)
- Neurofibroma

GI tract trauma

Haemoperitoneum

- Found in paracolic gutters and the pelvis
- CT attenuation values during intravenous contrast administration
  - Serum: 0–20 Hounsfield units
  - Fresh unclotted blood: 30–45 Hounsfield units
  - Clotted blood: 50–100 Hounsfield units
  - Active bleed: > 180 Hounsfield units
- 'Sentinel clot' sign indicates the highest attenuation value of blood clot and marks the site of injury

Hypovolaemia

Imaging features

CT
- Collapsed IVC (anteroposterior diameter < 9 mm) at three levels
  - Intrahepatic IVC with a halo of fluid (non-specific)
  - At the renal artery level
  - 2 cm below renal artery level
- Heterogenous hepatic enhancement, typically 25 Hounsfield Units less than the spleen, with intensely enhancing intrahepatic vessels and periportal oedema; differential diagnosis is fatty liver
- Small, hypodense spleen (non-specific)
- Small aorta (< 13 mm at levels 2 cm above and 2 cm below the renal arteries)
- Pancreatic enhancement (20 Hounsfield Units greater than the liver)
- Peripancreatic oedema in addition to mesenteric and retroperitoneal fluid collections
- Intense and prolonged nephrogram (non-specific)
- Intense adrenal enhancement greater than those of the IVC
- Mucosal enhancement of the gallbladder
- Manifestations of shock bowel
- Increased enhancement of small bowel mucosa (greater than the psoas muscle)
- Mural thickening of small bowel (> 3 mm)

- Small bowel dilatation (> 2.5 cm) or a fluid-filled small bowel
- Presence of focal thickening and enhancement of the bowel wall with free fluid is suspicious of bowel perforation

Blunt trauma to the bowel

- Causes include road traffic accident, bicycle handlebar injury and child abuse
- The jejunum distal to the ligament of Treitz is the commonest location, followed by the duodenum, the ascending colon at the ileocaecal valve, and the descending colon

Imaging features

CT
- Bowel discontinuity is primary finding but is rarely seen
- Extraluminal oral contrast is 100% specific but its sensitivity is low
- Extraluminal air or pneumoperitoneum has a sensitivity of 40–50% and is more often seen in the setting of duodenal perforation or injury
- Extraluminal air and intramural gas indicates a full-thickness injury to bowel
- Bowel wall thickening is seen in 75% of transmural injuries to the bowel and is very sensitive
- Isolated mesenteric lacerations may also give this sign
- A combination of focal or disproportionate and circumferential thickening of the bowel wall with adjacent normal bowel is usually an indicator of injury
- Bowel wall enhancement more than that of the psoas muscle together with the signs above is more specific for injury
- Mesenteric stranding, predominantly on the mesenteric border, is an ancillary sign
- Haemoperitoneum is a common finding with intraperitoneal bowel or mesenteric lacerations
- Haematoma in the mesentery at the site of bowel wall thickening, as in the case of a periduodenal haematoma, is also fairly specific for bowel injury

- Free fluid on three contiguous sections suggests significant bowel or mesenteric injury
- Interloop fluid in the mesentery is associated with bowel wall injury
- 5% of hepatic lacerations and splenic lacerations are associated with major bowel injury
- Other findings are focal discontinuity of the bowel wall, focal thickening of the bowel thickening, intramural haematoma, mesenteric haematoma, extravasation of oral contrast and free fluid

Malrotation

- Abnormal position of the gut secondary to narrow mesenteric attachment
- Caused by arrest in embryological development of gut rotation and fixation
- Complications include midgut volvulus and duodenal obstruction

Imaging features

Barium meal
- Evaluates the position of peritoneal fixation
- In normal situation, barium flows through the 'C'-shaped configuration of duodenum; in addition, barium must pass to left of the spine

CT
- Superior mesenteric vein is seen to the left the superior mesenteric artery (in 80% of cases)

Hernia

External hernia

- Bowel extends outside the abdominal cavity
- Ventral hernias
  - Postoperative
  - At a trocar site (the commonest type)
  - Umbilical
  - Epigastric
  - Spigelian (ventrolateral hernia through a defect in the aponeurosis of the transverse and rectus muscles)

- Diaphragmatic hernias
  - Bochdalek's hernia
  - Morgagni's hernia
- Lumbar hernias
  - Grynfelt's hernia
  - Petit's lumbar triangle
- Pelvic floor hernias
  - Obturator (between the pectineus and external obturator muscles)
  - Sciatic notch
  - Perineal
- Groin hernias
  - Inguinal (a direct inguinal hernia is caused by a defect in Hesselbach's triangle, medial to the inferior epigastric vessels; an indirect hernia passes through the inguinal canal lateral to the inferior epigastric vessels)
  - Femoral
  - Richter's (entrapment of the antimesenteric border of the bowel in the hernia orifice most commonly seen in older women with a femoral hernia)

Internal hernia

- Herniation of bowel through a developmental or surgically created defect in the peritoneum, omentum or mesentery or herniation through an adhesive band
- Paraduodenal hernias are associated with a congenital defect in the descending mesocolon
- Lesser sac hernias are through the foramen of Winslow in a retrogastric location
- Hiatus hernia: 99% are sliding hernias, in which the gastro-oesophageal junction remains in chest; in 1% of cases the paraoesophageal portion of the stomach is superiorly displaced into the thorax with gastro-oesophageal junction remaining subdiaphragmatic

Duodenum
Duodenal diverticulum

- Primary: mucosal prolapse through the muscularis propria
- Secondary: involves all layers of the duodenal wall; a complication of duodenal inflammation

- Usually occur in the first part of the duodenum
- Complications include perforation, bowel obstruction, biliary obstruction, bleeding and diverticulitis

Causes of 'cobblestone duodenal cap'

- Big cobblestones
  - Hypertrophy of Brunner's glands
  - Oedema
  - Crohn's disease
  - Varices
  - Carcinoma
  - Lymphoma
- Small cobblestones
  - Food residue
  - Duodenitis
  - Nodular lymphoid hyperplasia
  - Heterotropic gastric mucosa

Causes of decreased or absent duodenal folds

- Amyloidosis
- Crohn's disease
- Cystic fibrosis
- Scleroderma
- Strongyloidiasis

Causes of thickened duodenal folds

- Inflammatory causes
  - Crohn's disease
  - Duodenitis
  - Pancreatitis
  - Zollinger–Ellison syndrome
- Neoplasia
  - Metastases
  - Lymphoma
  - Infiltrations
  - Eosinophilic enteritis
  - Amyloidosis
  - Mastocytosis
  - Whipple's disease
- Vascular causes
  - Intramural haematoma
  - Ischaemia
- Oedematous causes
  - Hypoproteinaemia
  - Venous obstruction

- Lymphatic obstruction
- Angioneurotic oedema
- Infestations
  - Worms
  - Giardiasis

Causes of a dilated duodenum

- Mechanical obstruction
  - Bands
  - Atresia/webs/stenosis
  - Annular pancreas
  - Superior mesenteric artery syndrome
- Paralytic ileus
- Scleroderma

Intestinal lymphoma

- Commonest malignant small bowel tumour
- Commonest cause of intussusception in children aged > 6 years
- Incidence is 4–20%; 10% have bowel involvement
- Median age at time of onset is 60 years
- Risk factors include coeliac disease, AIDS, systemic lupus erythematosus, Crohn's disease and chemotherapy
- Seen as a large, cavitating, ulcerating or nodular mass with aneurysmal dilatation of the bowel lumen
- Primary lymphoma of the bowel can be localised or diffuse, and is associated with coeliac disease
- Secondary lymphoma of the bowel occurs in generalised systemic disease
- Areas of spread (in descending order are the stomach (2.5% of all gastric neoplasms), the small bowel (20% of malignancies), the rectum, the colon and the oesophagus

Pathology

- Hodgkin's lymphoma
- Non-Hodgkin's lymphoma (T cell or B cell)
  - High-grade and intermediate-grade tumours carry a poor prognosis
  - Low-grade tumours carry a good prognosis
  - Low grade B-cell tumours are MALT lymphomas
  - Can be secondary to *Helicobacter pylori* gastritis

Imaging features

- Polypoidal or nodular tumour in 47% of cases
- Diffuse infiltrating disease in 11%: hose-like thickening with reduced peristalsis
- Ulcerative tumour in 42% of cases, which can perforate

CT staging

- Stage I: tumour confined to the bowel wall
- Stage II: local nodes
- Stage III: widespread nodes
- Stage IV: disseminated to the liver, marrow or other sites

Lymphoma of the stomach

- 2.5% of all lymphomas present with gastric neoplasms
- Commonest site of extranodal spread
- Arises from the lamina propria after *Helicobacter pylori* infection
- Extends to the pancreas, spleen, transverse colon and liver
- Diffuse mucosal thickening with or without ulcers in 50% of cases
- Smooth nodular mass with or without mucosal thickening (segmental involvement is seen in 25% cases)
- Ulcers, which may be single or multiple, in 8% of cases
- Linitis-like picture with thickened wall and reduced motility
- May be seen as a duodenal ulcer associated with a gastric mass, as an ulcerated mass

Lymphoma of the small intestine

- Multiple sites of involvement
- Commonest cause of intussusception
- 51% are located in the ileum, 47% in the jejunum and 2% in the duodenum
- Arise from Peyer's patches
- Types
  - Single or multiple polypoidal masses: seen as cobblestoning; associated with ulceration and intussusception
  - Infiltrating lymphoma involving < 5 cm of the bowel wall: associated with a desmoplastic response, thickened valvulae and aneurysmal dilatation
  - Mesenteric or retroperitoneal lymphoma: may be single or multiple extraluminal masses, in a 'cake' configuration engulfing multiple bowel loops or a 'sandwich' configuration in which a mass surrounds mesenteric vessels that are separated by perivascular fat; can also occur as a mesenteric and retroperitoneal mass
  - Endoexoenteric lymphoma: a large mass with small intramural component, which can cause fistulas

Lymphoma of the colon

- Mainly affects the caecum (in 85% of cases)
- Can be seen as a single mass, as diffuse infiltration or as a polypoidal lesion
- Focal soft tissue thickening

Carcinoid tumour

- Commonest primary malignant tumour of the small bowel
- 33% occur in the small bowel; 45% occur in the appendix
- 33% of patients have a second primary malignancy
- Distribution of GI carcinoid: 81% ileum, 7% jejunum, 2% duodenum, 10% gastric
- Arises from neuroendocrine cells of the submucosa
- Secretes a variety of products, including 5-hydroxyindoleacetic acid (5-HIAA), adrenocorticotropic hormone (ACTH), histamine and serotonin

Gastric carcinoid

- Usually solitary lesions located in the gastric fundus or body and show metastasis at presentation in 50–70% of cases
- Best seen on double-contrast upper GI examination as smoothly marginated mural multifocal lesions with/out mucosal ulceration. They may be seen as thickened mucosal folds. There may be flocculation of contrast due to fluid in the stomach
- Mucosal or submucosal masses that enhance on CT, with mucosal ulceration

Duodenal carcinoid

- An intraluminal polypoid mass (in 50% of cases) or an intramural mass (in 40%)
- On upper GI series they are seen as well-defined, rounded masses
- On CT they enhance on the arterial phase of the scan and lose contrast on delayed images
- In the ampullary region they are found to enhance, whereas adenocarcinomas and adenomas do not

Jejunal and ileal carcinoid

- Account for the majority of cases
- Clinically presents with cramping abdominal pain or with features caused by local effects
- On small bowel meal or enema, they are seen as single or multiple mural lesions, which may cause the overlying mucosa to ulcerate
- Larger lesions are better seen on CT, but there may be bowel wall thickening and distortion
- Occlusion or invasion of the small bowel vessels may give rise to ischaemic changes
- If there is fibrosis of the tissues, there may be a kink in the small bowel, known as a 'hairpin turn', on CT
- Gadolinium-enhanced T1 fat-suppressed MRI may show these lesions in the wall of the small bowel

Metastases

- Common sites of metastases are the liver, lymph nodes, lung and bone
- 2% of tumours < 1 cm metastasise; 85% of tumours > 2 cm metastasise
- Rare in carcinoid of the appendix; commoner in carcinoid of the ileum

Adenocarcinoma

- Solitary
- Located in proximal small bowel
- Imaging features include ulceration, annular constriction with shouldering and marked desmoplastic reaction, and polyps

Coeliac disease

- Chronic disease that interferes with the digestion and absorption of nutrients
- Strong hereditary component
- Immune-mediated, inflammatory response in the mucosa, resulting in maldigestion and malabsorption
- Bimodal age distribution: 1–3 years in children and 30–50 years in adults
- Females are twice as commonly affected as males
- Most prevalent in western Europeans; rare in Africans and Asians
- Primarily involves the mucosa of the small intestine
- The submucosa, muscularis and serosa are usually not involved
- Villi are atrophic or absent, and crypts are elongated
- Cellularity of the lamina propria is increased, with a proliferation of plasma cells and lymphocytes
- Disease progresses in a proximal-to-distal fashion, with more severe disease in the jejunum than in the ileum
- Jejunal atrophy causes secondary hypertrophy of the ileum, resulting in a reversal of fold patterns
- Patients cannot tolerate gluten, a protein commonly found in wheat, rye and barley
- Most patients tolerate oats, but should be monitored closely
- Clinical features
  - Gastrointestinal symptoms include diarrhoea, steatorrhoea and flatulence
  - Extraintestinal features include anaemia, bleeding, osteopenia, neurological symptoms (resulting from hypocalcaemia), skin disorders (including dermatitis herpetiformis), hormonal disorders (including amenorrhoea, delayed menarche, infertility and impotence)
- Complications
  - Ulcerative jejunoileitis: multiple ulcers that are usually fatal
  - Peptic duodenitis
  - Intussusception
  - Cavitary mesenteric lymph node syndrome
  - Hyposplenism and splenic atrophy (in 30–50% of cases)
  - Small bowel lymphoma

- Adenocarcinoma of the small bowel, rectum or stomach
- Squamous cell cancer of the oesophagus
- Endocrine diseases, seen in up to 10% of cases, including autoimmune thyroiditis and Sjögren's syndrome
- Management is by a gluten-free diet

Imaging features

- Investigated radiologically by a small bowel series or a small bowel enema (best imaging test and suggestive of the diagnosis in 75% of cases)
- Upper endoscopy with duodenal biopsy is considered the criterion standard
- Jejunoileal fold reversal is diagnostic; in addition at least three of the following need to be seen
  - Fold thickening
  - Jejunal atrophy: three folds or fewer per 2.5 cm in the first loop of the jejunum, with a concomitant increase in the number of folds in the ileum, are highly diagnostic
  - Mosaic pattern of mucosa is maintained in the jejunum in 10% of cases
  - Dilatation of bowel
  - Barium flocculation: a sign of hypersecretion and malabsorption, seen in 20–30% of cases
  - Jejunisation of the ileum (hypertrophy of ileum with thickening of folds)
- Gastric metaplasia in the duodenum may give rise to mucosal nodules (the 'bubbly bulb' sign)

Whipple's disease

- Systemic disease caused by infiltration of tissues by the Gram-positive bacterium *Tropheryma whippelii*
- Disordered host response
- Seen in immunocompromised patients
- Males predominate, roughly in a ratio of 8:1 or 9:1
- Affects the small bowel, joints, central nervous system and cardiovascular system
- Clinical presentation: muscle wasting, arthralgia, arthritis, fever, diarrhoea, pericarditis
- Diagnosis is by macrophages that stain

positive with periodic acid–Schiff (not pathognomonic)
- Almost universally fatal after 1 year in patients who are not diagnosed and who do not receive therapy with antibiotics, e.g. ceftriaxone followed by oral trimethoprim-sulfamethoxazole

Imaging features

Barium study
- Minimal bowel dilatation
- No ulceration
- Thickening of duodenal or jejunal folds

CT
- Thickening of the small bowel wall thickening and bulky hypodense abdominal nodes
- Associated systemic or articular disease is in favour of the diagnosis

Radiation enteritis

- Radiation injury, either in an acute form or chronic form
- Injury follows a dose 45–60 Gy for the small intestine and colon and 55 80 Gy for the rectum
- Acute injury is a function of the fraction of the dose, field size and the type of radiation
- Chronic injury is a function of the total dose of radiation
- Injury results in an inability to repopulate the surface epithelium as well as in collagen deposition and fibrosis, leading to bowel wall thickening, obliterative endarteritis and neural injury, all of which lead to impaired mucosal and motor function
- Acute injury occurs within 6–24 months of the initial radiation therapy
- Risk factors include hypertension, diabetes mellitus, atherosclerosis, adhesions, peritonitis, previous abdominal surgery, pelvic inflammatory disease and combination radiation–chemotherapy

Radiation injury of the stomach

- Usually occur with doses of 45–60 Gy given over 5 weeks

- Acute phase is seen 2–8 weeks after treatment
- Chronic phase occurs 4 weeks to 7 months after treatment
- Two main types seen, prepyloric or pyloric ulceration and antral narrowing
- Prepyloric or pyloric ulcers
  - More typical of the acute phase and indistinguishable from benign ulcers
- Antral narrowing
  - Seen with chronic injury
  - Appears as narrowing of the antrum and pylorus without ulceration
  - The mucosa is irregular and may mimic gastric cancer
  - Similar to linitis with little peristalsis
  - CT shows non-specific gastric wall thickening, loss or widening of the gastric folds and perigastric fat stranding
  - Associated duodenal injury may also be present

Radiation injury of the small intestine

- Although radiosensitive, because of its relative mobility the small bowel is less commonly affected by radiation changes
- Injury occurs with doses above 50–Gy over a 6-week period
- Three phases are seen
- Acute phase (during and immediately after therapy)
  - Hyperaemia, oedema and inflammation of the mucosa
  - Crypt abscess and sloughing of the mucosa
- Subacute phase (2–12 months after therapy)
  - Obliterative endarteritis of the small vessels
- Chronic phase (> 1 year after therapy)
  - Progressive fibrosis and serosal changes with adhesions and fistula formation
  - In order to evaluate small bowel changes, good distension and opacification of the bowel is needed
  - Loops of bowel that are thickened and matted with a serpentine appearance are indicative of irradiated bowel

- Discrete masses are not observed
- Mesenteric changes include increased attenuation and thickening of the mesentery
- The changes are non-specific, but correlation with history and radiation ports are important

Radiation injury of the colon and rectum

- The colon and rectum are commonly affected by irradiation to the pelvis in gynaecological malignancies
- Time interval to appearance of changes is similar to that seen with the small intestine
- Acute radiation colitis presents non-specifically as mucosal irregularity and submucosal thickening, resulting in cobblestone pattern on barium enemas
- Increase in the presacral space and thickening or effacement of the haustral folds or rectal valves of Houston may be seen
- The chronic form manifests itself as strictures that may be long or short and are generally tapered
- Fistulation can be seen
- Bowel obstruction may be seen
- Colonic hypoplasia is a rare complication in children

Imaging features

CT
- Increased attenuation of the prerectal fat and fibrous tissue, giving a halo effect
- Increase in the presacral space to > 1 cm in the anteroposterior diameter

MRI
- Early increase in signal on T2WI of the submucosa, with a normal low signal outer wall of the rectum
- Further injury results in the outer wall also becoming high signal, with loss of differentiation of the mucosa and muscle

Graft-versus-host disease

- Loss of haustrations
- Effacement of small bowel with tubular appearance
- Fold thickening

- Persistent coating of bowel mucosa by barium
- Reduced transit time

Causes of bowel obstruction

Small bowel obstruction

- Adhesions
- Hernias
- Intussusception
- Crohn's disease
- Gallstone ileus
- Ileus
- Tumour
- Foreign body (e.g. smuggled cocaine)

Large bowel obstruction

- Faeces
- Sigmoid volvulus or caecal volvulus
- Tumour
- Diverticulitis

Symptoms

- Anorexia, nausea, vomiting with relief
- Colicky abdominal pain with distension
- Constipation if distal obstruction
- Active, 'tinkling' bowel sounds

Imaging features

AXR
- Small bowel obstruction
  - Central gas shadows
  - Collapsed large bowel
- Large bowel obstruction
  - Gas proximal to the obstruction, collapsed bowel distally

Management

- Strangulation and large bowel obstruction → urgent surgery (within 1 hour)
- Paralytic ileus and incomplete small bowel obstruction can be managed conservatively initially

Causes of dilated small bowel

Normal folds seen on imaging

- Mechanical obstruction
- Ileus
- Scleroderma
- Iatrogenic
- Coeliac disease
- Tropical sprue
- Dermatitis herpetiformis

Thick folds seen on imaging

- Crohn's disease
- Ischaemia
- Lymphoma
- Radiotherapy
- Zollinger–Ellison syndrome
- Extensive small bowel resection
- Amyloidosis

Appendicitis

- Inflammation of the appendix
- Caused by luminal obstruction from faecolith (in 33% of cases), lymphoid hyperplasia, foreign body, parasites or a primary tumour
- Presents clinically with mild periumbilical pain that then localises to the right iliac fossa, anorexia, nausea, vomiting and low-grade fever
- Consider perforation if the temperature is > 38.3°C)
- Complications include perforation, abscess formation, peritonitis, sepsis, infertility and bowel obstruction

Imaging features

AXR
- Abnormalities seen in < 50% of cases
- May reveal a faecolith, a thickened caecum, small bowel obstruction or extraluminal gas

Ultrasound
- Graded compression ultrasound is 85% sensitive and 92% specific for appendicitis
- Mural wall thickness 2 mm or more

CT
- 87–100% sensitive and 89–98% specific for appendicitis
- Abnormal appendix (> 7 mm in diameter) with periappendicular inflammation

Meckel's diverticulum

- Persistence of the omphalomesenteric duct on the antimesenteric border of the ileum
- Commonest congenital abnormality of the gastrointestinal tract
- Contains ectopic mucosa (gastric, pancreatic and colonic) in 50% of cases
- The 'rule of twos': 2% of the population, 2 inches long, 2 feet from the terminal ileum,

symptomatic before the age of 2 years
- Asymptomatic in 20–40% of cases
- Complications include bleeding, diverticulitis, bowel obstruction secondary to intussusception, malignancy (carcinoma, carcinoid or sarcoma) and chronic abdominal pain

Imaging features

Technetium-99m pertechnetate scan
- 85% sensitive and > 95% specific
- Sensitivity drops after adolescence because adults are less likely than children to have gastric mucosa in the Meckel's diverticulum

Angiogram
- Identification of vitelline artery is pathognomonic

Chronic mesenteric ischaemia

- Cause by diffuse atherosclerotic disease in > 95% of cases
- All three major mesenteric arteries usually involved
- Clinical presentation is with weight loss, postprandial epigastric or periumbilical pain, a fear of eating and a history of vascular disease involving other risk factors
- Risk factors include smoking, hypertension, diabetes mellitus and hypercholesterolaemia
- Medical treatment involves primary prevention and anticoagulation
- Surgical treatment
  - Transaortic endarterectomy of the celiac or superior mesenteric artery
  - Retrograde bypass from the external iliac artery
  - Anterograde bypass, which provides the best orientation of the graft to the aorta
  - Mesenteric artery reimplantation, which has been performed but is not widely recommended because of the technical difficulties of the procedure

Imaging features

Arteriogram
- Arteriography is the criterion standard and will show occlusion and collateral flow

Ultrasound
- Mesenteric Doppler ultrasound is a non-invasive method of analysing vessel flow

Epiploic appendagitis

- Rare condition
- Inflammation of the epiploic appendage
- Cause
  - Primary epiploic appendagitis is caused by torsion or venous thrombosis
  - Secondary epiploic appendagitis is caused by inflammation of an adjacent organ
- Presents clinical with an abrupt onset of localised abdominal pain (in the right lower quadrant in 50% of cases); there is a palpable mass in 10–30% of cases
- Management is conservative

Imaging features

Ultrasound
- Solid, hyperechoic, non-compressible ovoid mass with a hypoechoic margin

CT
- Pericolic, oval-shaped, pedunculated mass 1–4 cm in diameter

Causes of small bowel strictures

- Adhesions
- Tumours, e.g. lymphoma, carcinoid, carcinoma, sarcoma, metastases
- Crohn's disease
- Radiation enteritis
- Ischaemia
- Enteric-coated potassium tablets

Causes of multiple small bowel nodules

- Inflammatory causes
  - Nodular lymphoid hyperplasia
  - Crohn's disease
- Infiltrative causes
  - Whipple's disease
  - Waldenström's macroglobulinaemia
  - Mastocytosis
- Neoplasia
  - Lymphoma
  - Polyposis
  - Metastases

- Infective causes
  - Typhoid
  - *Yersinia* infection

Causes of lesions in the terminal ileum

- Inflammatory causes
  - Crohn's disease
  - Ulcerative colitis
  - Radiation enteritis
- Infective causes
  - Tuberculosis
  - *Yersinia* infection
  - Actinomycosis
  - Histoplasmosis
- Neoplasia
  - Lymphoma
  - Carcinoid
  - Metastases
- Ischaemia

Causes of small bowel aphthoid ulceration

- Crohn's disease
- Polyarteritis nodosa
- *Yersinia* enterocolitis

Colon

Ischaemic colitis

- Non–occlusive ischaemic disease that reduces blood flow to 20% of normal
- Acute and rapid onset
- Reperfusion injury is likely when blood flow is re-established
- Causes include bowel obstruction, thrombosis and trauma; it may also be idiopathic
- Presents clinically with an abrupt onset of lower abdominal pain, rectal bleeding and diarrhoea
- Prognosis
  - Transient ischaemia resolves in 1–3 months (76% of cases)
  - Stricturing ischaemia leads to incomplete and delayed healing
  - Overall mortality is 10–30%
- Affected segments
  - Griffith's point (80% of cases): the junction between the superior

mesenteric artery and the inferior mesenteric artery at the splenic flexure
  - Sudeck's point: the anastomotic plexus between the inferior mesenteric artery and the hypogastric supply at the rectosigmoid junction
  - The right colon is involved in 30% of cases, the left colon in 45–90%

Imaging features

AXR
- Segmental 'thumb-printing'

Barium enema
- Thickening of the bowel wall, loss of haustrations and 'thumb-printing'

CT
- Segmental thickening
- Enhancement of the colon wall
- Portal or mesenteric air
- Thrombus in the superior mesenteric artery or the superior mesenteric vein
- Haemorrhage

Angiogram
- Mild acceleration of arteriovenous transit time
- Small tortuous ecstatic draining veins

Pseudomembranous colitis

- Results from a disturbance of the normal bacterial flora of the colon, colonisation with *Clostridium difficile* and release of toxins that cause mucosal inflammation and damage
- *Clostridium difficile* is a Gram-positive, anaerobic, spore-forming bacillus
- Pathogenic strains of *Clostridium difficile* produce two distinct toxins: toxin A is an enterotoxin and toxin B is a cytotoxin
- *Clostridium difficile*-associated diarrhoea can be a serious condition with a mortality rate of up to 25% in elderly, frail patients
- Risk factors include advanced age (> 60 years) and hospitalisation
- 20% of hospital patients *Clostridium difficile* during their hospital stay, and more than 30% of these patients develop diarrhoea
- The commonest antibiotics implicated in *Clostridium difficile* colitis include

cephalosporins (especially second- and third-generation agents), ampicillin, amoxicillin and clindamycin
- Disease distribution
  - Pancolitis in 50% of cases
  - Right-sided colitis in 27% of cases
  - Isolated rectosigmoid disease in 12% of cases (the rectosigmoid area is spared in 67% of cases)
- Stool cytotoxin test has high sensitivity (94–100%) and high specificity (99%), and is the test of choice
- Endoscopy may demonstrate the presence of raised, yellowish–white plaques 2–10 mm in diameter (pseudomembranes) overlying an erythematous and oedematous mucosa
- Medical care:
  - Most patients recover, even without specific therapy
  - The decision to treat *Clostridium difficile* infection and the type of therapy may depend on the severity of the disease
  - No treatment is necessary for asymptomatic carriers
  - Cessation of the causative antibiotic is essential when possible
  - Patients with more severe diarrhoea or colitis should receive antibiotic therapy directed at *Clostridium difficile*, e.g. metronidazole or vancomycin
- Complications include fulminant colitis (in 3% of cases), toxic megacolon, colonic perforation and peritonitis
- Persistent diarrhoea may be debilitating and can last for several weeks

Imaging features
CT
- Non-specific mural thickening with bowel dilatation and a paucity of pericolonic inflammation

Diverticular disease
- Diverticula are small mucosal herniations protruding through the intestinal layers and smooth muscle along the natural openings created by the vasa recta or nutrient vessels in the wall of the colon
- Diverticula can occur anywhere in the gastrointestinal tract but are usually observed in the colon and most often affect the rectosigmoid region
- Associated with a low-fibre diet, constipation and obesity
- Affect 70–80% of people aged 80 years

Diverticulitis (inflammation of one or more diverticula)
- Faecal material or undigested food particles may collect in a diverticulum
- Obstruction of the neck of the diverticulum results in distension of the pouch secondary to mucous secretion and overgrowth of normal colonic bacteria
- The thin-walled diverticulum, consisting solely of mucosa, is susceptible to vascular compromise and subsequent microperforation or macroperforation
- 10–25% of people with colonic diverticular disease develop diverticulitis
- Once the inflamed mucosa has healed, colonoscopy or contrast enema is important to rule out a malignancy masquerading as diverticular bowel thickening, phlegmon or postinflammatory stricture
- Complications
  - Abscess
  - Intestinal fistula (in 14% of cases)
  - Intestinal perforation
  - Intestinal obstruction
  - Peritonitis
  - Sepsis and septic shock
  - Bleeding (more common in diverticulosis than diverticulitis)

Imaging features
CT
- Modality of choice
- Pericolic fat stranding
- Colonic diverticula and thickening of the bowel wall
- Soft tissue inflammatory masses or phlegmon
- Abscesses or fistula formation may also be seen

Colonic polyps
- Slow-growing overgrowths of the colonic mucosa that carry a small risk (< 1%) of becoming malignant
- Can occur as part of inherited polyposis

syndromes, in which their number is greater and the risk for malignant progression is much greater
- 30% of middle-aged and elderly people have colonic polyps
- Management
  - Colonoscopic polypectomy for solitary pedunculated polyp
  - Repeat colonoscopy in 5 years after complete removal of a low-risk adenomatous polyp
  - Repeat colonoscopy in 3 years if the polyp has high-risk features

Types of polyp

- Hyperplastic polyps
  - Account for 90% of all polyps
  - Benign protrusions
  - Usually < 0.5 cm in diameter
  - Most commonly occur in the rectosigmoid area
  - Possess some malignant potential in the setting of the hyperplastic polyposis syndrome
- Adenomas
  - Account for 10% of polyps
  - Most (approximately 90%) are small, usually < 1.5 cm in diameter, and have a very small potential for malignancy
  - The remaining 10% of adenomas are > 1.5 cm in diameter and have about a 10% chance of containing invasive cancer
  - Traditionally divided into three subtypes: tubular, tubulovillous and villous
  - Tubular adenomas are the commonest subtype

Polyposis syndromes

- Hereditary conditions, including familial adenomatous polyposis, Gardner's syndrome, Turcot's syndrome, Peutz–Jeghers syndrome, Cowden's disease, familial juvenile polyposis and hyperplastic polyposis
- Complications include bleeding, diarrhoea, intestinal obstruction and progression to cancer
- Colonic resection remains the only feasible treatment option

---

Imaging features

Air-contrast barium enema
- Detects larger polyps (> 1 cm in diameter) but can miss smaller ones
- Low false-positive rate

CT virtual colonoscopy
- Detects more than 80% of large polyps

Colonoscopy
- Preferred test to detect colonic polyps, obtain biopsies, and/or perform endoscopic resection
- 80–90% sensitivity for large polyps

Colorectal carcinoma

- Commonest cancer of the GI tract
- Risk factors
  - Family history or personal history of colonic adenoma (5% tubular, 30–40% villous)
  - Carcinoma
  - Inflammatory bowel disease
  - Prominent lymphoid follicular pattern
  - Pelvic irradiation
  - Ureterosigmoidostomy
  - Diet low in fibre and high in fat and animal protein
  - Obesity
  - Asbestos exposure
  - Lynch's syndrome (hereditary non-polyposis colorectal cancer syndrome)
- Staging (modified Dukes' staging)
  - Stage A: limited to the mucosa
  - Stage B: involvement of the muscularis propria
  - Stage C: lymph node metastases
  - Stage D: distant metastases
- Location
  - Rectum (in 30% of cases)
  - Sigmoid (in 30% of cases)
  - Descending colon (in 10% of cases)
  - Transverse colon (in 10% of cases)
  - Ascending colon (in 10% of cases)
  - Caecum (in 10% of cases)
- Metastasises to the liver (in 75% of cases), the adrenal glands (in 10% of cases), the lung (in 5–50% of cases), the ovary (in 5% of cases), bone (in 5% of cases) and the brain (in 5% of cases)
- 5-year survival depends on disease stage
  - Stage A: 85%
  - Stage B: 70%

- Stage C: 33%
- Stage D: 5%
- Peritoneal involvement is present in 25% of cases and is a poor prognostic sign
- Recurrence occurs in 33% of cases: 50% recur within 1 year and of these 60% recur locally
- 5% of recurrent tumours are endoluminal and 50% are extraluminal
- Preoperative radiotherapy reduces local recurrence
- Complications include bowel obstruction, perforation, intussusception, abscess formation and fistula formation

Sigmoid volvulus

- Sigmoid colon twists on the mesenteric axis
- Seen as greatly distended, paralysed loop of bowel with fluid–fluid levels mainly on the left side, extending to the diaphragm
- Distinct midline crease ('coffee bean' sign)
- Management is with a flatus tube

Causes of colonic strictures

- Neoplasia
  - Carcinoma
  - Lymphoma
- Inflammatory causes
  - Ulcerative colitis
  - Crohn's disease
  - Pericolic abscess
  - Radiotherapy
- Infective causes
  - Tuberculosis
  - Amoeboma
  - Schistosomiasis
  - Lymphogranuloma venereum
- Cathartic colon
- Ischaemia
- Extrinsic masses
  - Inflammatory masses
  - Tumours
  - Endometriosis

Causes of pneumatosis intestinalis

- Primary pneumatosis intestinalis accounts for 15% of cases
- Secondary pneumatosis intestinalis accounts for 85% of cases
  - Necrotising enterocolitis

- Colitis and enteritis
- Collagen disorders
- Leukaemia
- Corticosteroids and other immunosuppressive therapy

Causes of colonic aphthoid ulceration

- Crohn's disease
- Ischaemia
- Amoebic colitis
- *Yersinia* enterocolitis
- Behçet's disease

Causes of anterior indentation of the rectosigmoid junction

- Tumours
- Haematoma
- Hydatid
- Abscess
- Ascites
- Endometriosis
- Previous surgery

Causes of a widened retrorectal space (> 1.5 cm at the S3–S5 level)

- Normal variant
- Neoplasia
  - Rectal carcinoma
  - Rectal metastases
  - Sacral tumours
- Inflammatory causes
  - Crohn's disease
  - Ulcerative colitis
  - Abscess
  - Radiotherapy
  - Diverticulitis
- Pelvic lipoma
- Anterior sacral meningocoele
- Enteric duplication cysts

Crohn's disease

- Uncertain aetiology
- Pathologically the disease affects the bowel in a transmural pattern and can affect any part of the GI tract from the mouth to the anus
- Early mucosal involvement consists of longitudinal and transverse aphthous ulcers

- Progression to fissuring and fistulation follows, eventually resulting in communication with adjacent segments of bowel
- Risk factors include a positive family history, smoking and oral contraceptives
- Complications
  - Sinus tracks (in 15% of cases)
  - Bowel obstruction (in 20% of cases)
  - Fistula formation (in 50% of cases)
  - Malignant transformation; cancer is a leading cause of death (the majority of malignancies are adenocarcinomas)

Imaging features

AXR
- Main role is to assess for obstruction or perforation

Contrast studies
- Used to diagnose and differentiate disease
- Characterised by aphthoid ulcers, which are separated by normal bowel but which can become more confluent and give rise to serpigenous and linear ulcers affecting the mesenteric borders
- Cobblestoning is seen with transmural inflammation, giving a reticular pattern
- As transmural inflammation increases, there is eventual narrowing of the lumen, giving rise to the 'string sign'

CT
- Used in the context of an acute abdomen in Crohn's disease to assess for complications and for surgical planning and postoperative management
- Ulceration and mucosal oedema can be seen on thin-section CT, although contrast examinations are better for this
- Associated mesenteric stranding is not reliable in evaluating active disease because it is also found during periods of remission
- Identification of abscess and fistula formation is useful for management

Ulcerative colitis

- Involves the mucosa with formation of crypt abscesses
- Severe cases affect the other layers of the large bowel wall

- Most cases occur in the rectum and travel proximally
- May involve the terminal ileum (back-wash ileitis caused by an incompetent ileocaecal valve)
- Risk of colorectal cancer increases by 0.5 to 1% per year after 10 years of the disease
- Toxic megacolon occurs in 2% of cases

Imaging features

AXR
- Colonic dilatation
- Dilatation >9 cm in the caecum and 10 cm in the transverse colon means that there is a toxic megacolon, which carries a high chance of perforation and is a surgical emergency
- Colon may demonstrate 'thumb-printing'

Barium enema
- Usually performed in the quiescent phase
- Left colon is usually involved and the disease is segmental but skip lesions are not seen
- Mucosal oedema is seen with a fine granular pattern
- In more advanced disease, ulceration is seen, characteristically 'rose thorn' ulcers
- Other types of ulcers include 'collar button' ulcers (with undermining of the edges) and longitudinal ulcers
- Confluent ulceration is seen as a coarse, granular appearance
- Symmetrical haustral thickening resulting from oedema produces the impression of 'thumb printing'
- Pseudopolyps are seen in severe cases and result from normal mucosa adjacent to areas of ulceration
- Recurrent inflammation leads to narrowing and shortening of the colon
- Rectal narrowing is seen as an increase in the presacral space
- Benign strictures occur in 10% of patients with long-standing disease

CT
- Now become the primary imaging modality
- Circumferential, symmetrical thickening of the bowel well, with thickened haustral folds

- Target sign (alternating high and low attenuation of the colonic wall, caused by oedema)
- Submucosal fat deposition is seen in ulcerative colitis more often than Crohn's disease
- Main use of CT is to identify the complications of ulcerative colitis, including perforation, abscess formation, obstruction secondary to strictures and malignant change, as well as for surgical planning and postoperative imaging

Ultrasound
- Used to diagnose ulcerative colitis but is operator-dependent
- Thickening of the bowel wall is seen as a hypoechoic wall, but it may become inhomogeneous as a result of fatty deposition
- Haustral folds are lost and there is reduced peristalsis and compressibility
- Ultrasound can differentiate between Crohn's disease and ulcerative colitis: Crohn's disease is a transmural disease whereas ulcerative colitis affects the superficial layers

Chapter 4

Genitourinary system, adrenal gland, obstetrics and gynaecology, and breast

Anatomy

- The kidneys develop from the pronephros, mesonephros and metanephros of which the pronephros and mesonephros regress; some segments of the mesonephros develop into segments of the genital system
- The ureteric bud develops as an outgrowth from the mesonephric duct proximal to the cloacal entry. The ureter, renal pelvis, calyces and collecting tubules develop from the ureteric bud
- The metanephric blastema arises from the caudal part of the nephrogenic cord. Physical contact with the ureteric bud induces its development. The excretory part of the kidney develops from the ureteric bud
- The kidneys originally develop in the upper sacral region but migrate cranially receiving successively higher branches from the aorta. The final adult position is reached by 8 weeks of gestation. Renal maturation continues until the age of 5 years and hence the kidneys are prone to scarring until this age

Imaging

Ultrasound

- Normal renal cortex is hypoechoic compared with normal liver
- Renal medulla is hypoechoic compared with cortex
- Arcuate arteries may be seen as punctate echogenic foci at the corticomedullary junction and should not be mistaken for a calculus
- Renal sinus is hyperechoic, mainly due to the presence of fat

Radionuclide imaging

- Technetium-99m is the isotope most commonly used
- High gamma photon energy (140 keV)
- Short half-life of 6 hours with even shorter biological half-life due to renal excretion
- Iodine-123 or iodine-131 are the other commonly used isotopes
- ^{99m}Tc-DTPA (diethylene triamine penta-acetic acid) is used to assess renal blood flow and urinary excretion
- ^{99m}Tc-MAG3 (mercapto acetyl tri-glycine) is used to assess renal function
- ^{99m}Tc-DMSA (dimercaptosuccinic acid) is used to depict focal renal parenchymal lesions
- ^{99m}Tc-MAG3 is the agent of choice for urinary tract obstruction, but DTPA is an alternative agent
- ^{99m}Tc-sulphur colloid is the agent of choice for demonstrating vesicoureteric reflux

Autosomal dominant polycystic kidney disease

- Hereditary disorder in which there is variable enlargement of the kidneys with multiple cysts
- Progressive renal failure and hypertension
- Usually presents in the third or fourth decade of life

Clinical symptoms and signs

- Flank pain, haematuria,
- Pyelonephritis, urolithiasis, hypertension, renal failure

Pathology

- Cysts develop anywhere along the nephron and are variable in size
- Intracystic haemorrhage may occur
- Intracystic calcifications may also be seen
- Strong penetrance (nearly all who inherit the gene develop the disease)
- Extrarenal abnormalities are common
- Liver cysts occur in up to 50% of patients
- Berry aneurysms occur in up to 15% of patients

Diagnostic criteria

- Two or more cysts in both kidneys detected with ultrasound in at-risk patients < 30 years
- Two or more cysts in each kidney detected with ultrasound in patients aged 30–60 years
- Patients > 60 years must have at least four detectable cysts in each kidney

Nephrocalcinosis

- Radiologically detectable diffuse calcium deposition within the renal substance
- Mechanism of calcium deposition can be metastatic (in morphologically normal kidneys), dystrophic (in injured tissue) or due to urine stasis (as in medullary sponge kidney)

Causes

- Primary and secondary hyperparathyroidism
- Metastatic carcinoma to bone
- Hypercalcaemia of malignancy
- Prolonged immobilisation
- Sarcoidosis
- Milk-alkali syndrome
- Hypervitaminosis D
- Renal tubular acidosis
- Medullary sponge kidney
- Hyperoxaluria
- Bartter's syndrome
- Prolonged furosemide (frusemide) administration, e.g. in premature infants
- Nephrotoxic drugs
- Papillary necrosis

Imaging features

- Extent of parenchymal calcification is variable
- In hypercalcaemic states, only a few scattered punctate densities in the medullary portions of the kidneys may be seen
- In renal tubular acidosis, often very dense and extensive calcification of the medulla is seen

Medullary sponge kidney

- Dysplastic cystic dilatation of papillary and medullary portions of the collecting ducts
- Symptoms can occur secondary to stasis but condition is often asymptomatic
- Bilateral in 75%
- Medulla appears echogenic on ultrasound due to the medullary calcification
- Intravenous urogram: 'striated' nephrogram phase, 'bunch of flowers' appearance may also be seen

Renal sinus cysts (parapelvic cysts)

- Benign extraparenchymal cysts located within the renal sinus
- Most likely lymphatic in origin
- May be uni- or multilocular
- May be bilateral
- Differential diagnoses include pelviureteric junction obstruction, multicystic dysplastic kidney

Imaging features

Ultrasound
- Features of a simple cyst: anechoic, thin wall, post acoustic enhancement
- No communication with the pelvicalyceal system
- Intravenous urogram
- Soft tissue density in the renal sinus that causes focal displacement and smooth effacement of the adjacent pelvicalyceal system

CT
- Homogeneous, near water density and non-enhancing
- Displacement of renal pelvis and calyces
- Surrounding halo of renal sinus fat is a characteristic feature
- MRI: water signal intensity lesion (low T1 and high T2 signal) surrounded by high-signal renal sinus fat

Acquired cystic kidney disease

- Development of multiple renal cysts in patients with chronic renal failure (uraemia) but without a history of inherited renal cystic disease
- 90% of patients with end-stage renal disease, > 5–10 years of dialysis and 8–13% patients not on dialysis
- Usually asymptomatic
- Diagnosis based on detection of 3–5 cysts in each kidney in a patient with chronic renal failure not caused by an inherited cystic disease
- Affected kidneys are usually small, but due to progression, nephromegaly eventually develops

- Haemorrhagic cysts occur in 50% of patients with acquired cystic kidney disease
- Renal cell carcinoma develops in up to 7% of patients
- Subcapsular and perinephric haematomas can occur due to rupture of haemorrhagic cysts

Imaging features

CT
- High attenuation values may be seen within cysts as a result of haemorrhage
- Lack of enhancement post-contrast

Ultrasound
- Multiple simple cysts

MRI
- Haemorrhagic cysts display high signal on T1WI and T2WI in the subacute phase
- No enhancement following gadolinium

Renal haemorrhage

- May be suburothelial, intraparenchymal, subcapsular, perinephric, pararenal or in the renal sinus

Causes

- Trauma
- Shock wave lithotripsy
- Spontaneous: anticoagulation, blood dyscrasias (usual cause for suburothelial and renal sinus haemorrhage)
- Renal infarction
- Polyarteritis nodosa
- Renal aneurysms and arteriovenous malformations
- Tumours: renal cell carcinoma (commonest cause of spontaneous subcapsular and perinephric haemorrhage)
- Renal vein thrombosis
- Rupture of a haemorrhagic cyst

CT features

Suburothelial haemorrhage
- Thickened wall of renal pelvis and upper ureter by high attenuation blood

Subcapsular haematoma (limited by capsule)
- Recent haemorrhage is of higher attenuation than adjacent parenchyma
- Flattening of kidney
- Elevation of capsule
- Medial displacement of collecting system
- May eventually calcify
- Large chronic subcapsular haematoma can cause hypertension (Page kidney)

Perinephric haematoma (involves fat between capsule and fascia)
- Can simulate a subcapsular haematoma, but usually extends below the kidney margin
- If CT reveals no cause for haemorrhage angiography is recommended

Renal infarction

Causes

- Renal artery thrombosis or embolism
- Vasculitis, e.g. polyarteritis nodosa
- Trauma
- Sickle cell disease
- Aortic dissection

CT features

- Depends upon extent and age of infarct

Global renal infarction (main renal artery occlusion)
- Non-enhancing kidney with high-density cortical rim from perfusion by collateral vessels

Large branch occlusion
- Sharply demarcated hypodense wedge-shaped defect with the base of the wedge on the renal capsule and apex towards the renal hilum
- Cortical rim may enhance

Small vessel occlusion (emboli, vasculitis, sickle cell)
- Multiple, often bilateral, focal infarcts
- Multiple 'slit-like' areas of low attenuation (sickle cell)
- Main differential diagnosis is acute pyelonephritis (cortical rim is not usually seen with pyelonephritis)

Renal artery stenosis

- Accounts for 1–5% of hypertension in young adults
- Causes:
  - Atherosclerosis (up to 90%)
  - Fibromuscular dysplasia

Imaging features

CT
- Prolonged corticomedullary differentiation in comparison with normal kidney on a conventional dynamic CT is suggestive of significant stenosis
- Multidetector CT angiography has improved spatial resolution compared with magnetic resonance angiography and can be used to evaluate renal vascularity when imaged in the arterial phase

MRI
- Gadolinium-enhanced magnetic resonance angiography has a high sensitivity for detection of proximal renal artery stenosis

Catheter angiography
- Gold standard test
- In renal artery stenosis secondary to atherosclerosis the ostium or proximal 2 cm of the renal artery is affected
- In fibromuscular dysplasia the mid/distal main renal artery is involved and characteristically has a 'string of beads' appearance
- Cannot be used to assess haemodynamic significance of lesion

Colour Doppler ultrasound
- Peak systolic velocity > 150 cm/sec
- Post stenotic spectral broadening and/or flow reversal
- Parvus tardus waveform of interlobar artery
- Acceleration time > 0.07 sec

Acute cortical necrosis

- Ischaemic necrosis of the renal cortex with sparing of the medulla

Causes

- Haemorrhage (classically in third trimester of pregnancy)
- Septic abortion
- Severe trauma with shock
- Transfusion reaction
- Severe dehydration
- Haemolytic–uremic syndrome
- Acute aortic dissection
- Toxins including snake venom
- Usually bilateral

CT features

- Acute phase: zone of unenhanced cortex between enhancing medulla and subcapsular cortical rim
- Chronic phase: small smooth kidneys. The cortex may calcify

Renal vein thrombosis

Causes

- Extrinsic occlusion by an adjacent neoplasm
- Direct extension of a renal or adrenal carcinoma
- Primary renal disease: membranous glomerulonephritis (most common in adults) also systemic lupus erythematosus and amyloidosis
- Secondary renal vein occlusion from thrombosis of the inferior vena cava
- In infants: sickle cell disease, haemoconcentration states such as diarrhoea and sepsis, hypoxia in cyanotic congenital heart disease and hypercoagulable states and maternal history of diabetes
- Clinical consequences depend on the rapidity of development of obstruction and development of collateral circulation
- If completely occluded acutely, renal infarction occurs, eventually causing a small, smooth non-functioning kidney

Imaging features

Intravenous urogram
- Large and smooth kidney
- Variable contrast excretion
- Attenuation of the collecting system by swollen parenchyma
- Increasingly dense nephrogram in some cases
- Medullary striations on intravenous urogram and CT have been described

- Cortical rim sign may be seen as in acute arterial infarction
- Varices can cause indentation of the renal pelvis and ureter

Doppler ultrasound
- Loss of normal low-resistance pattern of renal artery waveform
- Visualisation of thrombus within the renal vein

CT
- Prolonged corticomedullary differentiation
- Focal areas of non-enhancement where infarction has occurred
- Retroperitoneal haemorrhage
- Expansion and enlargement of renal vein with low-attenuation thrombus
- Fine linear densities radiating from the kidney to the perirenal space are characteristic and enhance on contrast administration
- Enlargement of the kidney in acute renal vein thrombosis
- No contrast flow may occur in acute cases

Renal artery occlusion

Causes
- Embolism
- Thrombosis
- Dissection
- Trauma
- Involvement of the main artery or major branches occur only in a small number of cases

Signs and symptoms
- Variable and can be asymptomatic
- Abrupt onset of severe abdominal or flank pain, nausea, vomiting, haematuria and albuminuria
- Fever and leucocytosis
- Enlarged tender renal mass

Imaging features

Intravenous urogram
- Non-opacified, normal to enlarged kidney, with a normal pelvicalyceal system is characteristic

CT
- 'Cortical rim' sign on nephrogram phase

Acute bacterial pyelonephritis

- Imaging is indicated if severe and/or refractory to treatment
- Aim is to determine complications and diagnose any predisposing abnormalities

Imaging features

Intravenous urogram
- Usually normal
- Abnormal in 30%, but with non-specific features
- Enlargement of the kidney, delayed or poor excretion of contrast and a striated nephrogram may be seen
- Hydroureteronephrosis can occur secondary to the effect of bacterial endotoxins

CT
- 'Striated nephrogram': discrete rays of alternating attenuation extending to the cortex (better demonstrated on CT than intravenous urogram)
- Diffuse renal involvement: poor contrast enhancement, delayed/absent excretion of contrast, global renal enlargement
- Unifocal or multifocal renal involvement may be seen, with areas of apparently normal renal parenchyma
- Wedge-shaped areas of decreased attenuation with straight borders, widest at the periphery of the kidney, represent the abnormal areas
- Low-attenuation masses with bulging of the renal surface in severe inflammation (do not enhance following contrast administration)
- Liquefaction (central low attenuation) in involved regions suggests abscess formation

Renal abscess

- Acute pyelonephritis can progress to tissue necrosis and abscess formation
- Small abscesses may respond to antibiotics
- Larger abscesses and perinephric involvement require drainage (may be performed under ultrasound or CT guidance)

CT features

- Attenuation value of around 30 HU
- Distinct rounded margins and thick enhancing walls
- Non-enhancing contents
- Occasionally gas bubbles may be seen
- Focal thickening of the adjacent renal fascia and perinephric stranding
- Perinephric abscess if infection extends through the capsule

Emphysematous pyelonephritis

- Life-threatening infection of renal parenchyma by gas forming organisms
- Most patients are diabetic
- *Escherichia coli* is the most common bacterial species involved

Emphysematous pyelonephritis

Type 1
- Destruction of more than one third of parenchyma
- Mortality rate approximately 70%
- Streaky mottled gas radiating peripherally
- May require nephrectomy if conservative measures fail

Type 2
- Destruction of less than one third of the parenchyma
- Renal or perirenal fluid collection with locules of gas within the collecting system
- Mortality rate approximately 20%

Utility of CT
- Most sensitive modality for diagnosis
- Can identify gas in the collecting system, parenchymal or perinephric tissue

Pyonephrosis

- Accumulation of pus in an obstructed pelvicalyceal system

- Often associated with severe sepsis
- Treatment with percutaneous nephrostomy or ureteric stenting to bypass the obstruction is first line

CT features

- Thickening of renal pelvic wall
- Inflammatory changes in perinephric fat
- Rarely, layering of contrast medium anterior to pus in a dilated renal pelvis
- Pelvicalyceal system gas in the absence of instrumentation
- CT may be able to demonstrate the site of obstruction

Xanthogranulomatous pyelonephritis

- Chronic inflammatory disease associated with indolent bacterial infection
- Inflammatory process begins in the renal pelvis and extends into the renal medulla and cortex
- Lipid-laden macrophages replace the renal parenchyma
- Usually diffuse but can be focal
- Typical patients are middle-aged females
- *E. coli* or *Proteus mirabilis* are frequently cultured from urine

Symptoms

- Malaise, fever, chills and weight loss
- Flank pain, frequency, dysuria and nocturia

CT features

Diffuse form
- Diffuse reniform enlargement with ill-defined central low attenuation
- Apparent cortical thinning
- Staghorn calculus in up to 70% of cases
- Absence or decrease of contrast excretion on affected side
- Less commonly a small contracted kidney with replacement lipomatosis
- Multiple fluid-density, rounded areas almost completely replacing the kidney
- Rim enhancement of the low-density areas
- Extrarenal extension is common
- Perinephric and psoas muscle abscesses are common

Focal form
- Poorly enhancing mass in one pole or adjacent to a calyx
- May be associated with calculus
- Sometimes misdiagnosed as a neoplasm

Renal trauma

- Can be caused by blunt or penetrating injuries

Renal trauma

Category I
- 75–85%
- Contusions and small corticomedullary lacerations that do not communicate with collecting system
- Clinically insignificant
- Managed conservatively

Category II
- 10%
- Laceration through the renal cortex extending into the medulla or collecting system with or without urinary extravasation
- May be managed conservatively

Category III
- 5%
- Multiple deep lacerations and injury to the renal pedicle

Category IV
- Rare
- Pelviureteric junction avulsion
- Laceration of the renal pelvis

Subcapsular and perinephric haematomas may occur with any of these grades but when isolated are categorised as category I

Symptoms and signs
- Gross haematuria
- Absence of haematuria does not preclude serious injury
- Absence of haematuria is reported in 24% of renal artery thrombosis and one third of pelviureteric junction injury

CT features
- Contrast-enhanced CT is modality of choice
- Scans are obtained at 70 seconds and 3 minutes after the start of contrast injection

Contusion
- Amorphous interstitial extravasation of blood and oedema
- Unenhanced CT: focal swelling and irregular high-density infiltrates
- Enhanced CT: ill-defined rounded or ovoid areas of low attenuation
- Small interstitial accumulations of contrast material on delayed images

Laceration
- Superficial: limited to cortex
- Deep: extends to medulla
- Contrast extravasation is often seen into the perinephric tissues

Infarction
- Focal area may be caused by thrombosis or laceration of the segmental arteries
- Typically appears as non-enhancing peripherally based wedge-shaped areas

Haematoma
- Can be intrarenal, subcapsular or perinephric

Main renal artery injuries
- Absence of contrast medium enhancement
- Cortical rim sign may or may not be seen
- Haematoma surrounding the renal hilum may be seen
- Abrupt cut-off of contrast-filled renal artery

Acute renal vein occlusion
- Enlarged kidney
- Thrombus visualised in the renal vein
- Venography may be performed if injuries to the renal vein and inferior vena cava are suspected

Pelviureteric junction injuries
- Rare
- Excellent excretion of contrast material in the intrarenal collecting system
- Medial perinephric urinary extravasation
- Circumrenal urinoma may be seen

Simple renal cyst

- Most common renal masses
- Frequency increases with age
- Usually asymptomatic
- May cause pressure symptoms or symptoms due to haemorrhage or infection
- Solitary or multiple and commonly bilateral

Ultrasound features

- Sharp margination and demarcation from surrounding parenchyma
- Smooth and thin walled
- Homogeneous anechoic content

Bosniak classification

- **Category 1:** classical 'simple cysts'
- **Category 2:** thin (< 1 mm) septae, fine calcifications in cyst wall or septa or high density. Can be monitored with serial imaging. MRI may be helpful to characterise high-density lesions
- **Category 3:** thick irregular mural or septal calcification, numerous or thick irregular septae, Uniform or slightly nodular wall thickening. These lesions shall be explored surgically unless contraindicated
- **Category 4:** clearly malignant lesions with cystic components

Renal adenoma

- Solid lesion < 3 cm in size detected on ultrasound or CT
- Previously considered to be benign but is now considered to be renal carcinoma in evolution and treated by partial nephrectomy

Oncocytoma

- Solid epithelial neoplasm with a generally benign course
- Represents 10–15% of small (< 3 cm) solid renal neoplasms
- Arises from proximal tubular epithelium

Imaging features

CT features

- Well-defined masses with smooth rounded margins
- Occasionally contain calcifications
- May be multiple and bilateral
- Small oncocytomas are usually displayed homogeneous enhancement and may be impossible to distinguish from small slow-growing renal cell carcinomas
- 25–33% of large oncocytomas have central, sharply defined stellate scar which strongly suggests the diagnosis
- 'Spoke wheel' enhancement pattern in larger lesions, but this does not reliably differentiate from renal cell carcinoma

Catheter angiography

- Homogeneous blush
- Cannot reliably distinguish from renal cell carcinoma

MRI

- Iso/hypointense to normal parenchyma on T1-weighted image (T1WI)
- Variable appearance on T2-weighted image (T2WI)
- Central scar
- Enhances less than normal renal parenchyma following gadolinium administration
- Fine-needle aspiration is helpful in discriminating between oncocytoma and renal cell carcinoma

Angiomyolipoma

- Benign hamartomas composed of blood vessels, smooth muscle and fat
- May be seen in isolation or in patients with tuberous sclerosis (usually multiple)
- Sporadic form (accounts for 80–90% of cases)
  - Typically seen in middle age
  - More common in females (4:1)
- Usually asymptomatic
- Large masses can cause flank pain, haematuria and anaemia, and carry a high risk of intratumoural or perinephric haematoma
- Conservative for lesions smaller than 4 cm with typical features

- Partial nephrectomy or selective catheter embolisation for masses larger than 4 cm is advocated
- Annual follow up with CT or ultrasound in asymptomatic patients with lesions approaching 4 cm in diameter; larger lesions are followed up more frequently

Imaging features

CT
- Unenhanced: fatty attenuation (values less than -10 HU)
- Around 5% do not contain fat and therefore cannot be differentiated from renal cell carcinoma
- Extensive intratumoural haemorrhage can obscure the presence of fat
- Well-circumscribed mass
- Vary in size from tiny nodules to large tumours
- Extensive bilateral involvement in patients with tuberous sclerosis
- Presence of intratumoural fat is almost diagnostic
- Retroperitoneal lymph node involvement may be seen
- Extrarenal extension may be seen
- Extension into the renal vein and inferior vena cava may be seen

MRI
- Presence of fat is demonstrated by chemical shift imaging

Von Hippel–Lindau disease

- Autosomal dominant with almost 100% penetrance
- Cysts are the most common renal manifestation
- 25–40% of affected patients develop clear cell renal carcinoma
- Often develop renal cell carcinoma in the fourth or fifth decade of life
- Synchronous and metachronous renal cell carcinomas are common
- Transformation of simple cysts to solid lesions is rare
- Complex lesions require follow up as solid elements may transform
- Predominantly cystic lesions with solid components are characteristic

- Pancreatic cysts, islet cell tumours, phaeochromocytomas, retinal angiomas and central nervous system haemangioblastomas are other features. Endolymphatic sac tumours, cystadenomas of the epididymis and broad ligament cysts and tumours are recognised manifestations
- Pancreatic cysts occur in around 30% of patients
- Pheochromocytomas occur in about 10% of patients (often multiple and ectopic; 50–80% are bilateral)
- Abdominal CT screening of first-degree relatives is sometimes advocated from the second decade of life

Tuberous sclerosis

- Autosomal dominant with variable penetrance
- More than half of cases are sporadic
- Classic triad: epilepsy, mental retardation and adenoma sebaceum
- Renal lesions are seen in 50% of patients
- Bilateral renal cysts
- Bilateral angiomyolipomas that may appear at an early age and grow faster
- Multiple renal angiomyolipomas are the sine qua non of tuberous sclerosis
- Occur in about 15% of patients, mostly females
- 1–2% of patients with tuberous sclerosis develop renal cell carcinoma
- Perirenal cystic collections or lymphangiomas
- Other associated abnormalities include subependymal nodules, giant cell astrocytoma, peripheral tubers, retinal hamartomas, cardiac rhabdomyomas, lymphangioleiomyomatosis, shagreen patches, subungual fibromas and bone cysts

Renal carcinoma

- Most common urological malignancy in adulthood
- Can occur at any age but most common in seventh and eighth decades

- Known risk factors: smoking, petroleum products, obesity, acquired cystic renal disease, Von Hippel–Lindau disease, tuberous sclerosis and hereditary papillary renal cancer
- Almost 50% are detected incidentally on imaging for symptoms other than haematuria or flank pain
- Most commonly metastasises to the lungs, bones and liver
- Less commonly to the adrenal glands, kidney, brain, pancreas, mesentery and abdominal wall

Imaging features

CT

- Unenhanced, corticomedullary and nephrographic phase imaging are necessary
- Corticomedullary phase is best for evaluating venous extension
- Nephrographic phase is best for evaluating the primary mass lesion
- Calcification in up to 30% of tumours (may be amorphous or curvilinear)
- Enhancement is usually less than that of the normal renal parenchyma
- Tumour haemorrhage or necrosis can cause heterogeneous enhancement
- Lobulated or irregular margin may be seen, though small tumours often have distinct smooth margins

MRI

- Hypo- to isointense to renal parenchyma on T1WI
- Heterogeneously hyperintense on T2WI
- Less enhancement than normal parenchyma after gadolinium
- Presence of fat, haemorrhage and necrosis affects signal intensity

Post-nephrectomy evaluation

- Recurrence in the renal bed occurs in about 5% patients after radical nephrectomy
- Renal bed recurrence is most likely within first 2 years following nephrectomy

Upper tract transitional cell carcinoma

- 10% of neoplasms of the upper tract
- Usually present as haematuria; can present as renal colic
- Multicentric
- 2–4% of cases are bilateral
- Most common sites of metastases are liver, bone and lungs

Imaging features

Intravenous urogram

- Calcification is uncommon (2–7%) and may mimic calculi
- Enlargement of the kidney with large infiltrating tumour or ureteric obstruction
- Filling defect in the collecting system or ureter
- 'Stippling sign' : tracking of contrast medium into the interstices of a papillary lesion
- Stricturing (if multiple can mimic tuberculosis)

Ultrasound

- Usually slightly hyperechoic compared with normal renal parenchyma
- Typically infiltrative and does not cause contour distortion

CT

- Typically hyperattenuating compared with renal parenchyma
- Sessile filling defect seen on the excretory phase of CT urography
- Centrifugally expanding mass causing compression of the renal sinus fat
- Pelvicalyceal irregularity, focal or diffuse thickening or focally obstructed calyx
- Reniform shape is typically preserved
- Ureteric lesion may manifest as hydronephrosis

MRI

- Not commonly used technique for assessment of transitional cell carcinoma
- Nearly isointense to renal parenchyma on T1WI and T2WI
- Moderate enhancement following gadolinium
- Static or dynamic MR urography may be employed

Renal lymphoma

- Usually secondary to systemic disease
- Bilateral in 75%
- More common in non-Hodgkin's lymphoma
- Seen in about 8% of patients with lymphoma

Imaging features

CT
- Five patterns are recognised:
  - Multiple renal masses (59%)
  - Solitary mass (3%)
  - Renal invasion (contiguous retroperitoneal spread) (28%)
  - Perirenal disease (10%)
  - Diffuse renal infiltration (rare)
- Homogenously enhancing nodule which are less dense than normal parenchyma on contrast-enhanced CT
- Renal arteries and veins remain patent despite tumour encasement (characteristic sign)
- Obstructive hydronephrosis may be seen when there is retroperitoneal lymphadenopathy

MRI
- Same morphologic features as on CT
- Hypointense relative to the cortex on T1WI and heterogeneously hypointense to isointense on T2WI
- Minimal enhancement following gadolinium

Renal metastases

- The kidneys are the fifth most common site of metastasis in the body
- Mainly haematogenous spread
- Lung, breast and contralateral kidney are the most common primary sites
- Usually discovered incidentally
- Some patients present with haematuria and flank pain

CT features
- Multiple discrete bilateral lesions are most common
- Usually homogeneous enhancement pattern
- Central necrosis may be seen with large lesions
- Occasionally solitary lesions, but if there are metastases in other regions a solitary renal lesion can be assumed to be metastasis
- Colonic metastases are commonly solitary and exophytic
- Melanoma metastases typically have perinephric extension

Chronic renal failure from diffuse parenchymal disease

- Also known as chronic medical renal disease
- Marked parenchymal atrophy with smooth reniform contour
- Hyperechoic on ultrasound

Renal papillary necrosis

- Chronic tubulointerstitial nephropathy
- Predominantly affects the renal medulla

Causes
- Diabetes
- Analgesic abuse or overuse
- Sickle cell disease
- Pyelonephritis
- Renal vein thrombosis
- Tuberculosis
- Obstructive uropathy

Imaging features
- Intravenous urogram
- Normal in the initial period of early ischaemic change
- Clefts extending from the fornices to the papillary tips
- Cavity in the papilla filled with contrast
- Sloughed papilla may calcify over the course of time

CT
- Nephrographic phase: poorly marginated areas of diminished enhancement at the tip of medullary pyramid in the early ischaemic phase
- Excretory phase: clefts and cavities filled with contrast medium
- Calyceal blunting at the papillary tip
- Scarring and atrophy of the kidney following healing
- Diffuse papillary calcifications

Genitourinary tract tuberculosis

- Second most common site of tuberculosis
- Usually haematogenous spread to the kidneys
- May be asymptomatic

Pathogenesis

- Begins as small tubercles and progresses to necrotic lesions/irregular cavities
- Cavities communicate with calyces, which can undergo structuring
- Usually bilateral asymmetrical renal involvement
- Unilateral in 25%
- If not appropriately treated, the kidney becomes atrophic scarred and densely calcified
- Ureteric involvement may occur secondary to renal involvement
- Mucosal granulomas form which eventually fibrose
- Upper and/or lower thirds of the ureters are usually involved
- Vesicoureteric reflux can occur from a fixed patulous vesicoureteric junction
- Bladder infection usually occurs secondary to renal infection
- Bladder mucosal ulceration can lead to scarring and fibrosis, resulting in a thickened contracted bladder
- Bladder wall calcification is uncommon
- Seminal vesicle involvement is usually haematogenous in nature; mucosal tuberculomas, ulceration and fibrosis can occur
- Prostatic infection is usually secondary to renal infection. Can cause fistulae into the surrounding tissues
- Can cause chronic epididymitis and epididymoorchitis
- Female genital tract involvement may be secondary to haematogenous or lymphatic spread. Can cause infertility

Clinical features

- Presentation is usually late
- Frequency, urgency and dysuria may occur with tuberculous cystitis
- Secondary infection of hydronephrosis cause symptoms
- Epididymitis, hydrocoele, palpable testicular mass, discharging scrotal or perineal sinuses may be the first presentation of male genital tract involvement
- Rectal or pelvic pain may be the presenting symptom of prostatic tuberculosis
- Pelvic pain, menstrual irregularity and sterility may be the presenting features of female genital tract involvement

Radiographic features

- Plain radiographs
- Signs of extrarenal tuberculosis (e.g. lung consolidation, lymphadenopathy)
- Active or healed pulmonary tuberculosis in 50%
- Dystrophic renal calcification may sometimes be seen

Intravenous urogram

Kidneys

- 'Smudged papillae' due to surface irregularity
- 'Moth-eaten' calyx
- Irregular tract formation from the calyx to the papillae
- Large irregular cavities
- Enlarged kidneys initially; later become atrophic
- Hydrocalyces with no pelvis dilatation or an atrophic pelvis is suggestive
- 'Hiked-up renal pelvis': cephalic retraction of the infero-medial margin of renal pelvis at the pelviureteric junction
- Stricture at pelviureteric junction can cause hydronephrosis or delayed function, clubbed calyces or no function
- Associated renal calculi seen in 20% of cases
- Autonephrectomy (small scarred non-functioning kidney with calcification)
- Renal calcification seen in 50% (amorphous granular associated with active infection; dense punctate associated with healed tuberculomas)

Ureters

- Usually unilateral (if bilateral appears asymmetrical)
- Intraluminal filling defects
- Irregularity of the mucosa

- Beaded or 'corkscrew' appearance from scarring alternating with dilatations
- Rigid, aperistaltic, shortened ureter
- Bilateral hydroureters

Bladder
- Small trabeculated bladder
- Vesicoureteric reflux
- Wall calcification rare
- Fistulae or sinus formation

Prostate
- Dense calcification in the prostatic bed

CT features
- Calyceal changes are better seen on intravenous urogram
- CT is superior for demonstrating calcification and extrarenal extension

MRI features
- Good for depicting tuberculous cavities, sinuses, fistulae, and extrarenal and extraprostatic spread

Ultrasound features
- Hypoechoic or cystic masses communicating with collecting system, representing excluded calyces
- Renal tuberculomas usually appear as a solid mass
- Calcifications may be seen as echogenic foci with post-acoustic shadowing
- Thick-walled small-volume bladder
- Enlarged heterogeneous epididymis, hypoechoic lesions in the testis or diffusely hypoechoic testis
- Thickening of scrotal wall and tunica albuginea, and moderate hydrocoele

Ureters

Anatomy and embryology

- The pelvicalyceal system and ureter develop from the ureteric bud which in turn arises from the mesonephric duct
- 10–25 calyces develop per kidney
- The ureters usually lie anterior to the transverse processes of the lumbar vertebrae
- In the pelvis the ureters cross the common iliac vessels
- The ureters enter the bladder from its posterolateral surface
- The ureters and pelvis are lined by transitional epithelium

Ureteral duplications

- Result from more than one ureteric bud forming from the mesonephric duct

Incomplete
- Usually not clinically significant

Complete
- Much less common than incomplete duplication
- Weigert–Meyer rule: ureter draining the upper moiety of the kidney inserts inferior and medial to the other ureter
- Upper moiety ureteric insertion can be extravesical
- The ureter draining the lower moiety of the kidney is prone to reflux
- The upper moiety ureter is prone to develop a ureterocoele
- May present with infection, incontinence or renal impairment from obstruction

Ectopic ureterocoele

- Submucosal dilatation of the intramural ureter at the vesicoureteric junction
- Most occur in association with duplication
- May project into the bladder lumen
- Can obstruct the other ureter if a duplex system is present
- Seen more commonly in females

Extravesical insertion of ureter

- Bladder neck, urethra or vagina in females

- Associated with incontinence (chronic leakage), normal voiding and infections
- Chronic infection can lead to fibrosis and stenosis of the ureter resulting in hydronephrosis of the upper moiety

Retroperitoneal fibrosis

- Rare fibrotic retroperitoneal process

Causes and associations

- Idiopathic form known as Ormond's disease (more common in men)
- Approximately two thirds are considered idiopathic
- Peak age fifth and sixth decades of life
- Often coexists with inflammatory bowel disease, sclerosing cholangitis, fibrosing mediastinitis, Riedel's thyroiditis, sclerosing mesenteritis and orbital pseudotumour
- Can occur secondary to aortic aneurysm, retroperitoneal metastasis from lymphoma, breast carcinoma or carcinoid tumour, retroperitoneal haematoma, abscess, urinoma, diverticulitis or appendicitis
- Drugs known to be associated are ergot alkaloids and hydralazine
- Typically originates below the aortic bifurcation and extends superiorly
- Fibrosis begins just lateral to the aorta
- Usually involves the left ureter before the right
- Fibrotic process extends to the aortocaval and pericaval region
- Usually does not extend between the aorta and vertebral bodies
- The ureter can be involved at any level, but L3–5 most common
- Usually does not encase the renal pelvis
- Limited anteriorly by the peritoneum

Symptoms and signs

- Dull back, flank and abdominal pain
- As ureters are most frequently involved, pain, oliguria, anuria and eventually renal failure may occur
- Lower extremity oedema, scrotal oedema or deep vein thrombosis from compression of the inferior vena cava

Imaging features

- Soft tissue layered around the aorta and inferior vena cava
- Usually does not lift the aorta off the vertebral bodies
- Encases ureteric wall, leading to loss of peristalsis of the involved segment
- Ureteric mucosa is always spared
- Absence of peristalsis leads to functional obstruction, while the lumen remains patent
- Degree of hydronephrosis does not correlate with degree of renal insufficiency
- Passage of ureteral stents is unusually easy
- Presence of other lymphadenopathy or metastatic disease, osseous destruction
- Variable enhancement characteristics

Malignant retroperitoneal fibrosis
- Ill-defined margin or inhomogeneity of plaque is suggestive
- Malignant lymphadenopathy usually lifts the aorta from the vertebral bodies and displaces the ureters laterally

MRI features
- T1WI: low to intermediate signal intensity
- T2WI:
  - Low signal: benign retroperitoneal fibrosis (mature fibrotic plaque)
  - High signal: early benign and malignant retroperitoneal fibrosis

Pelvic lipomatosis

- The true pelvis is infiltrated by unencapsulated benign mature adipose tissue
- African-American men are affected in two thirds of cases
- Peak age third and fourth decades

Symptoms

- Non-specific abdominal or low back pain
- Urinary frequency infections
- Urinary tract obstruction in 40% of cases
- Constipation
- Associated with proliferative cystitis, particularly cystitis glandularis (75% of cases)
- Increased risk of bladder adenocarcinoma

Imaging features

Intravenous urogram
- Bladder assumes an inverted pear shape, with narrowing most prominent in the centre or inferiorly
- Elevation of bladder base
- Reduction of bladder capacity
- Medial deviation of pelvic ureters
- Dilatation of proximal ureters may also be seen

Barium enema
- Elongation and narrowing of rectum and sigmoid colon
- Intact colonic mucosa
- Enlarged retrorectal space

CT
- Confirms the presence of fat in the pelvis, with mass effect on the pelvic organs

MRI
- Signal intensity of mature fat on all pulse sequences

Trauma to the ureter

- Penetrating injury is the most common mechanism
- Acceleration or deceleration trauma can cause avulsion of the ureter, the commonest site involved is the pelviureteric junction
- This type of injury is more common in children
- Imaging findings include urinoma formation, contrast extravasation and discontinuity of the ureter

Ureteritis cystica

- Associated with chronic urinary tract infections
- Sterile submucosal fluid collections caused by intramural inflammation
- Leads to encystment and submucosal extension of transitional epithelium
- Typically multicentric smooth and round
- Seen as filling defects in the ureter on intravenous urography (intramural haemorrhage can have a similar appearance)

Bladder and urethra

Embryology

- The bladder develops from the anterior urogenital sinus of the cloaca
- It communicates with the allantois through the urachus
- The urachus becomes obliterated and forms the median umbilical ligament
- Most of the female urethra, the prostatic and membranous portions of the male urethra develop from the urethral part of the urogenital sinus
- A small portion of the urethra and vestibule in the female and the penile urethra in the male develops from the phallic part of the urogenital sinus.

Schistosomiasis

- *Schistosoma haematobium* infestation causes bladder and ureteric disease
- The eggs of the fluke cause a foreign body reaction in the bladder mucosa or distal ureter
- Affects men more commonly than women
- Symptoms include haematuria, dysuria, frequency and urgency
- Major differential diagnosis is tuberculosis
- High incidence of associated squamous cell carcinoma

Imaging features

- Plain film: calcification in bladder wall and distal ureters may be seen
- Intravenous urogram: mucosal irregularity, ureteritis cystica, ureteral dilatation and stricture (mostly limited to distal ureters)
- Persistent filling/beading in lower ureters
- Linear or parallel calcification in distal ureters
- Mucosal irregularity and reduced bladder capacity
- Bladder wall calcification can completely encircle the bladder (initially seen at the bladder base)
- Even though fibrotic the bladder still remains distensible and retains normal volume
- Calcifications are better delineated with CT and are more common on the anterior bladder wall

Inflammatory pseudotumour

- Non-neoplastic proliferation of myofibroblastic spindle cells and inflammatory cells with myxoid components
- Symptoms: haematuria, iron deficiency anaemia, fever
- Can mimic malignancy clinically and at cystoscopy and imaging

Imaging features

- Single bladder mass that may be exophytic or polypoid and may be ulcerated
- Intramural solid and cystic variants
- Tends to spare the trigone
- Invasion through the bladder wall and extravesical extension is possible
- Contrast enhancement on CT and MRI
- Internal vascularity may be seen on colour Doppler sonography

Endometriosis

- Bladder is the most common site of urinary tract involvement
- Prevalence of 1–5% in women with endometriosis
- Reported in premenopausal women only
- Cyclic haematuria occurs in only 20% of cases
- Asymptomatic or symptoms of cyclic pain, dysuria, urgency and pain
- Bladder endometriosis is deeply infiltrating
- Most lesions are found in the posterior wall of the bladder above the trigone or at the dome

Imaging features

- Can be non-specific
- Lesion location is most helpful for diagnosis
- Posterior and may be inseparable from the anterior aspect of the uterus
- MRI: haemorrhagic foci with high signal intensity on fat suppressed and non-fat suppressed T1WI
- High signal intensity on T2WI may be seen
- Contrast enhancement can be either homogeneous or peripheral

Nephrogenic adenoma

- Benign reactive process to chronic irritation

- Involves the lamina propria but spares the muscular layer
- Not premalignant
- May recur after resection in up to 63% of cases
- Symptoms: irritative voiding symptoms or haematuria
- Imaging features are nonspecific
- Polypoid or sessile masses or simply mucosal irregularity

Malacoplakia

- Chronic granulomatous condition, most frequently affecting the bladder
- Predominantly seen in women
- Peak occurrence in middle age
- More common in diabetics or immunocompromised patients
- Highly associated with *E. coli* infection
- Symptoms: gross haematuria, signs of urinary tract infection

Imaging features

- Multiple, polypoid, vascular, solid masses or circumferential wall thickening
- Can be extremely aggressive, invading the perivesical space or even bone destruction

Cystitis

- Cystitis cystica and cystitis glandularis (chronic reactive inflammatory disorders
- Can occur at any age
- Symptoms: frequency, dysuria, urgency, haematuria

Imaging features

- Filling defects at urography
- Hypervascular polypoid mass on CT and MR
- Low signal on T1WI; predominantly low signal on T2WI with central branching high signal
- Muscle layer is intact

Malignant tumours of the bladder

- Accounts for 4% of all malignancies
- Peak age sixth and seventh decade
- More common in men (3:1)
- 95% are carcinomas
- The most common non-epithelial malignancy is leiomyosarcoma
- Other pelvic malignancies can infiltrate into the bladder
- Stomach and breast cancers may metastasise to the bladder

Anatomy

- Ovoid in shape
- 3.5–4.0 cm in length
- Covered by a fibrous capsule called the tunica albuginea
- Mediastinum testis: vertical invagination of the fibrous capsule in the posterosuperior portion of the testis (spermatic cord enters testis here)
- Multiple lobules form each testis, the apices of which converge into the mediastinum
- The seminiferous tubules in each lobule coalesce and enter the mediastinum testis
- These form 12–20 efferent ductules after multiple anastomosis

Epididymis

- Continuation of the ductal system of the testis
- Lies posterolateral to testis
- Head of the epididymis (globus major) is lateral to the upper pole of the testis (normally 7–8 mm in diameter)
- The body and tail of epididymis extend inferiorly and continue as the vas deferens

Vas deferens

- Ascends on posterior aspect of spermatic cord
- Leaves spermatic cord at deep inguinal ring
- Extends anterior to internal iliac artery
- Descends between the posterior surface of bladder and the superior pole of the seminal vesicle
- Forms ejaculatory duct by joining seminal vesicle at base of prostate
- Ejaculatory duct opens into urethra adjacent to veru montanum and prostatic utricle

Spermatic cord

- Composed of the vas deferens and vessels, lymphatics and nerves
- Internal spermatic (testicular) artery, external spermatic (cremasteric) artery and artery to the vas are the arteries in the cord
- The pampiniform plexus drains the scrotum into the ipsilateral testicular vein
- The cremasteric nerve, genital branch of the genitofemoral nerve and the testicular sympathetic plexus are the nerves in the cord
- Lymphatic vessels ascend with the testicular vessels and drain into the lateral and preaortic nodes

Scrotum

- Wall is derived from the layers of the abdominal wall
- The tunica vaginalis is in continuity with the peritoneal processus vaginalis. The tunica vaginalis is reflected on itself forming a visceral and parietal layer. The visceral layer is closely applied to the testis, epididymis and posterior scrotal wall. The parietal layer is in contact with the scrotal wall
- The dartos is a highly vascularised muscle layer of the scrotum

Embryology

- Genital ridges extend from the sixth thoracic to the second sacral segments
- Coelomic epithelial cells migrate into and proliferate to form primitive sex cords
- Germ cells in the wall of the yolk sac migrate into the sex cords through along the hindgut and dorsal mesenteric root
- In the presence of a Y chromosome, primitive sex cords form the seminiferous tubules
- The migrated germ cells form the spermatogonia
- The mesenchyme between the seminiferous tubules forms the Leydig's cells
- The tunica albuginea forms along the surface of the primitive testis
- At about 8 weeks the Leydig's cells begin to secrete testosterone
- Under hormonal influence, the mesonephric ducts develop into the epididymis, vas deferens, seminal vesicles and ejaculatory ducts

- The paramesonephric ducts regress
- Between 7 and 8 weeks the testes descend into the pelvis and remain near the deep inguinal ring until the seventh month
- The testes descend through the inguinal canal into the scrotal sac

Acute epididymitis

- Commonest acute scrotal pathology in postpubertal age group
- Retrograde infection from the urethra or prostate is thought to be the cause
- Symptoms: presents as acute or subacute pain and fever, dysuria
- Signs: scrotal erythema, pyuria
- Orchitis develops a complication in 20% of patients

Ultrasound features

- Swollen epididymis (> 5 mm thickness)
- Usually hypoechoic (rarely hyperechoic)
- Thickening of the scrotal skin and/or hydrocoele
- Increased vascularity on colour Doppler is suggestive of inflammation
- Hyperaemia may be the only sign in up to 20% of patients
- Hyperaemia may be focal
- Complex fluid collection around the testis is suggestive of pyocoele
- Hypoechoic area in the testis may indicate orchitis

Chronic epididymitis

Imaging features

Ultrasound
- Swollen epididymis which may be hyperechoic on ultrasound

MRI
- Epididymal inflammation as evidenced by increase in size, increased signal on T2WI, sympathetic hydrocoele, increased number of vessels seen with signal voids
- Patchy areas of low signal intensity may be seen in areas of orchitis. Normal testis is of high signal intensity

Varicocoele

- Compressible tangle of veins in the scrotum measuring > 2 mm in diameter
- Abnormal dilatation of pampiniform venous plexus
- Results from incompetent valves of the internal testicular vein; rarely caused by venous obstruction
- Commonest treatable cause of male infertility
- More common on left side (95%)
- Ultrasound: compressible, tortuous vessels, made more prominent by standing up or Valsalva manoeuvre. Colour Doppler demonstrates flow

Orchitis

- Infection of the testis
- Most common complication of mumps infection in postpubertal males
- Mumps orchitis is more commonly unilateral

Imaging features

Ultrasound
- Diffuse enlargement of the testis
- Homogeneously hypoechoic
- Can also appear normal or have a diffusely inhomogeneous texture
- Vascularity may be increased especially when compared with the normal side
- Epididymis or scrotal skin may be abnormal
- Testis may return to normal once the inflammation resolves or may atrophy
- Atrophy is usually detectable within 6 months
- Unilateral atrophy in one third of patients with mumps orchitis and bilateral in 10%
- Focal orchitis is difficult to distinguish from cancer, but usually does not distort the contour of the testis
- Discrete intratesticular fluid collection, which is typically complex
- Gas if present will produce 'dirty' acoustic shadowing

Malignant testicular neoplasm

- Approximately 1% of all male malignancies
- Commonest malignancy in 15- to 30-year-old males
- Usually presents as painless scrotal swelling
- Infarction or haemorrhage into the tumour can mimic torsion or epididymoorchitis

Classification

- Primary germ cell
- Primary non-germ cell
- Metastatic
- Germ cell tumours constitute 95%, of which 40% are seminomas and 40% have mixed histology (teratocarcinoma is the commonest among mixed)
- Non-seminomatous germ cell tumours are more aggressive. These include embryonal cell carcinoma, teratoma, choriocarcinoma and yolk sac carcinoma
- Serum alpha-fetoprotein levels are increased in 60% patients with testicular cancer
- Serum beta-human chorionic gonadotropin levels are increased in 50% patients with testicular cancer
- Pure seminomas do not cause increase in alpha-fetoprotein
- Non-germ cell tumours are usually benign
- Leydig cell tumours may produce testosterone and 30% may be associated with precocious virilisation or feminisation. Sertoli cell tumours can produce oestrogen and can present with gynaecomastia
- Lymphoma is the most common tumour in older men and may be bilateral
- Prostate, lung, kidney, gastrointestinal tract, myeloma and leukaemia are other recognised primary sites that metastasise to the testis (lymphatic and haematogenous spread)
- Haematogenous spread does not occur before lymphatic spread
- Sentinel lymph node group for a left testicular cancer is the left renal perihilar group, immediately below the left renal vein
- A right testicular cancer first metastasises to the paracaval lymph node group at or below the right renal vein
- Paralumbar nodes below the renal hilum and thoracic sites are involved later
- If local spread into the epididymis or scrotum has occurred, iliac and inguinal lymph nodes may become involved
- Choriocarcinoma is prone to early haematogenous metastasis
- Haematogenous spread is most common to the lungs
- Liver, bone and brain are other sites involved
- Brain metastases are common with choriocarcinoma
- Germ cell tumour metastases may have histology characteristics different from those of the original tumour

Imaging features

Ultrasound

- Most tumours are hypoechoic

Seminoma

- Uniform decreased echogenicity
- Usually focal but may be diffuse
- May cause bulging of tunica albuginea if focal and peripheral
- Usually sharp interface with normal parenchyma
- Generalised hypoechoic appearance in diffuse infiltration

Lymphoma or metastatic disease

- Usually focal hypoechoic mass
- Mixed histology and non-seminomatous germ cell tumours
- Heterogeneous due to cystic areas or hyperechoic foci
- Less distinct tumour margin
- Contour of the testis may be lobulated

Differential diagnosis for a focal intratesticular mass

- Orchitis
- Haematoma
- Abscess

- Enlargement of the epididymis, scrotal skin thickening and hydrocoele are more commonly associated with inflammatory processes
- Small hydrocoele may be seen in about 10% of tumours

Staging (TNM)

- **Low-stage disease:** tumour confined to the testis, epididymis or spermatic cord (T1–T3) and mild to moderate adenopathy (N1and N2)
- **Advanced-stage disease:** tumour that invades the scrotal wall (T4), significant retroperitoneal adenopathy (N3), or visceral metastasis (M1)

Testicular calcifications and microlithiasis

- Large calcifications may be seen with tumours (teratocarcinoma, seminoma, embryonal cell carcinoma, and Sertoli and Leydig cell tumour)
- Large irregular calcifications seen with teratoma
- Treated cancers, old infections, haematomas and infarcts can also calcify
- Microlithiasis (tiny, 1–2 mm), diffuse calcifications in the seminiferous tubules
- May be bilateral but asymmetrical
- Seen also in cryptorchid or atrophic testis

Testicular cysts

- Benign cysts: simple cysts, tubular ectasia, epidermoid cyst, tunica albuginea cyst
- Intratesticular varicocoele, abscess and haemorrhage
- Malignant cyst: teratoma

Tunica albuginea cyst
- Mean age at presentation: 40 years
- 2–5 mm in diameter
- Location—upper anterior or lateral aspect of testis
- Uni- or multilocular
- If palpable, firm to palpation

Simple cysts
- Tend to occur in men 40 years or older
- Usually 2 mm to 2 cm in diameter
- More often arise near mediastinum testis
- Usually not palpable (when palpable are not firm)
- Usually single but can be multiple
- Imperceptible wall on ultrasound with through transmission

Epidermoid cysts
- Germ cell origin (so called keratocysts)
- Non-tender and usually palpable
- Age usually 20–40 years
- Size usually 1–3 cm

Ultrasound
- Varies with cyst content
- A solid mass with an echogenic rim and onion ring appearance
- Avascular

Undescended testis

- Root of scrotum (50%)
- Within inguinal canal (20%)
- Abdominal: any location between lower pole of the kidney and internal ring (10%)
- Bilateral (10%)
- Ultrasound is useful to identify the testes in extra-abdominal location (it is essential to identify the mediastinum testis)
- Laparoscopy and MRI are used for locating the testes within the abdomen

Testicular trauma

- Intratesticular: may need surgical intervention
- Extratesticular: usually managed conservatively
- Ultrasound readily distinguishes between the two types

Testicular torsion

- Also termed torsion of the spermatic cord
- Causes obstruction of the blood supply to the testis

Extravaginal
- Occurs in fetuses and neonates

- The testis, epididymis and tunica vaginalis twist in the spermatic cord

Intravaginal

- More common in the peripubertal period
- Associated with bell clapper deformity (tunica completely surrounds the testis) and seen in around 12% of males

Clinical features

- Acute onset of severe scrotal pain and associated nausea and vomiting
- Scrotal swelling and erythema
- Difficult to palpate the testis
- 10% may be bilateral
- Spontaneous detorsion may occur

Ultrasound

- Grey scale is sensitive but not specific
- Colour Doppler ultrasound approaches 100% specificity

Differential diagnoses

- Acute epididymitis
- Epididymo-orchitis
- Testicular abscess
- Torsion of testicular appendix
- Incarcerated hernia
- Scrotal haematoma
- Ruptured varicocoele
- Scrotal tumour (rarely)

Anatomy

- Derived from the urethral epithelium
- Prostatic utricle develops from the epithelium of the urogenital sinus, Wolffian ducts and Müllerian ducts

Benign prostatic hyperplasia

- Unusual below 40 years
- Affects 50–75% of men over 60 years
- More common in Afro-Caribbean patients and in patients with diabetes and hypertension

Symptoms

- Usually results from obstruction of the urethra at the level of the prostate
- Hesitancy, diminution in the strength of the urinary stream, post-void dribbling, sensation of incomplete emptying
- Frequency and urgency from uninhibited contractions of the detrusor muscle
- Overflow incontinence and nocturia with increasing volumes of residual urine
- Chronic urinary retention

Pathology

- Involves the glandular tissue surrounding the prostatic urethra, in the transitional zone
- Commonly situated closer to the proximal end of veru montanum

Imaging features

Intravenous urogram
- 'J-hook' configuration of the distal ureters
- Visualisation of the entire ureter in a single film
- Dilatation of the ureter and tortuosity of the ureter if obstruction is long standing
- Pelvicalyceal dilatation with renal cortical thinning if obstructive nephropathy has developed
- Trabeculation of the bladder and diverticula formation
- Prominent prostatic impression on the bladder

Transrectal ultrasound
- Usually possible to differentiate the central and transitional zones
- Adenomatous nodules may appear as hyper- or hypoechoic areas; biopsy is required to exclude cancer

MRI
- Glandular hyperplastic nodules are of high signal intensity on T2WI
- Low or high signal intensity on T1WI
- Stromal proliferation gives decreased signal on T1WI and T2WI

Prostatitis

- Usually presents with pain
- Imaging is not usually indicated
- MRI: low signal intensity on T2WI (in peripheral zone) without focal mass or capsular irregularity
- Chronic inflammation can appear similar to cancer

Prostate carcinoma

- Most common malignancy in men
- Tumour differentiation and size are important for predicting behaviour and prognosis

Gleason grading system

Grades 1–5 depend on tumour differentiation:
- Grade 1 well differentiated, grade 5 poorly differentiated
- Grades 4 and 5 have potential for lymphatic spread

Grades of the two predominant histologic patterns in any specimen are summed to give the Gleason score:
- 2–4 is well differentiated
- 5–7 moderately differentiated
- 8–10 poorly differentiated

Size: larger tumours are more often associated with metastases

- 85% are located in the peripheral zone

Staging

- A: Occult cancer
- B: Confined to the capsule; suitable for radical surgery
- C: Extracapsular spread; non-surgical therapy
- D: Distant metastasis

Imaging features

Transrectal ultrasound

- Round or oval hypoechoic lesion in the peripheral zone (classic appearance)
- Iso- or hyperechoic lesions can also occur
- Distortion of the regular contour of the prostate is used to direct biopsy

MRI

- Transaxial T1WIs are used to assess periprostatic extension
- Axial and sagittal T2WIs are also routinely acquired
- Foci of low signal in the peripheral zone (fibrosis, prostatitis and calcification) can also cause a similar appearance
- Haemorrhage after biopsy can cause low or high signal on T2WI (high signal on corresponding T1WI will also be seen)

- Mucinous adenocarcinoma and small infiltrating cancers may be very difficult to detect

Patterns of metastases

- Nodal metastasis to local lymph nodes
- Obturator, internal iliac and external iliac groups
- More than 80% of patients with lymph node metastases develop bone metastases within 5 years

Osseous metastasis

- Majority are osteoblastic
- 5% are purely lytic
- 10% are mixed osteolytic and osteoblastic
- The pelvic bones, lumbar spine, femur, thoracic spine and ribs are involved, in descending order of frequency
- Prostate-specific antigen levels > 58 ng/ml are indicative of bone metastasis

Intrathoracic metastasis

- 6% of patients at first diagnosis have intrathoracic metastasis
- 25% of patients with stage D cancer have lung or pleural involvement
- Lymphangitis carcinomatosis is more common pattern than lung nodules

Anatomy

- The adrenal gland is 4–6 cm in length. Its limbs are 3–6 mm thick. It has two parts—cortex and medulla
- Blood supply is via the inferior, middle and superior adrenal arteries
- Cortex is derived from mesoderm—forms about 90% of the gland
- Cortex is subdivided into zona glomerulosa (aldosterone), zona fasciculata (cortisol) and zona reticularis (epiandrosterone)
- Medulla is derived from the neuroectoderm and secretes adrenaline and noradrenaline (epinephrine and norepinephrine)
- Right gland is posterior to the inferior vena cava and lateral to the right crus of diaphragm
- Left gland is lateral to the aorta and left crus of diaphragm
- Venous drainage from the right adrenal gland is to the inferior vena cava. The left adrenal gland drains into the superior aspect of the left renal vein, hence adrenal vein sampling may be used to localise the side of the abnormality in the case of a functioning adenoma not detected by imaging

Imaging

- Abdominal X-ray: calcifications may be detected
- Ultrasound: normal glands are often not visible
- Scintigraphy:
  - Iodine-131 labelled 6 beta-iodomethyl-19-norcholesterol used to investigate adrenocortical pathology
  - Iodine-131 labelled meta-iodobenzylguanidine/indium-111 octreotide used to investigate functional lesions of the adrenal medulla
  - Fluorine-18 labelled fluorodeoxyglucose (FDG) positron emission tomography (PET) is useful in differentiating benign from malignant pathology

- CT: contrast washout properties can be used to help characterise adrenal masses
- MRI: T1WI, T2WI and chemical shift imaging is employed for characterisation of masses
- Angiography: only used in certain specific conditions

Adrenal adenomas

- 2–10% normal people at autopsy and 1% of patients undergoing abdominal CT
- In the absence of known malignancy, adrenal masses < 1.5 cm are almost always adenomas
- Adenomas remain stable in size over time
- The majority are non-functional (non-secreting)

Imaging features

- Attenuation values < 10 HU at unenhanced CT (71% sensitive and 98% specific for adenoma)
- Contrast material washout occurs rapidly in adenomas, resulting in 60% or more washout (< 30 HU) at 15-minute delayed-phase imaging

MRI
- Characteristic high-signal rim on fat-saturated SE sequence
- Non-functioning adenomas: isointense to liver on T1WI and iso- or hyperintense on T2WI with relative loss of signal intensity on out-of-phase imaging

Adrenal myelolipoma

- Uncommon, benign, encapsulated lesion
- Incidental detection; may be large at presentation
- No malignant potential
- Large tumours can bleed spontaneously and become centrally necrotic
- Always non-functioning

Imaging features

- Hallmark on imaging is the demonstration of lesional fat
- Ultrasound: increased echogenicity

- CT: heterogeneous; foci of calcification in 20% (especially if haemorrhage has occurred)
- MRI: high signal on T1WI in areas of fat and previous haemorrhage. Chemical shift artefact on out-of-phase imaging

Adrenal cyst

- 45% endothelial cysts; 40% pseudocysts (secondary to previous haemorrhage, infarction or cystic degeneration)
- May be large (> 3 cm) at presentation

Imaging features

- Peripheral or curvilinear calcification in 15%
- Thick irregular walls and septations may be seen with pseudocysts

Adrenal haemorrhage

- Acute haemorrhage can be spontaneous, post-traumatic (more common on right side) or due to coagulation disorders
- Metastases (e.g. melanoma) are prone to spontaneous haemorrhage
- Up to 20% of haemorrhage is bilateral: this requires assessment for adrenal insufficiency
- Spontaneous haemorrhage should become smaller on follow up

Imaging features

- MRI: varying signal intensity depending on age of bleed
- Calcifications may develop beyond 1 year

Phaeochromocytoma

- Rule of tens: 10% extra-adrenal, 10% malignant, 10% extra-abdominal, 10% familial and 10% bilateral
- Catecholamine-secreting tumours, derived from chromaffin cells of the adrenal medulla
- 90% of phaeochromocytomas are located within the adrenal glands
- 98% occur in the abdomen
- Usually unilateral and benign
- Extra-adrenal phaeochromocytomas are considered to be paragangliomas; up to 40% of these are malignant. Most common extra-adrenal site is the organ of Zuckerkandl situated at the aortic bifurcation
- Can occur as part of a syndrome: multiple endocrine neoplasia (MEN) types 2 and 3, neurofibromatosis, von Hippel–Lindau syndrome, Sturge–Weber syndrome, Carney's triad and tuberous sclerosis
- Clinical features: headaches, palpitations, excessive sweating, tremor, anxiety, hypertension
- Occasional hypertensive crisis can be induced by contrast medium

Imaging features

- Usually > 3 cm
- Characteristically solid and hypervascular. Central necrosis, calcification and cystic changes may rarely be present
- MRI: low, intermediate or high signal intensity on T2WI
- Atypical features such as areas of fat density and contrast washout may be encountered
- Scintigraphy: meta-iodobenzylguanidine (mIBG) and octreotide uptake. FDG avid
- Laboratory: increased vanilmandelic acid levels in 24-hour urine sampling

Adrenal carcinoma

- Very rare; can be functioning or non-functioning
- Associated with MEN type 1
- Two peaks: one in paediatric population; other in fourth and fifth decades of life
- Large tumour size (> 12 cm), intratumoural haemorrhage and high mitotic rates are predictors of poor prognosis
- Cushing's syndrome and virilisation are frequently present
- Metastasises by haematogenous and lymphatic spread

Imaging features

- Calcification seen in 20–30% of cases
- CT: large inhomogeneous mass with heterogeneous enhancement pattern

Adrenal metastasis

- 1–2% of patients have incidental adrenal masses on cross-sectional imaging

- In patients with known cancer of any type, 38–57% of detected adrenal nodules are metastatic
- Lung, breast, renal and melanoma are commonest primary sites
- Metastases are commonly larger; heterogeneous and poorly marginated
- Frequently bilateral. Thick irregularly enhancing rim may be seen

Imaging features

- CT: delayed contrast washout
- PET: considered positive if FDG uptake greater than or equal to liver uptake
  - False positives occur in around 5% of adenomas, especially those that are functional
  - Phaeochromocytoma, inflammatory conditions and cysts may also cause false positive PET results
  - False negatives can occur with lesions < 1 cm, metastasis from carcinoid and bronchioloalveolar carcinoma, haemorrhage, necrosis and metastasis from clear cell renal carcinoma
- PET-CT has better diagnostic accuracy than either dynamic CT or MRI
- Chemical shift MRI: most metastatic lesions do not show signal dropout unlike adenomas. False positives can occur with 'fat poor' adenomas and phaeochromocytomas

Adrenal lymphoma

- Most commonly occurs in patients with non-Hodgkin's lymphoma
- Bilateral involvement is common (70%)
- Diffuse glandular enlargement or more discrete solid masses
- Commonly associated with lymphadenopathy

Cushing's syndrome

- Due to a chronic excess of circulating glucocorticoids
- Clinical features: obesity, plethora, bruising, striae, muscle wasting, diabetes mellitus (10–15%), osteoporosis, hypertension

Causes

- 70% due to adrenocorticotropic hormone (ACTH) secreting pituitary adenoma
- 5% due to ectopic ACTH secretion by lung, islet cell pancreatic or ovarian tumours
- 20% due to adrenal adenomas (usually 2–4 cm in size)
- 5% due to adrenal cortical carcinoma (only 10% of these cause Cushing's syndrome)

Imaging features

- CT is the modality of choice in corticotropin-independent Cushing's syndrome
- Cortisol-producing adenomas have a characteristic low density and the remainder of the glands becomes atrophic due to ACTH-induced suppression of activity
- In adrenal hyperplasia due to excess ACTH secretion, diffuse bilateral enlargement without a focal lesion is the most commonly encountered pattern
- Adrenal venous sampling is a useful additional test if no cause is identified on CT

Conn's syndrome

- Results from hypersecretion of aldosterone
- Causes hypertension, hypokalaemia, polyuria and hypernatremia
- Female predilection with peak incidence in the fourth and fifth decade
- 70% due to aldosterone-secreting adenoma
- Remainder mostly due to adrenal cortical hyperplasia
- Usually < 2 cm in size if caused by an adenoma

Imaging features

- CT: solitary adenomas are usually small, with low attenuation and eccentrically situated
- In adrenal hyperplasia, the gland is mildly enlarged with an irregular outline (limb of adrenal > 10 mm, but shape is maintained)
- Up to one third of patients will have morphologically normal glands
- If the CT appearance is normal, venous sampling can be useful as the tumour can be very small

Adrenal hypofunction

- Primary: results from destruction of the cortex
- Secondary: results from inadequate stimulation by the pituitary gland

Causes of primary adrenal cortical failure

- Autoimmune disorders
- Infection (fungal or tuberculous); glandular enlargement when acute; calcifications if chronic
- Drug induced
- Bilateral adrenal haemorrhage
- Metastases
- Sarcoidosis
- Haemochromatosis
- Amyloidosis

Multiple endocrine neoplasia

- Conditions in which tumour or hyperplasia of two or more endocrine organs occur. There are three main types. All are autosomal dominant

  - **MEN type 1:** adrenal cortical nodules or functioning adenoma, parathyroid hyperplasia or adenoma, pancreatic islet cell tumour, pituitary adenoma and carcinoid tumour. Multiple lipomas and thyroid nodules may also occur
  - **MEN type 2A:** phaeochromocytomas, medullary carcinoma of the thyroid and parathyroid hyperplasia or adenoma
  - **MEN type 2B:** phaeochromocytomas of the adrenal medulla and thyroid medullary carcinoma, soft tissue neuromas, ganglioneuromatosis of the intestine and Marfanoid features
- Increased incidence of extra-adrenal phaeochromocytomas in MEN Type 2
- **Carney's triad:** gastric leiomyogenic neoplasms, extra-adrenal phaeochromocytomas or paragangliomas and pulmonary chondromas

Adrenal collision tumour

- Co-existing histologically different tumours within the same gland as in MEN syndromes (both benign and malignant in the same gland)

Anatomy

- Inner mucosa called the endometrium
- Middle muscular layer called the myometrium
- Outer serosal layer called the perimetrium
- Internal os divides the uterus into corpus and cervix
- Fallopian tubes enter the uterus at the cornua
- Fundus is located superior to the cornua
- Cervix projects into the vagina
- Bladder lies anteriorly and rectum posteriorly
- Broad ligaments are peritoneal folds that extend from the lateral sides of the uterus to the pelvic side walls
- Fallopian tubes and uterine arteries run in the broad ligaments
- Size of uterus and endometrial thickness vary with age and menstrual cycle

Hysterosalpingography

- Radiographic evaluation of uterus and fallopian tubes
- Best method for visualising and evaluating fallopian tubes

Indications

- Infertility
- Recurrent spontaneous abortions
- Postoperative evaluation following reversal of tubal ligation or tubal ligation
- Preoperative evaluation prior to myomectomy

Contraindications

- Pregnancy
- Active pelvic infection

Technique

- Performed between days 7 and 12 of the menstrual cycle
- Water-soluble contrast material is used

Complications

- Bleeding
- Infection
- Contrast medium reaction
- Uterine injury
- Potential for irradiation of a very early, unsuspected pregnancy

MRI of the uterus and ovaries

- T2WI demonstrates the zonal anatomy very well in the reproductive age group
- Endometrium is of high signal intensity
- Junctional zone is of low signal intensity
- Peripheral myometrium has intermediate signal intensity (higher than striated muscle)
- Cervical zonal architecture is also well seen on T2WI
- Epithelium and mucus are seen as central high signal intensity
- The fibrous stroma in the middle has low signal intensity
- The peripheral myometrium has medium signal intensity
- Zonal anatomy becomes indistinct post-menopause

Ovary in the reproductive age group (T2WI)

- Low signal stroma
- High signal follicles

Congenital anomalies (see box opposite)

- Prevalence of 2–3%

Female infertility

Causes

- Ovulatory dysfunction in 30–40% cases
- Hyperprolactinaemia due to drugs or prolactin-producing pituitary tumours
- Polycystic ovarian syndrome
- Disorders of fallopian tubes in 30–40% of cases
- Damage or obstruction to the tubes
- Peritubal adhesions
- Adenomyosis
- Leiomyoma
- Endometriosis

American fertility society classification of anomalies

- **Class I (absence of Müllerian ducts)**
  Agenesis of the vagina, uterus or uterine tubes, either alone or in combination

- **Class II**
  Agenesis or incomplete development of one Müllerian duct, e.g. unicornuate uterus

- **Class III**
  Complete lack of fusion of the Müllerian ducts (uterus didelphys)

- **Class IV**
  Partial failure of Müllerian duct fusion (bicornuate uterus)

- **Class V**
  Septate uterus (commonest uterine anomaly). A fibrous septum may divide the endometrial cavity alone (partial septate) or extends into the endocervical canal

- **Class VI**
  Arcuate uterus (considered a normal variant)

- **Class VII**
  Uterine anomalies associated with diethylstilbestrol exposure

Gestational trophoblastic disease

- Chorionic tissue that undergoes hydropic change but retains the capacity to produce chorionic gonadotrophins
- Consists of a spectrum of diseases: hydatidiform mole, chorioadenoma destruens (invasive mole) and malignant choriocarcinoma
- Complete or classic hydatidiform mole: hydropic enlargement of chorionic villi, resulting in multiple vesicles of varying size
- Rarely associated with fetal tissue
- The majority of hydatidiform moles are complete moles
- Presents with heavy painless vaginal bleeding in the first trimester
- Hydropic placental tissue may be passed per vaginum
- Severe hyperemesis gravidarum may be the presenting feature
- Uterine size is usually large for gestational age
- Ovarian cysts (theca lutein) are common
- Partial or incomplete moles present with a dysmorphic, frequently triploid, fetus
- Chorioadenoma destruens is locally invasive, but nonmetastatic (represents < 10% of gestational trophoblastic disease)

Ultrasound features

- Enlarged uterus
- Multiple small anechoic areas (3–10 mm diameter) in uterine cavity

Differential diagnoses

- Hydropic placental degeneration after incomplete abortion
- Myxoid degeneration of a leiomyoma
- Retained products of conception
- Endometrial proliferative disease

Choriocarcinoma

- Need not necessarily follow a pregnancy
- Can arise in the ovary or testis
- Pathologically there are no recognisable villous structures
- Syncytial and cytotrophoblasts are interspersed between areas of haemorrhage and necrosis
- Haematogenous dissemination to the lungs, liver, kidneys, brain and gastrointestinal tract can occur

Ultrasound features

- Sonographic appearance is similar to hydatidiform mole
- Myometrial invasion and metastases may be evident
- Theca lutein cysts that fail to resolve 3–4 months after evacuation of the uterus are suggestive of residual or metastatic disease

Pelvic inflammatory disease

- Multibacterial infectious diseases of the genital tract, ovary or pelvic peritoneum
- Symptoms: lower abdominal pain, vaginal discharge, cervical motion tenderness, adnexal tenderness, dyspareunia
- Usually begins as cervicitis
- Secondarily involves the endometrial cavity and fallopian tubes
- Tubal spillage results in local peritonitis and oophoritis
- Adnexal adhesions can result causing fusion of the tube and ovary
- Necrosis of the inflamed mass can result in tubo-ovarian abscess

Imaging features

- Variable appearance depending on extent and severity of involvement and development of complications

Ultrasound

- Up to one third of patients have normal examination
- Enlarged and ill-defined uterus
- Excessive fluid in the endometrial cavity
- Indistinct central endometrial echo complex
- Tubes visible with thick echogenic walls
- Hydro- or pyosalpinx visualised as cystic adnexal masses
- Loculated collections in the adnexa or pouch of Douglas

CT

- Nonspecific features
- Bilateral low-attenuation adnexal masses with thickened walls representing tubo-ovarian complex
- Enlarged ill-defined uterus
- Hydrosalpinx may appear as fluid-filled multicystic mass
- Increased density of pelvic fat
- Thickening of uterosacral ligaments
- Pelvic ascites

Uterine tuberculosis

- Commonly involves the fallopian tubes

Hysterosalpingogram features

- Almost always bilateral and asymmetrical
- Flask-shaped dilatation of fallopian tubes due to obstruction at the fimbria
- Tubes may not be seen if the obstruction is at the uterine end
- Tubal sacculation with infiltration of contrast material around the fallopian tube
- Focal irregularity and areas of tubal calcification
- Rigid shortened fallopian tubes
- Synechiae in the uterine cavity
- Complete obliteration of the uterine cavity may occur in late-stage disease

Endometrial hyperplasia

- Overgrowth of normal endometrium due to unopposed persistent oestrogen
- May occur during periods of infrequent ovulation, administration of exogenous oestrogens and oestrogen-producing ovarian neoplasms
- Tamoxifen therapy can cause endometrial hyperplasia
- Low risk of progression to endometrial carcinoma

Endometrial polyp

- Polypoid mass originating in the endometrium
- May be a true polyp, submucosal fibroid or endometrial carcinoma
- Can cause bleeding
- In postmenopausal women, 10% of endometrial polyps are malignant

Endometrial carcinoma

- Most common gynaecological malignancy
- Predominantly affects postmenopausal women
- Prolonged unopposed oestrogen activity is a major risk factor
- Usually presents with abnormal vaginal bleeding
- 85% are adenocarcinomas
- Histologic grade of neoplasm, depth of myometrial invasion and presence of metastatic lymphadenopathy influence prognosis
- Local invasion, lymphatic spread to aortocaval and pelvic lymph nodes, and haematogenous metastasis to liver, lungs or brain are common routes of spread

Ultrasound features

- Thickening of the endometrial stripe > 8 mm (postmenopausal), > 15 mm (premenopausal)
- Thinning of the inner myometrium adjacent to the echogenic endometrium is suggestive of myometrial invasion
- Obliteration of the hypoechoic layer suggests deep myometrial invasion

Endometriosis

- Primarily affects women of reproductive age (mean age at diagnosis 25–29 years)
- 24% of women with pelvic pain may have endometriosis, 20% of women undergoing laparoscopy for infertility investigation may have endometriosis
- Obstructive Müllerian duct anomalies of the uterus or vagina account for most cases of endometriosis in girls aged < 17 years
- Around 5% of cases occur in postmenopausal women
- Caused by functioning endometrium located outside the uterus
- Ovaries are the most common sites involved
- May also involve the gastrointestinal tract, urinary tract, chest and soft tissues
- Endometriosis of the gastrointestinal tract occurs in 12–37% patients with endometriosis (rectosigmoid colon is most common site involved)
- Pathologic findings depend on duration of disease and depth of penetration of lesions
- Mature endometriotic tissue initiates an inflammatory response with areas of haemorrhage, fibrosis and adhesion formation

Symptoms

- Some patients are asymptomatic
- Others may present with pelvic pain, dysmenorrhoea, dyspareunia, infertility, adnexal masses or rectal discomfort
- Symptoms may not correlate with the severity of the disease

Diagnosis

- Laparoscopy is the gold standard for diagnosis

Complications

Gastrointestinal implants
- Double-contrast barium enema: variable appearance. Often asymmetrical, with a puckered or crenulated appearance to the affected wall
- Adhesions: difficult to define radiologically (fixed pelvic organs are suggestive)

Cyst rupture
- Uncommon (can occur during pregnancy)

Malignant transformation
- Rare (< 1%)
- 75% arise from endometriosis of the ovary
- Endometrioid carcinoma is the most common

Imaging features

Ultrasound
- Indicated for diagnosis of endometriotic cysts
- Majority of cysts exhibit diffuse low-level internal echoes
- Classic endometrioma is a homogeneous, hypoechoic focal ovarian lesion
- Some cysts are anechoic an can mimic a simple ovarian cyst
- May be unilocular or multilocular
- Thin or thick septations may be seen
- Solid wall nodules may be seen and mimic neoplasia
- Hyperechoic foci in the wall may be seen and is predictive of endometrioma
- Lesions that resolve on follow-up examinations are unlikely to be endometriomas

> **Differential for ultrasound appearances in endometriosis**
> - Dermoid cyst
> - Haemorrhagic cyst
> - Cystic neoplasm

MRI
- T1, T2 and fat-suppressed T1WI are routinely performed
- Homogeneous high signal on T1WI

- Contrast enhancement is not particularly useful and it should be reserved for cases suspicious of malignancy
- Degenerated blood products may give high signal on T1WI and T2WI
- Loss of signal (shading) seen on T2WI is an important feature
- Shading can range from faint, dependent layering to complete signal void
- The fibrous nature of the cyst wall gives a low signal on both T1WI and T2WI
- Other high signal intensity lesions on T1WI include dermoids, mucinous cystic neoplasms and haemorrhagic masses
- Dermoid cysts demonstrate chemical shift artefact and signal dropout on fat suppression
- Signal intensity of mucinous tumours is less than that of fat or blood
- Haemorrhagic corpus luteal cysts have similar appearance to endometriomas, however these are usually unilocular and unilateral. Haemorrhagic cysts do not exhibit shading and resolve with time

Adenomyosis

- Presence of endometrial tissue and stroma in the myometrium
- Induces overgrowth of surrounding smooth muscle
- Typically presents in women aged 40–50 years
- Two thirds present with menorrhagia or dysmenorrhoea

Focal and diffuse forms

- Diffuse form is more common, distributed asymmetrically in the uterus
- Difficult to differentiate from leiomyomas on ultrasound
- Adenomyosis is less well defined than leiomyomas
- Always contiguous with the junctional zone
- Margins appear 'shaggy'
- Minimal mass effect on the endometrial canal

MRI features

- Short axis measurement of the junctional zone ≥ 12 mm
- Thickness of 8–12 mm is considered indeterminate
- Hyperintense 2–4 mm foci in the thickened junctional zone on T2WI
- Often oriented parallel to the endometrial strip

Fibroid uterus (leiomyoma)

- Common benign neoplasm, occurring in 20–40% of women
- Derived from myometrial smooth muscle
- Most women are asymptomatic
- May present as palpable abdominal masses or with pelvic pain, abnormal bleeding or infertility or with symptoms related to pressure on the bladder or rectum
- Can be subserosal, submucosal or intramural
- May undergo degeneration, necrosis or calcification
- Variable appearance on imaging depending on location and degeneration
- Coarse dystrophic calcification is a relatively specific feature

Imaging features

Ultrasound

- Majority appear as focal hypoechoic masses
- Increased echogenicity may be seen in some fibroids
- Distortion of the endometrial cavity may be seen with submucosal fibroids

MRI

- Low signal intensity on T2WI
- One third of leiomyomas demonstrate a high signal intensity rim on T2WI
- Well circumscribed with well-defined margins
- Subserosal exophytic fibroids demonstrate a 'bridging-vessel sign' (presence of flow voids on T1WI and T2WI from branches of the uterine artery located between the mass and the uterus)

Cervical carcinoma

- Invasive cervical cancer is the third most common gynaecological malignancy in the UK
- Peak age 35–50 years
- Vaginal bleeding is commonest presenting symptom
- Most are of squamous cell type
- Locally invasive neoplasm
- Lymphatic spread occurs initially to parametrial, obturator and presacral nodes followed by internal, external and common iliac nodes
- Haematogenous spread to liver, lung and bone occurs in late-stage disease

Anatomy

- Ovoid intraperitoneal structures, variable in size depending on age, hormonal status and menstrual cycle
- Volume around 3 ml before menarche, 10 ml in menstruating women and 6 ml when postmenopausal
- Mesovarium anchors ovary to posterior surface of broad ligament
- Ovarian ligament anchors ovary to uterus
- Suspensory ligament anchors ovary to pelvic side wall
- Position of ovaries is highly variable
- Internal iliac artery and the ureter lie posterior to the ovary
- External iliac vein lies superiorly and anteriorly
- Ovarian artery originates from the abdominal aorta below the renal artery
- Left ovarian vein drains into left renal vein
- Right ovarian vein drains into inferior vena cava

Ovarian tumours (general features)

Imaging features suggestive of a benign tumour

- Diameter < 4 cm
- Entirely cystic components
- Wall thickness < 3 mm
- Lack of internal structure
- Absence of ascites/adenopathy

Imaging features suggestive of a malignant tumour

- Thick irregular wall
- Thick septa
- Papillary projections
- Large soft tissue component with necrosis
- Pelvic organ invasion
- Peritoneal, mesenteric or omental implants
- Ascites
- Lymphadenopathy

Serous and mucinous tumours

- Can be uni- or multilocular
- Varying amounts of solid tissue

Benign serous cystadenoma

- Can be uni- or multilocular
- Homogeneous CT attenuation or MR signal intensity in all locules,
- Thin regular wall or septum
- No endo/exocystic vegetations

Benign mucinous cystadenoma

- Almost always multilocular; locules of varying intensity/density, smooth walls/septae
- Mucinous cystadenomas tend to be larger than serous cystadenomas at presentation

Endometrioid carcinoma

- 10–15% of all ovarian carcinomas
- 15–30% associated with endometrial carcinoma/endometrial hyperplasia
- Most common malignant neoplasm arising from endometriosis
- Bilateral involvement in 30–50%

Clear cell carcinoma

- 5% of ovarian tumours
- Majority are stage I at time of presentation
- Nearly all patients have previous endometriosis
- A large endometrioma with solid components suggests malignancy

MRI features

- Unilocular or large cyst with solid protrusions
- Smooth cyst margin
- Low to high signal intensity on T1WI

Brenner tumour

- Usually small and discovered incidentally

- Rarely malignant
- Associated with other ovarian tumours in 30% of cases

Imaging features
- Multilocular cystic mass or a small mostly solid mass
- Solid components may enhance to a mild or moderate extent
- MRI: low signal intensity (similar to fibroma)
- CT: extensive amorphous calcifications may be seen

Germ cell tumours

- 15–20% of all ovarian tumours
- Mature and immature teratomas, dysgerminomas, endodermal sinus tumour, embryonal carcinoma and choriocarcinoma
- Only mature teratoma is benign, but it is the most common type
- Elevated serum alpha-fetoprotein and human chorionic gonadotropin is seen with the malignant germ cell tumours

Mature teratoma

- Most common benign ovarian tumour in women < 45 years of age
- Composed of mature tissue from two or more embryonic germ cell layers
- Cystic teratomas are unilocular
- 88% of tumours are filled with sebaceous material and lined by squamous epithelium
- Usually there is a raised protuberance projecting into the cavity called a Rokitansky nodule
- Complications: torsion, rupture, malignant degeneration

Imaging features
- Can be purely cystic, cystic–solid, solid
- Sebaceous material, hair, bone or fat appears as echogenic material on ultrasound
- CT: fat attenuation with or without mural calcification is diagnostic of mature cystic teratoma
- MRI: sebaceous component is high signal on T1WI

Immature teratoma

- Contains immature tissue from all three germ layers
- Occurs in first two decades of life
- Large complex mass with cystic and solid components and scattered calcifications
- Rapid growth
- Perforation of capsule is frequently demonstrated

Dysgerminoma

- Occurs predominantly in young women
- Ovarian counterpart of seminoma of the testis
- Calcification may be present (typically with a 'speckled' pattern)

Ultrasound features
- Multilobulated, solid masses with prominent fibrovascular septa
- Necrosis and haemorrhage may appear as anechoic, low signal intensity or low attenuation areas

Endodermal sinus tumour

- Second decade of life
- Large complex pelvic mass that extends into the abdomen
- Both solid and cystic components
- Mature teratomas may coexist with the tumour
- Rapid growth and poor prognosis

Sex cord-stromal tumours

- Derived from granulosa cells, theca cells, fibroblasts, Leydig's cells and Sertoli's cells
- Affects all age groups
- Represent 8% of all ovarian neoplasms
- Most are benign or confined to the ovary at the time of diagnosis

Granulosa cell tumour
- Most common malignant sex-cord stromal tumour
- Most common oestrogen-producing ovarian tumour
- Occurs predominantly in peri- and postmenopausal women

- The hyperoestrogenaemia can cause endometrial hyperplasia, polyps or carcinoma
- Endometrial carcinoma is associated with 3–25% of these tumours

Imaging features

- Wide range of appearances
- Solid or multiloculated cystic tumours
- Intratumoural bleeding, infarcts and fibrous degeneration may be seen
- Usually confined to the ovary

Fibrothecoma

- Lipid-rich thecoma demonstrates oestrogen activity
- Occurs in both pre- and postmenopausal women
- Fibroma is the most common sex-cord tumour
- Appears as solid mass mimicking malignant tumours
- Associated with ascites or Meigs' syndrome (unilateral pleural effusion)

Imaging features

Ultrasound
- Homogeneous hypoechoic mass with posterior acoustic shadowing

CT
- Homogeneous solid tumour with delayed enhancement
- Dense calcifications

MRI
- Low signal intensity on T1WI and very low signal intensity on T2WI

- Scattered high signal areas represent oedema or cystic degeneration

Sclerosing stromal cell tumour

- Benign tumour occurring predominantly in young women
- Large mass with both cystic and solid components
- Early peripheral enhancement with centripetal progression on contrast-enhanced dynamic studies

Sertoli and Leydig cell tumour

- Low-grade malignancy occurring predominantly in young women
- Most common virilising tumour
- Composed of heterologous tissue
- Well-defined, enhancing solid mass with intratumoural cysts

Ovarian metastases

- Colon and stomach are the most common primary sites
- Breast, lung and contralateral ovary are the other frequent primaries
- Represent 10% of all ovarian tumours and develop during the reproductive years
- Imaging findings are non-specific

Kruckenberg's tumour

- Contains mucin-secreting signet ring cells, usually originating in the gastrointestinal tract
- Bilateral complex masses with hypointense solid components on T1WI and internal hyperintensity on T2W1

Anatomy and embryology

- Modified skin gland
- Can extend from clavicle to 8th rib and sternum to midaxillary line
- Formed by about 20 lobes which in turn are formed of lobules
- The immediate branches of a major duct and its lobule form the terminal duct lobular unit—the terminal duct is thought to be where breast cancer originates
- Fibrous tissues support the glandular tissue, which is progressively replaced by fat with advancing age
- Develop from the mammary ridge which in the early stages extend from the upper limb bud to the lower limb bud ventrally; only the mid portion of the upper third of the ridge develops into mammary tissue
- Accessory breast tissue may be seen anywhere along the mammary ridge

Arterial supply, venous drainage and lymphatics

- Axillary artery through the lateral thoracic artery supplies the upper outer quadrant
- Internal mammary artery supplies the central and medial portions
- Intercostal arteries supply the lateral breast tissue
- Venous drainage through axillary, internal mammary and intercostal veins
- Lymphatic drainage is primarily to the axillary nodes
- Small percentage into the internal mammary nodes and the upper abdomen

Investigations

Ultrasound

- Usually high-frequency transducers are used
- Is not useful as a screening tool
- Can be used to characterise some lesions detected on mammography
- May be used to clarify lesions seen on only one mammographic view
- Can be used to guide needle placement in aspirations/biopsies

- Cancers are usually hypoechoic and cause acoustic shadowing
- Implant rupture gives snow storm appearance if extracapsular and step ladder pattern if intracapsular

Mammography

- Most widely used screening tool for the detection of breast cancer
- Needs dedicated equipment

Anode and filters

- Molybdenum anode is used to produce low-energy photons (17.9 and 19.5 keV)
- A molybdenum filter is used to filter out the photons of energy > 20 keV
- X-ray tube windows used in mammography are made of beryllium to reduce the amount of filtration of the low-energy photons

Purpose of breast compression

- Hold breast away from chest wall
- Reduce motion blur
- Reduce radiation dose by reducing thickness
- Further reduce dose and motion by shorter exposure times
- Separate out overlapping structures
- Improve resolution by keeping the object closer to the detector
- Reduce scatter
- Permit more uniform exposure by providing more uniform thickness

Breast calcifications

- Large calcifications with popcorn appearance—involuting fibroadenoma or less commonly, a papilloma
- Fine curvilinear calcifications delineating the walls of a round or oval mass—usually benign cyst
- Dense lucent centred calcifications in fat necrosis
- Vascular calcifications are linear and parallel
- Calcified rods in secretory disease

- Pleomorphic calcifications < 0.5 mm when associated with a mass are of concern—intraductal cancer
- Fine linear calcifications in comedocarcinoma
- Magnification mammography is used to further analyse calcifications
- Benign and malignant processes may produce similar calcifications

Breast MRI

- Breast coils are designed to image patients in a prone position
- Small lesions are better detected with three-dimensional sequences than two-dimensional
- If possible MRI of the breast is best done between days 7 and 14 of the menstrual cycle because physiological enhancement is most pronounced before and immediately after the menstruation
- Almost all assessments need intravenous contrast
- Almost all invasive cancers enhance
- Normal tissue and benign pathology also may enhance
- Round or oval lesions with non-enhancing septations are almost always fibroadenoma
- Heterogeneous enhancement is more common in malignant lesions
- Peripheral enhancement is more common with malignant lesions
- Inflammatory lesions that show peripheral enhancement have thinner rims
- Cancers are low in signal intensity in T2WI
- Implant ruptures can be evaluated well with MRI

> ### Lesions that enhance on contrast MRI
>
> - Breast cancer
> - Fibroadenomas
> - Fibrocystic change including sclerosing adenosis
> - Fat necrosis
> - Radial scars
> - Mastitis
> - Atypical hyperplasia
> - Lobular neoplasia
> - Normal breast tissue

Breast cysts

- Peak prevalence 30–50 years
- Most represent dilatation of the lobular acini
- Some are distended ducts
- Solitary or often multiple
- Carcinoma is rarely found in cysts; when found most are papillary
- Intracystic cancer is found in < 0.2% of cysts
- Pericystic leak of fluid can cause inflammation and fibrosis
- May resolve spontaneously

Imaging features

Mammography
- Multiple, rounded densities
- May be lobulated
- Usually well defined with circumscribed margins
- Margins may be obscured especially with pericystic fibrosis from inflammation
- A lucent halo may be seen around (Mach effect)
- Does not distort normal breast architecture
- Cyst wall may calcify—egg-shell thin rim
- Milk of calcium (concave crescent) when viewed tangentially in the upright lateral projection and concomitant amorphous dots of calcium when seen en face in the caudocranial projection

Ultrasound
- Round, ovoid, flattened or lobulated
- Sharply marginated with no internal echoes
- Enhanced through transmission of sound
- Bleeding into a cyst give rise to internal echoes and other complex appearance
- Complicated cysts (with internal echoes, septations or solid areas) need close follow up or aspiration cytology of the fluid

MRI
- Round, oval or lobulated, well defined
- High signal on T2WI
- May demonstrate rim enhancement following contrast (unusual and due to pericystic inflammation)

Fibroadenoma

- Most common benign solid lesion of the breast
- Common in teenage women
- Freely movable
- Mammography
- Sharply circumscribed
- Round, ovoid or smoothly lobulated
- A thin lucent halo may be seen
- May have one or more flattened surface
- Can be multiple and bilateral
- May calcify—popcorn-shaped large calcifications are pathognomonic; but fine and irregular calcification as in malignancy may be seen
- Cancer can develop in a fibroadenoma or can engulf it

Imaging features

Ultrasound
- Extremely variable appearance
- Typically well-circumscribed, ovoid, hypoechoic lesions
- Lateral wall refractive shadowing may be seen
- Homogeneous or irregular internal echo pattern
- Occasionally isoechoic to surrounding parenchyma and can be barely visible
- Frequently posterior acoustic enhancement is seen
- Posterior acoustic shadowing can occur with lesion having more fibrosis

MRI
- Almost always enhances
- Gross morphology as described before
- Non-enhancing septations may be virtually diagnostic

Phyllodes tumour (cystosarcoma phyllodes)

- Unusual, usually benign stromal tumour
- 25% recur locally if incompletely excised
- 10% can metastasise; metastasis is by haematogenous route
- Peak prevalence between 30–50 years
- Rapidly enlarges
- Smooth lobulated contours
- Relatively mobile even when large
- Malignant tumours contain sarcomatous elements
- Mammography
- Generally well defined
- Spiculation does not occur
- Microcalcification is not a feature
- A halo may be seen
- Tumours > 3 cm are likely to be malignant

Imaging features

Ultrasound
- Large well-circumscribed lesions
- Variable low-amplitude internal echoes
- Posterior acoustic attenuation or enhancement can occur

MRI
- Enhance rapidly
- Indistinguishable from fibroadenoma

Gynaecomastia

- Non-neoplastic enlargement of the male breast
- If breast enlargement is purely due to fat deposition, it is pseudogynaecomastia
- With true gynaecomastia, the ducts increase in number and may become dilated
- May be unilateral or bilateral

Associations/causes

- Endogenous hormonal imbalance, exogenous hormone use, hormone-producing tumours, hepatic disease, renal disease and hyperthyroidism
- Drugs: reserpine, cardiac glycosides, spironolactone, cimetidine, thiazides, marijuana
- Testicular tumours: seminoma, choriocarcinoma and embryonal cell carcinoma
- Klinefelter's syndrome (also associated with increased risk of breast cancer)
- Lung cancer

Intraductal papilloma

- One of the most common causes of serous or bloody nipple discharge
- Benign proliferation of the ductal epithelium that projects into the lumen of the duct and has a fibrovascular stalk

- Usually solitary but may be multiple
- Solitary papillomas are usually in the subareolar region, and multiple papillomas in the smaller ducts peripherally
- Solitary papillomas are more common in peri- and postmenopausal years
- Multiple peripheral papillomas are less common, usually in younger women and there is an increased likelihood for atypical changes and carcinoma
- Imaging features cannot differentiate between benign and malignant process

Imaging features

Mammography
- Most are not visible
- Occasionally seen as lobulated lesion forming a fairly well-circumscribed mass
- When visible, almost always located in the anterior part of the breast
- When seen within a cyst, the cyst may be evident on the mammogram
- Occasionally can produce a non-specific cluster of microcalcifications
- 'Shell-like', lucent-centred, calcific densities in the subareolar region
- May be seen as filling defects on ductography

Ultrasound
- Solid, hypoechoic, usually lobulated masses when large enough to be seen
- Occasionally located within a cystically dilated duct
- When seen within a cystic structure, the frond-like structure may be more obvious

MRI
- May enhance with contrast

Lipoma

- Generally superficial, found around the periphery of the parenchyma and always encapsulated
- Freely movable and soft
- Mammography:
  - Typically radiolucent
  - Thin capsule
- May cause distortion of the surrounding architecture by displacement or themselves become moulded by the surrounding parenchyma

- Occasionally contains typical spherical calcification of fat necrosis

Imaging features

Ultrasound
- Hypoechoic and similar to subcutaneous fat
- Specular reflection from the capsule may be seen
- Calcifications may be present

MRI
- Similar appearance to breast fat
- Incidental finding on MRI

Focal fat necrosis

- May produce a palpable mass and can be extremely hard if oil cysts are formed

Mammography
- Round or oval, lucent lesion defined by its capsule
- Cysts may calcify
- Irregular clustered deposits of calcium can occur similar to malignancy

Galactocoele

- Milk-containing cystic structure
- Usually associated with lactation

Imaging features

Mammography
- Indistinguishable from other fat-containing rounded lesions
- Usually appears radiolucent surrounded by dense lactating breast tissue
- Fat-fluid levels may be seen

Ultrasound
- Varied appearance
- Thin well-defined walls
- May contain low-level echoes
- May cause shadowing

Hamartoma (fibroadenolipoma)

- Proliferation of fibrous and adenomatous nodular elements in fat surrounded by a capsule of connective tissue

Imaging features

Mammography
- Sharply marginated
- May look like lipomas with fibroglandular tissue within
- Capsule may be evident if there is fat outside the lesion

Ultrasound
- Sharply defined
- Displaces surrounding structures
- Heterogeneous echo pattern

Radial scar

- Idiopathic process that produces as scar-like lesion
- Should be biopsied to establish diagnosis

Imaging features

Mammography
- Appearance is indistinguishable from cancer
- Area of architectural distortion with speculations radiating from a central point
- Microcalcifications may be seen
- Generally do not have a central mass

Ultrasound
- Appearance is indistinguishable from cancer
- Irregularly shaped hypoechoic poorly defined tissue

MRI
- May have similar appearance to cancer

Duct ectasia

- Primarily affects the major ducts in the subareolar region
- Non-specific dilatation of one or more ducts that may be palpable or visible on mammography
- Ducts become thicker due to periductal collagen deposition from inflammation

Imaging features

Mammography
- Tubular serpentine structures converging on nipple in subareolar region
- Rod-shaped calcifications may be seen that may be thick continuous solid deposits; rarely branch

- Rods with central lucency
- Spherical or globular densities with central lucencies

Ultrasound
- If there is fluid in the distended duct, tubular anechoic branching structure is seen
- Duct filled with debris produces fairly homogeneous solid tubular structure

Breast abscess

- Results from infection in the breast
- More common in young, nursing mothers
- Painful and associated with signs of inflammation

Imaging features

Mammogram
- Rarely indicated
- Round and well circumscribed or irregular and ill defined
- Skin and trabecular thickening

Ultrasound
- Can look like a cyst or solid mass
- Ultrasound-guided aspiration is generally needed to make the diagnosis
- Ultrasound-guided wide-bore needle aspiration is therapeutic

Ductal carcinoma

- Cancers with cellular features similar to ductal epithelium
- 90% of breast cancers
- Called ductal carcinoma in situ when confined to the duct
- Called invasive or infiltrating ductal carcinoma when the basement membrane of the duct is breached

Ductal carcinoma in situ

- Considered to be a precursor of invasive ductal carcinoma
- 30–50% of cases progress to invasive cancer if not treated
- Heterogeneous calcification along the duct lines
- May extend through large volumes of the breast

Imaging features

Mammography
- Fine linear branching calcifications are very characteristic
- Calcifications can be heterogeneous or granular

Ultrasound
- A mass may or may not be seen
- Calcifications may be seen as bright reflections in hypoechoic tissue

MRI
- Not always evident on MRI
- Extensive ductal carcinoma in situ can be seen as pronounced segmental enhancement, but can be lost in the background enhancement

Invasive ductal carcinoma

- Causes desmoplastic response with cicatrisation and fibrosis
- A hard palpable mass may be found
- If left untreated the lesion can ulcerate through the skin

Imaging features

Mammography
- Irregular mass with spiculated margin
- Lobulated contours are common
- Calcifications in association with a typical tumour mass are diagnostic
- Distortion of surrounding architecture
- Skin or nipple retraction
- The tumour may be undetectable on mammography if the surrounding breast tissue is of the same density as the tumour

Ultrasound
- Irregular hypoechoic structure that produces retrotumoural shadowing
- Tends to be vertically oriented relative to skin
- Can be irregular and lobulated
- Varying internal echotexture
- Ultrasound is used to guide needle positioning for interventional procedures

MRI
- Irregularly shaped mass with contrast enhancement
- Typical pattern of contrast enhancement

is a rapid increase followed by a plateau or rapid washout
- Peripheral enhancement may be seen

Paget's disease

- Ductal carcinoma that involves the nipple
- Usually no tumour mass is evident
- Generally favourable prognosis due to early presentation

Imaging features

Mammography
- There may be no mammographic abnormality
- Occasionally a mass with malignant characteristics
- Microcalcification in the subareolar region directed towards the nipple
- Diffuse pattern of ductal calcification

Ultrasound
- Not indicated when there is nipple abnormality

Tubular cancer

- Well-differentiated form of invasive ductal carcinoma
- Sometimes palpable
- Frequently detected on mammography
- Slow growing

Mammography
- Small spiculated lesion
- Some contain microcalcification
- Axillary lymph-node metastases are rare

Papillary carcinoma

- A form of ductal malignancy
- Epithelium proliferates into villous projections and eventually fills lumen
- Frequency increases with age
- Slow growth rate
- Can infiltrate but not aggressively infiltrative
- Generally well circumscribed and not particularly hard

Imaging features

Mammography

- May not be evident when small
- Fairly well-circumscribed masses
- Lucent halo surrounding the mass may be seen
- When within a cyst, appearance similar to cyst
- If the cancer bleeds, the cyst will be very dense on mammogram

Ultrasound
- When intracystic, multiple fronds projecting into the lumen of the cyst
- Complex mass with cystic or solid properties

Colloid or mucinous carcinoma

- Form of ductal carcinoma with more mucinous differentiation
- When pure, better prognosis
- Frequency increases with age

Imaging features

Mammography
- No differentiating features from other cancers
- Tends to be better circumscribed
- Small lobulations in the contour may be seen
- Density may be less than more scirrhous forms

Ultrasound
- Nonspecific appearance
- Hypoechoic lesions

MRI
- Lobulated tumours with slowly enhancing contrast pattern
- High signal intensity on T2WI

Medullary carcinoma

- Relative frequency rises in third decade of life then decreases steadily
- Frequently grows quite large
- Relatively soft on physical examination and tends to be freely movable

Imaging features

Mammography
- Fairly well-circumscribed smooth, round or ovoid masses

- Frequently has somewhat ill-defined margin

Ultrasound
- Well circumscribed, frequently lobulated
- Hypoechoic
- Low-amplitude internal echoes that may be heterogeneous
- Posterior acoustic enhancement is not unusual

MRI
- Round with fairly well-defined borders
- Diffuse enhancement

Inflammatory carcinoma

- Warmth, erythema and peau d'orange appearance on clinical examination
- Appearance can be mimicked by benign inflammatory disease
- Painless
- Peak incidence around 30 years of age

Imaging features

Mammography
- Unusual to find a mass or calcifications
- Skin thickening
- Diffuse increase in density on the affected side due to diffuse trabecular thickening

Ultrasound
- Non-specific skin thickening

MRI
- No distinctive findings
- Requires needle biopsy for confirmation

Lobular carcinoma

- Neoplastic cells are similar to cells lining the lobule
- Lobular carcinoma in situ if confined to the lobule
- Invasive lobular carcinoma if invades beyond the lobule
- Women with LCIS in one breast are at high risk for developing invasive lobular carcinoma in both breasts

---

Lobular carcinoma in situ

- Lower risk of progressing to invasive cancer than ductal carcinoma in situ
- Found more commonly in younger women than ductal carcinoma
- More common found in women with radiographically dense breasts

---

Imaging features

Mammography
- No lesions are usually seen
- Calcification in adjacent benign tissue is common

Ultrasound
- Not well characterised

Invasive lobular carcinoma

- More often bilateral
- Insidious in onset
- Less desmoplastic response than ductal cancers
- Tends to be large at diagnosis

Imaging features

Mammography
- Difficult to detect early
- Asymmetrical density without definable margins
- Area of progressively increasing density in a dense breast

Ultrasound
- Hypoechoic tissue with varying degrees of posterior acoustic shadowing

MRI
- Enhancement pattern similar to invasive ductal carcinoma

Mimics of breast cancer on mammography

- Post-surgical scarring
- Fat necrosis
- Radial scars
- Extra-abdominal desmoid tumours (very rare)
- Granular cell tumours (very rare)

Breast biopsy

- Palpable lesions can be biopsied without imaging guidance
- Any lesion that is visible by imaging can be biopsied under guidance
- Lesion that is only visible on mammography can be biopsied under stereotactic guidance
- For lesions that need surgical excision biopsy, hook wire localisation can be done under ultrasound/mammography guidance
- MRI can also be used to guide percutaneous biopsy

Chapter 5

Paediatrics

Neonatal cranial ultrasound

Probes

- At least 5 mHz for term infants and 7 mHz for premature infants

Standard views

Coronal views

- Anterior to the frontal horns of the lateral ventricles
- At the level of anterior horns and sylvian fissure
- At the level of the third ventricle and the intraventricular foramen, to include the thalamus
- At the posterior horns to include the choroid plexuses
- Posterior and superior to the lateral ventricles (parenchyma)

Sagittal views

- Midline through the third ventricle, cavum septum pellucidum and cerebellum
- Medial to the ventricles for the caudothalamic groove
- Through the lateral ventricles to include frontal, occipital and temporal horns
- Lateral to each ventricle to include frontal and parietal white matter

Normal variants and pitfalls

- The cavum septum pellucidum disappears by 2 months of age in 85% of infants
- However, its absence in the preterm baby is always associated with structural abnormalities
- The choroid plexus extends from the temporal horns to the foramen of Monro and then caudally into the third and fourth ventricles
- The ventricles in preterm infants appear fuller than at term, when they appear slit-like
- Thin-walled frontal horn cysts must not be confused with periventricular leukomalacia

Germinal matrix haemorrhage

Four grades of germinal matrix haemorrhage

- Subependymal, no long-term abnormalities
- Intraventricular, no ventricular dilatation
- Intraventricular with dilatation
- Intraparenchymal haemorrhage

- The thin microvasculature of the germinal matrix is susceptible to rupture
- Neonates born at 32 weeks' gestation or earlier and those born with birth weight < 1500 g are at particular risk
- Germinal matrix normally involutes at 34 weeks; it is unusual to find germinal matrix haemorrhage or intraventricular haemorrhage in infants born after 34 weeks' gestation
- Intracranial bleed associated with prematurity
- Commonest site is the caudothalamic groove
- 90% of periventricular haemorrhages occur in the first 3 days of life

Imaging features

Ultrasound

- Acute blood, < 7 days (old blood appears hyperechoic)
- The haematoma becomes less echogenic over time, beginning from the central portion
- Subsequent to eventual clot retraction, a subependymal cyst may develop or a linear echo may result
- Intraparenchymal haemorrhage
  - Usually located in the frontal and parietal lobes
  - Appears acutely as an echogenic homogeneous 'mass'

– As the haemorrhage evolves, an echogenic rim with an echo-poor centre forms
– After 2–3 months, a porencephalic cyst (if the lesion communicates with a ventricle)
– Pitfalls
– Intraventricular haemorrhage may blend imperceptibly with the choroid plexus, which has a similar echo texture
– Asymmetric thickness of the choroid plexus should be viewed with suspicion
– A lack of abnormality on ultrasound does not exclude the possibility of later neurodevelopmental problems

Periventricular leukomalacia

- Results from perinatal asphyxia
- Most common in premature infants born at less than 32 weeks' gestation with a birth weight < 1500 g
- Most commonly affects the white matter adjacent to the frontal horns of the lateral ventricles
- Associated with seizures, spasticity and movement disorders
- Seen acutely and subacutely as hyperechoic changes around the margins of the ventricles
- With time, these areas become progressively less echoic and finally hypoechoic with the development of cystic changes

Imaging features

Ultrasound

- On cranial ultrasound the earliest feature is increased echotexture in the periventricular white matter
- The abnormal periventricular echotexture of periventricular leukomalacia usually disappears at 2–3 weeks
- Periventricular cysts appear after 2–3 weeks
- Initial cranial ultrasound findings may be normal in some patients who actually go on to develop clinical and delayed imaging findings of periventricular leukomalacia

Choroid plexus cyst

- Most common at 16 weeks' gestation, when about 2% of fetuses will demonstrate this finding; almost always disappear by 26 weeks
- These cysts may be detected antenatally or postnatally
- Known association with trisomy 18
- Small cysts (< 10 mm in diameter) are known to resolve spontaneously
- Rarely, these cysts may obstruct the foramen of Monro causing hydrocephalus

Craniosynostosis

- Premature fusion of one or multiple cranial sutures
- Sporadic and familial forms are known
- The sagittal suture is the most commonly affected (in 50–60% of cases), followed by the coronal suture (20–30%), the metopic suture (4–10%) and the lambdoid suture (2–4%)
- May result from a primary defect of ossification (primary craniosynostosis) or, more commonly, from a failure of brain growth (secondary craniosynostosis)
- Craniosynostosis that involves more than one suture and also be associated with other body deformities, and is termed syndromic craniosynostosis
- Craniosynostosis is sometimes associated with sporadic craniofacial syndromes such as Crouzon's syndrome, Apert's syndrome, Chotzen's syndrome, Pfeiffer's syndrome or Carpenter's syndrome
- Secondary craniosynostosis typically results from systemic disorders
  – Endocrine disorders, e.g. hyperthyroidism, hypophosphatemia, vitamin D deficiency, renal osteodystrophy, hypercalcaemia, rickets
  – Haematological disorders that cause bone marrow hyperplasia, e.g. sickle cell disease, thalassemia
  – Inadequate brain growth, including microcephaly and its causes and shunted hydrocephalus

- Types of craniosynostosis
  - Scaphocephaly: early fusion of the sagittal suture
  - Anterior plagiocephaly: early fusion of one coronal suture
  - Brachycephaly: early bilateral coronal suture fusion
  - Posterior plagiocephaly: early closure of one lambdoid suture
  - Trigonocephaly: early fusion of the metopic suture

Widened cranial sutures

> **Widened cranial sutures are pathological in the following contexts**
>
> - > 10 mm at birth
> - > 3 mm at 2 years of age
> - > 2 mm at 3 years of age
>
> Complete closure occurs at 30 years of age

- Causes
  - Normal variant
  - Metabolic bone disease, e.g. hyperthyroidism, hypothyroidism, osteogenesis imperfecta
  - Raised intracranial pressure
  - Infiltration of sutures: leukaemia, lymphoma
  - Recovery from chronic illnesses and prematurity

Agenesis of the corpus callosum

- The corpus callosum forms from the commissural plate at the seventh week of gestation
- The genu is formed before the truncus and splenium
- The anterior parts, splenium and rostrum are completely formed by the 20th week of gestation

> **Associations of agenesis of the corpus callosum**
>
> - Dandy–Walker cyst
> - Interhemispheric arachnoid cyst
> - Hydrocephalus
> - Arnold–Chiari malformation type 2

Imaging features

MRI

- The corpus callosum and cingulum are typically absent or malformed
- High-riding third ventricle that is usually open superiorly to the interhemispheric fissure. This is seen as a 'candelabra' on coronal imaging
- The sulci and gyri on the medial hemispheric surface have a radial or 'spoke-like' configuration around the third ventricle
- Probst's bundles are longitudinal white matter tracts that indent and invaginate into the superomedial aspect of the lateral ventricles
- Three types of midline cysts are associated with agenesis or hypogenesis of the corpus callosum:
  - Type 1 is a large midline cyst that communicates with third ventricle and the lateral ventricles
  - Type 2 is similar to type 1 but associated with cortical anomalies (e.g. polymicrogyria, gray matter heterotopia, schizencephaly)
  - Type 3 involves complex, multilocular cysts that are asymmetric and independent of the ventricles. Cortical malformations are uncommon. With large cysts, the ipsilateral lateral ventricle may be compressed, and the contralateral ventricle may be obstructed and enlarged (hydrocephalus).

Paediatric brain tumours

Classification

- Supratentorial tumours
  - Account for one third of cases
  - Most often low-grade (I or II) astrocytomas
  - Pleomorphic xanthoastrocytoma
- Infratentorial tumours
  - Account for two thirds of cases
  - Medulloblastoma
  - Juvenile pilocytic astrocytoma
  - Ependymoma
  - Brainstem glioma

> Astrocytoma is the most common brain tumour in children

Medulloblastoma

- Commonest childhood posterior fossa tumour
- A primitive neuroectodermal tumour (PNET)
- Two age peaks
  - 75% occur in first decade of life: midline location (in the vermis or the roof of the fourth ventricle)
  - 25% occur in third decade of life: a parasagittal location in the cerebellar hemispheres
- Fast-growing, aggressive tumour (grade IV)
- Leptomeningeal 'drop' metastases are found in 40% of cases at the time of diagnosis; these metastases can seed anywhere along the neuroaxis but are commonest over the cerebral convexities and in the lumbosacral region
- Bone metastases (osteoblastic) are found in 5% of cases at the time of diagnosis
- Treatment is with surgical resection and full neuroaxis irradiation

Imaging features

CT
- Non-contrast CT shows a large hyperdense midline mass

- Hydrocephalus as a result of ventricular obstruction is seen in 90% of cases
- Dense homogeneous contrast enhancement
- Atypical features
  - 10% are calcified
  - 10% have haemorrhagic components
  - 10% have cystic components
  - 10% are non-enhancing

MRI
- Less specific imaging features than with CT
- Typically low T1 and high T2 signal
- Most sensitive modality for detecting 'drop' metastases
- FLAIR and T1-weighted images (T1WI) post-contrast are the best sequences
- Nodular surface enhancement, which follows the gyral contours
- Besides identifying the primary lesion, MRI is beneficial in detecting metastatic lesions
- To rule out drop metastases, MRI of the spine is obligatory when medulloblastoma is either considered or diagnosed
- Imaging of the spine is best performed before surgery in order to avoid postoperative artefacts, which may be interpreted as tumour metastases
- Metastases can occur in the basal cisterns
- Both recurrent lesions and metastases show sparse enhancement

> **Paediatric causes of 'drop' metastases**
>
> - Medulloblastoma
> - Ependymoma
> - Germinoma
> - Pineoblastoma

Juvenile pilocytic astrocytoma

- Second commonest posterior fossa tumour in children
- Slow growing (grade I)
- Peak age is 10 years
- Associated with neurofibromatosis type 1

- Commonest location is the cerebellar hemispheres
- Presents with headaches and ataxia
- Can occur, but rarely, in the optic nerves or the hypothalamus
- High survival rate after resection

Imaging features

CT
- Well-defined, cystic mass with an avidly enhancing mural nodule
- Very similar in appearance to cerebellar haemangioblastoma
- 10% calcify

MRI
- Cyst is low signal on T1WI and high signal on T2-weighted images (T2WI)
- Mural nodule displays prominent enhancement

Ependymoma

- Arises from ependymal cells lining the ventricles
- 70% occur in the brain; more commonly seen in children
- 30% occur in the spine; more commonly seen in adults
- Commonest location in the brain is within the fourth ventricle in children and within the lateral ventricles in adults
- Slow-growing (grade II) tumour
- Does not invade through the ventricular walls
- Fourth ventricle tumours typically extend through foramina of Luschka and Magendie

Imaging features

CT
- Large, low-attenuation midline tumour obliterating the fourth ventricle
- Non-communicating hydrocephalus
- 50% contain calcifications
- 50% contain cystic elements

MRI
- Heterogeneous signal on T1WI and T2WI
- Solid components enhance

CT features of ependymoma versus medulloblastoma

- High attenuation (ependymoma); low attenuation (medulloblastoma)
- Rarely calcified (ependymoma); commonly calcified (medulloblastoma)
- Rarely cystic (ependymoma); commonly cystic (medulloblastoma)

Brainstem glioma

- Three distinct anatomical locations: diffuse intrinsic pontine tumours, tectal tumours and cervicomedullary tumours
- Commonest location is the pons
- High-grade aggressive tumour with a poor prognosis
- Intrinsic pontine gliomas carry a particularly grave prognosis; longer survival is associated with the tectal and cervicomedullary gliomas
- Present early with cranial nerve palsies
- Hydrocephalus uncommon at time of diagnosis

Imaging features

MRI
- Cranial MRI is the diagnostic test of choice
- Typical appearance of a brainstem glioma is an expansile, infiltrative process with low-to-normal signal intensity on T1WI and heterogeneous high-signal intensity on T2WI, with or without contrast enhancement
- Can delineate the extent of infiltration of the leptomeninges and the surrounding structures
- High midbrain tumours, especially those arising in the tectum, are typically low-grade lesions by histological criteria and commonly appear hypointense on T1WI and hyperintense on T2WI even without contrast enhancement

CT
- Appearance of brainstem gliomas is variable
- CT is less sensitive than MRI and less useful for characterising the tumours

- Calcifications, cystic changes and displacement of the ventricular system can be identified; however, lower brainstem lesions are often not apparent on CT scan

Giant cell astrocytoma

- Subependymal tumour located at the foramen of Monro
- Tumour enlarges, causing hydrocephalus
- Can transform into a high-grade astrocytoma
- 15% of all paediatric brain tumours
- Other associations include tuberous sclerosis, cardiac rhabdomyomas and bone cysts

Imaging features

MRI
- Tumour is isointense on T1WI and hyperintense on T2WI
- Tumour avidly enhances

Retinoblastoma

- Commonest ocular malignancy of childhood
- One third are hereditary, and are usually bilateral
- Two thirds occur sporadically, and are usually unilateral
- Clinically patients have leukocoria (white pupil)
- Tumour mass arises from posterior aspect of the globe
- Propensity for extension along the optic nerve
- Meningeal metastases can occur via the subarachnoid space

Causes of leukocoria

- Retinoblastoma (50% of cases of leukocoria)
- Retinopathy of prematurity
- Coats' disease
- Persistent hyperplastic vitreous
- Toxocara infection
- Congenital cataract

Imaging features

Ultrasound
- Echo-bright mass
- Foci of calcification (in 80% of cases)
- Retinal detachment (in 100% of cases)

MRI
- Modality of choice
- Appears as a contrasting mass
- On T1WI, the vitreous humour is dark and the tumour is bright
- On T2WI, the vitreous humour is bright and the tumour is dark
- Calcifications are seen as areas of signal void

Poor prognostic signs in retinoblastoma (> 50% mortality)

- Invasion of the choroidal layer
- Lack of calcifications
- Extension along the optic nerve
- Contrast enhancement

Arnold–Chiari malformations (1 and 2)

Arnold–Chiari malformations type 1

- Presents clinically in adults
- Small posterior fossa
- Cerebellar tonsils > 5 mm below a normal-sized foramen magnum
- Elongated fourth ventricle, but in a normal position
- Obliterated cisterna magna
- Associations
  - Syringomyelia (in 25% of cases)
  - Hydrocephalus (in 25% of cases)
  - Fused cervical vertebrae (Kippel–Feil syndrome)
  - Fused atlanto-occipital junction
  - Platybasia
  - No myelomeningocele
  - No supratentorial abnormalities

Arnold–Chiari malformations type 2

- Presents in newborns with respiratory distress
- Small posterior fossa
- Wide foramen magnum with variable herniation of tonsils, vermis, medulla or pons
- Scalloped clivus and petrous ridges
- Dysplasia of membranous skull, which disappears by 6 months age
- Fourth ventricle may be elongated and low-lying or obliterated
- Obliterated cisterna magna
- Associations
  - Myelomeningocele (in 95% of cases)
  - Non-communicating hydrocephalus (in 95% of cases)
  - Syringomyelia
  - Tethered cord
  - Supratentorial anomalies: thinning of the tentorium with a wide incisura, upward herniation of the cerebellum, dysgenesis of the corpus callosum, a large massa intermedia with a small third ventricle, small gyri

Dandy–Walker malformation

- A sporadic condition
- Dysembryogenesis of the fourth ventricle
- Risk in subsequent pregnancies < 5%
- Associated anomalies seen in 90% of cases
  - Lipoma or agenesis of the corpus callosum
  - Holoprosencephaly
  - Klippel–Feil syndrome
- 50% mortality quoted in first year of life

Imaging features

- Large posterior fossa
- Large posterior fossa cyst connected to the fourth ventricle
- Elevated tentorium cerebelli

- Key feature is agenesis of cerebellar vermis with small and widely separated cerebellar hemispheres
- Non-communicating hydrocephalus in 75% of cases

Vein of Galen malformation

- Central arteriovenous malformation and resulting varix of vein of Galen
- Prenatal diagnosis with MRI and ultrasound
- Brain hypoperfusion ensues from increased pressure in the central veins
- Congestive heart failure develops as a result of the high cardiac output
- Treatment is with glue embolisation

Tuberous sclerosis

- Autosomal-dominant condition (70% are new mutations)
- Clinically presents with epilepsy and mental retardation

Skin abnormalities

- Adenoma sebaceum (butterfly distribution)
- Shagreen patches
- Ash-leaf macules
- Periungual fibromas
- Café-au-lait spots

Renal abnormalities

- Multiple angiomyolipomas
- Multiple renal cysts
- Renal cell carcinoma

CNS abnormalities

- Multiple cortical hamartomas (in 90% of cases); the majority calcify but there is no malignant potential
- Subependymal nodule
- Subependymal giant cell astrocytoma

Cardiac abnormalities

- Cardiac rhabdomyoma (single or multiple)

Imaging features

MRI
- The tubers are isointense on T1WI, hyperintense on T2WI and very rarely enhance

Heterotopic grey matter islands

- Caused by abnormal neuronal migration
- Lesions are of grey matter signal intensity
- Typically seen as curvilinear bands radiating out from the ventricles
- May calcify and approximately 20% enhance with contrast.

Neonatal spine

- Hypoechoic central tubular structure with parallel echogenic walls
- Conus is at the T12–L1 level and is continuous with the echogenic filum
- CSF pulsation is a normal finding on imaging

Tethered spinal cord

- Associated with spinal dysraphism, fibrolipoma and a thickened 'tight' filum (> 2 mm)
- MRI is confirmatory

Oesophagus

Tracheoesophageal fistula and oesophageal atresia

- Presents at birth, usually after failure to pass a nasogastric tube, or with excessive oral secretions, choking and at times cyanosis
- Incidence is 2.4 per 10,000 births
- Classification
  - Oesophageal atresia without a fistula
  - Oesophageal atresia with a proximal fistula
  - Oesophageal atresia with a distal fistula (commonest type)
  - Oesophageal atresia with a fistula to both pouches
  - H-type fistula without atresia (usually presents later in childhood with recurrent chest infections)
- Associations include VACTERL (vertebral defects, anorectal malformations, cardiovascular defects, tracheo-oesophageal defects, renal anomalies, limb deformities) and in 5% of cases a right-sided aortic arch
- No known association with pulmonary hypoplasia

Imaging features

- Blind, air-filled upper oesophageal pouch causing anterior displacement and compression of the tracheal air shadow is typical
- Gas in the bowel indicates a distal fistula
- Aspiration typical with H-type fistula
- Contrast examination, if performed, is done with the child prone

Duplication cyst

- Congenital cysts caused by abnormal embryological development leading to sequestration of cells from the primitive foregut
- Difficult to distinguish from bronchogenic cysts but duplication cysts usually lie more posteriorly, anywhere along the length of the oesophagus
- Associations include pulmonary cystic malformations, oesophageal atresia and vertebral defects

Gastro-oesophageal reflux

- A normal intermittent phenomenon, common after meals
- Termed GORD when the above becomes symptomatic with or without oesophagitis
- Most cases of infantile reflux resolve by the age of 1–2 years

Imaging features

- Retrograde flow of contrast during contrast studies
- Presence of a hiatus hernia
- Technetium-99m sulphur colloid scan offers direct evaluation of gastric emptying and reflux, with or without swallowing dysfunction, strictures and Schatzki's rings

Small intestine

Pyloric stenosis

- Incidence is one in 300 live births
- Four times as common in males as females
- Most commonly seen in first-born male children
- Peak age is 3–4 weeks, and it is never after 3 months of age
- Causes a hypochloraemic metabolic alkalosis
- The adult form is associated with peptic ulcer disease and chronic gastritis
- Associations include tracheo-oesophageal fistula, trisomy 18, Turner's syndrome, rubella and erythromycin ingestion

Imaging features

Plain X-ray
- Stomach > 7 cm
- Gastric pneumatosis is seen, secondary to increased pressure

Ultrasound
- Performed in the right posterior oblique position, without emptying the stomach
- Target sign on transverse section
- Pyloric muscle thickness > 3.5–4 mm
- Pyloric canal length > 15–18 mm

Contrast study
- Indented antrum ('shoulder' sign)
- Narrow elongated pylorus ('string' sign)
- Compression of the duodenal bulb

Duodenal atresia or stenosis

- Commonest cause of upper bowel obstruction in neonates
- Common locations are in the second or third part of the duodenum or in the region of the ampulla of Vater
- Strong association with Down's syndrome
- Other associations include annular pancreas, malrotation, congenital heart diseases, absence of the gallbladder, situs inversus, preduodenal portal vein

Imaging features

Plain X-ray
- Distended stomach and proximal duodenum
- 'Double bubble'
- In atresia, there is no distal gas; in distal stenosis, gas is present
- A diagnosis of isolated duodenal atresia can only be made once midgut volvulus has been excluded

Annular pancreas

- Ring of pancreatic tissue encircling the duodenum
- Child presents with nausea, vomiting, epigastric pain and jaundice
- Classical 'double-bubble' sign on plain films
- Seen in the second part of the duodenum in 85% of cases
- Associated with gastric or duodenal ulceration in up to 50% of cases and recurrent pancreatitis in 15–30% of cases

Meconium ileus

- Obstruction of the distal small bowel by thick, tenacious meconium
- A typical feature of cystic fibrosis

Imaging features

Plain X-ray
- Dilated loops of bowel
- Bubbly lucencies in the right lower abdominal quadrant
- Free gas when perforation has occurred
- Curvilinear calcifications on peritoneal surface or lining a pseudocyst
- Microcolon due to disuse may be seen

Contrast study
- Dilute water-soluble ionic contrast enema agents used
- Microcolon is seen
- Reflux contrast in the terminal ileum
- Meconium pellets in the terminal ileum

Malrotation and midgut volvulus

- Abnormal fixation of the small bowel mesentery leads to a short mesentery that is prone to twisting
- Twisting of the small bowel about the superior mesenteric artery is termed midgut volvulus
- Classically presents with bilious vomiting

Imaging features

- Confirm abnormal position of caecum by barium studies (follow-through or enema)
- In volvulus, expect a cork screw or 'Z'-shaped oesophagus that does not cross to the left of the midline
- Signs of perforation and ischaemia, as complications, may be present

Omphalocoele

- Herniation of the abdominal contents into the umbilical cord
- Predisposing factors
  - Babies born out of *in vitro* fertilisation
  - Obese mother
  - Mothers with bicornuate uterus
- Mostly contains liver and spleen
- Covered by peritoneum
- Associated with multiple-organ pathologies in about 50% of cases
  - Pulmonary hypoplasia
  - Pulmonary lobar collapse
  - Lumbar lordosis
  - Absent radial ray
  - Renal ectopia

- Hydronephrosis
- Aortic coarctation
- Absent inferior vena cava (IVC)

Gastroschisis

- Abdominal wall defect, off the midline and usually right-sided
- No peritoneal investment
- Does not contain liver
- Less common occurrence than omphalocoele
- Antenatal ultrasound demonstrates free floating loops of bowel in amniotic fluid

Intussusception

- Telescoping of the proximal bowel into a contiguous bowel segment
- Peak age is 2–20 years
- Commoner in males
- Ileocolic and ileoileocolic intussusceptions are the commonest forms

Imaging features

- Length of intussusception is crucial in determining management; > 3.5 cm is indicative of the need for surgical intervention
- Target or 'bull's eye' or pseudo-kidney sign is typical

Reduction of intussusception

- The 'rule of threes': bag 3 feet high, 3 minutes per try, 3 tries
- Dilute contrast medium is generally used; air reduction may also be attempted
- Continue reduction till there is free flow of contrast into the terminal ileum
- Contraindications to the procedure
  - Perforation
  - Peritonitis
  - Henoch–Schönlein purpura
- Success rate has been quoted at 18–90%
- Complications of the procedure
  - Perforation in 0.4% of cases
  - Recurrence in 10% of cases, half of which occur within 48 hours

Mesenteric adenitis

- Self-limiting lymphadenitis in the mesentery
- Three or more clustered nodes measuring > 5 mm are are diagnostic

- Important to demonstrate a normal appendix in these cases

Acute appendicitis

Imaging features

Plain film

- May be normal
- Appendicolith is seen in up to 10% of cases
- Air–fluid levels within the bowel in the right lower quadrant is a feature
- Loss of the right psoas margin may be shown

Ultrasound

- Graded-compression ultrasound with a high-frequency transducer is used
- Appendicolith, if present, is echogenic
- Appendix is a non-compressible, blind-ended tubular structure > 6 mm in diameter
- Fluid, phlegmon or abscess in the right lower quadrant

Necrotising enterocolitis

- Disease of premature babies. 10% of affected babies may be term
- Prevalence up to 2.4 cases per 1000 live births
- Child typically presents with abdominal distension, bloody diarrhoea, sepsis and increased gastric aspirates, typically in the first week of life
- Overall mortality is 20%

Imaging features

Plain X-ray

- Presence of pneumatosis is the best clue
- Asymmetric bowel dilatation with separated, dilated loops of bowel
- Commonest location is the right colon and the terminal ileum
- Portal vein gas present; its presence, however, is not associated with any higher mortality
- Pneumoperitoneum with perforation is an absolute indication for surgery

Contrast study

- Mucosal irregularity and ulceration, with widely separated bowel loops
- Mucosa becomes permeable to contrast media in the presence of necrosis, and

subsequent renal excretion of oral contrast is noted
- Enema is contraindicated in acute necrotising enterocolitis

Ultrasound
- Thickened, dilated loops of bowel
- Vascularity of the loops of bowel is increased when they are inflamed and decreased when they are ischaemic

Hirschsprung's disease

- Absence of parasympathetic ganglia in the submucosal and intramuscular colonic plexuses
- Strong male preponderance
- Associations include trisomy 21 and meconium ileus
- Extremely rare in premature infants
- Transition zone to normal ganglionic colon is located in the rectosigmoid in up to 80% of cases
- Total colonic aganglionosis is a familial variant in which male and females are equally commonly affected
- Complications include necrotising enterocolitis, caecal perforation, obstructive uropathy and enterocolitis

Imaging features

AXR
- Features of distal bowel obstruction
- Pneumoperitoneum with perforation is seen in 4% of cases

Contrast study with water-soluble medium
- Inverted cone like transition point is typical
- A rectosigmoid index < 1 is diagnostic
- Delayed radiographs should be done if the features are not typical

Anorectal malformation

- Occurs as a result of failure of descent and separation of the hindgut and the genitourinary system in the second trimester
- One in 5000 births
- Presents with failure to pass meconium or with meconium per vagina or per urethra
- High malformations (supralevator) are associated with genitourinary and cardiac anomalies
- Low malformations (infralevator) have a low association with other anomalies
- Associations include tethered cord, VACTERL, and duodenal and oesophageal atresia

Imaging features

Plain X-ray
- Low colonic obstruction
- Gas bubbles in the urinary bladder and the vagina
- Intraluminal calcification
- Fistulogram is performed to confirm the diagnosis

Liver and biliary system
Choledochal cyst

- Cystic dilatation of the extrahepatic bile duct with segmental aneurysmal dilatation of the common bile duct
- More common in females

Todani's classification
• **Type I:** segmental or diffuse fusiform dilatation of the common bile duct • **Type II:** cysts represent a diverticulum of the duct • **Type III:** cysts represent a choledochocoele occurring in the duodenal wall and protruding as a mass into the duodenal lumen • **Type IV:** multiple extrahepatic bile duct cysts • **Type V:** cystic dilatation of the intrahepatic ducts; also known as Caroli's disease

- Associations
  - Double gallbladder
  - Failure of union of left and right hepatic ducts
  - Polycystic liver disease
- Classical presentation triad as seen in 30% of cases
  - Intermittent obstructive jaundice

- Right upper quadrant pain
- Palpable mass
- Complications
  - Stones
  - Portal vein thrombosis
  - Cholangiocarcinoma
  - Hepatic abscess
  - Pancreatitis
  - Biliary cirrhosis

Imaging features

Ultrasound
- Porta hepatis cyst communicating with the common hepatic or intrahepatic ducts
- Dilatation of the intrahepatic duct

Hepatobiliary imino-diacetic acid (HIDA) scan
- Fills in 1 hour
- Prominent ductal activity

MR cholangiogram
- Helps in preoperative planning

Biliary atresia

- Severely deficient extrahepatic biliary tree
- Presents in the first week of life with conjugated hyperbilirubinemia
- Associations include trisomy 18, polysplenia and hepatocellular carcinoma
- Causes include hepatitis and sclerosing cholangitis, in some cases the cause is unknown
- Liver biopsy provides definitive histological diagnosis
- Correctable in 12% of cases, using Kasai's portoenterostomy (prompt diagnosis is essential)

Imaging features

Ultrasound
- Normal gallbladder in 20% cases
- Triangular cord sign
- Echogenic fibrous tissue above the bifurcation of portal vein
- No intrahepatic ductal dilatation

HIDA scan
- Non-visualisation of bowel at 24 hours
- Good hepatic visualisation at 5 minutes
- Increased renal excretion

Differential diagnosis

- Neonatal hepatitis
- Cystic fibrosis (inspissated bile in cystic fibrosis may be indistinguishable from biliary atresia)

MRI
- High-signal periportal fibrosis
- Absent hepatic ducts

Gastrointestinal tumours in children

Infantile haemangioendothelioma

- Commonest benign paediatric tumour
- Presents in infants < 6 months of age in 85% of cases
- Twice as common in girls
- There is a tendency to involute spontaneously over months or years
- Often followed with sequential ultrasound
- Association with cutaneous haemangioma (in 50% of cases)
- Complications
  - Arteriovenous shunts causing congestive heart failure
  - Intraperitoneal haemorrhage
  - Disseminated intravascular coagulation
  - Thrombocytopenia

Imaging features

Ultrasound
- Complex, hypoechoic mass

CT
- Low-attenuation mass in the liver
- Haemorrhage or calcification may alter the characteristics
- Contrast enhancement is variable

MRI
- T1WI: low signal compared with normal liver and spleen, with high-signal, intense haemorrhagic areas
- T2WI: typically high signal, but may be heterogeneous

Hepatoblastoma

- Commonest malignant primary tumour in children
- Median age of presentation < 2 years
- Commoner in males than females
- Commonest site is the right lobe of the liver
- Metastasises to lymph nodes, brain and lung
- Associated with Beckwith–Wiedemann syndrome and hemihypertrophy

Imaging features

Ultrasound
- Large mass with mixed echogenicity
- Calcification seen in 50% of cases
- May have 'spoke-wheel' appearance, owing to the presence of fibrous septa

CT
- Hypodense lesion with peripheral rim enhancement

Angiogram
- Hypervascular lesion
- No arteriovenous shunting

Hepatocellular carcinoma

- Second commonest tumour in children
- Presents in children aged > 3 years
- Associations
  - Glycogen storage disease
  - Galactosemia
  - Tyrosinaemia
  - Biliary atresia
- Difficult to distinguish radiologically from hepatoblastoma other than by clinical presentation, though it has a lower incidence of calcification than hepatoblastoma

Miscellaneous pathologies and tables

Peliosis hepatis

- Presence of multiple, blood-filled lacunar spaces in the liver
- Benign lesion but may cause complications, including liver failure, cholestasis, portal hypertension and liver rupture

- Associations
  - Chronic wasting diseases
  - Use of anabolic steroid medication
  - Sprue
  - Diabetes mellitus
  - Vasculitis
  - *Bartonella* species infection in HIV positive patients

Imaging features

CT
- Hypodense lesions with peripheral enhancement on non-enhanced scans
- Strong contrast enhancement on delayed imaging, with a branching appearance caused by the vascular component

Double-bubble sign (causes)

- Duodenal atresia
- Annular pancreas
- Duodenal diaphragm
- Midgut volvulus
- Preduodenal vein
- Superior mesenteric artery syndrome
- Duplication cyst
- Adhesions

Neonatal pneumoperitoneum (causes)

- Rupture in necrotising enterocolitis
- Rupture of the posterior urethral valves or the bladder
- Pneumopericardium (which may dissect downwards)
- Ruptured pneumatosis cystoides intestinalis

Cystic fibrosis

Imaging features

Plain X-ray
- Meconium ileus
- Dilated bowel loops with 'soap bubble' appearance in the right lower quadrant
- Peritoneal or scrotal calcifications and meconium pseudocyst formation seen, with intrauterine bowel rupture
- Meconium plug syndrome
- Dilated loops of bowel with distal obstruction
- Signs of constipation
- Intussusception

Contrast study

- Reflux
- Thickened duodenal folds
- Peptic ulceration
- Microcolon (small calibre but normal length) in meconium ileus

Ultrasound and CT

- Gallstones
- Fatty liver
- Atrophic pancreas
- Features of intussusception, if it is present
- Biliary cirrhosis
- Bowel wall thickening

Paediatric genitourinary system

Kidney and ureter

Renal agenesis

- Congenital absence of the kidneys
- Can be unilateral or bilateral
- Renal agenesis is associated with genital malformations
  - Hydrometrocolpos
  - Vaginal atresia and vaginal septum in girls
  - Cryptorchidism, hypospadias and absent testes in boys

Unilateral renal agenesis

- One in 500
- Failure of ureteric bud to induce metanephric bud
- Ipsilateral adrenal is present in 85% of cases
- Ipsilateral absence of the trigone and ureter

Bilateral renal agenesis

- Incompatible with life
- One in 8000
- Commoner in boys
- Associated with oligohydramnios, prematurity, Potter's facies with low set, floppy ears, prominent epicanthal folds, micrognathia and pulmonary hypoplasia

Horseshoe kidney

- Fusion of the lower poles prevents complete ascent of the kidneys
- Increased risk of adenocarcinoma, Wilms' tumour and hypertension
- Horseshoe kidneys are at particular risk of bleeding secondary to minor trauma
- Associations include caudal ectopia, vesicoureteral reflux and hydronephrosis

Pelvic kidney

- Ascent of kidneys is hindered by the inferior mesenteric artery
- Commoner on the left side
- Renal pelvis becomes anteriorly facing
- Blood supply to a pelvic kidney comes from the aorta or iliac vessels

Duplex kidneys

- Duplex kidneys have 2 collecting systems
- One in 125
- Duplex kidneys without dilatation do not need to be followed
- Duplex kidneys with dilatation should be evaluated by ultrasound and micturating cystourethrogram after the infant has been placed on prophylactic antibiotics

The Weigert–Meyer rule for duplex kidneys

- The rule states that the upper pole ureter inserts ectopically, medially and inferior to the normal position
- This ectopic ureter may terminate in a ureterocoele and can become obstructed, causing hydronephrosis
- The lower pole ureter may reflux and rarely it may cause hydronephrosis

Multicystic dysplastic kidney

- Most common cystic lesion of the kidney
- Results from early and complete obstruction of the ureteropelvic junction
- One in 4300 live births, more common in boys

- Non-functional kidney replaced by multiple cysts and dysplastic tissue
- There are no connections between the cysts and no normal renal parenchyma intervenes
- Contralateral kidney shows abnormalities in up to 50% of cases, including ureteropelvic junction obstruction, renal dysplasia, vesicoureteral reflux and multicystic dysplastic kidney

Autosomal-recessive polycystic kidney disease

- Autosomal-recessive disorder
- Bilateral symmetric cystic disease
- Medullary ductal ectasia is characteristic
- Kidneys have decreased concentrating ability and tubular atrophy, with systemic hypertension
- Associated with biliary duct hyperplasia and portal fibrosis
- Renal changes are inversely proportional to liver changes in terms of severity
- Normal number of glomeruli

Patterns of autosomal-recessive polycystic kidney disease

- Perinatal: 90% of tubules affected, death in <–30 days
- Neonatal: 50% of tubules affected, live up to 9 months
- Infantile
- Juvenile

Imaging features

Ultrasound
- Bright, bilateral nephromegaly
- Poor corticomedullary differentiation
- Tiny punctuate, hyperechoic foci develop with time and correlate with renal failure

Intravenous urogram
- Prolonged pyelogram, brush-like tubules and linear contrast streaks

CT
- Nephromegaly
- Trapping of contrast in dilated tubules
- May be diffusely microcystic
- Small bladder

Bilateral echo-bright kidneys in neonates

Never a normal variant

Causes include
- Acute tubular necrosis
- Renal vein thrombosis
- Autosomal-recessive polcystic kidney disease
- Autosomal-dominant polcystic kidney disease
- Tuberous sclerosis
- Cytomegalovirus infection
- Congenital syphilis
- Bilateral nephroblastomatosis

Vesicoureteral reflux

- Occurs in up to 15% of all children
- Primary reflux is due to immaturity or maldevelopment of the ureterovesical junction

Grades of reflux
- Grade I: distal ureteral reflux
- Grade II: reflux into the ureter and pelvis, with normal calyces
- Grade III: reflux into a mildly dilated ureter and renal pelvis, with blunt calyces
- Grade IV: reflux into a moderately dilated, tortuous ureter, with significant blunting of the calyces
- Grade V: loss of papilla

Indications for a micturating cystourethrogram

- Thick bladder wall
- Antenatally detected hydronephrosis
- All boys < 1 year of age with a urinary tract infection
- All boys < 3 years of age with a small kidney
- Terminal haematuria
- Sibling refluxing
- Ureteric dilatation in infants

Megaureter

- Primary megaureter represents an obstructive dilatation of the ureter above an aperistaltic segment near the ureterovesical junction
- Resolves spontaneously
- However, prophylactic antibiotics should be given

Urethra

Posterior urethral valve

- Only boys are affected
- Abnormal mucosal folds between the urethral wall and the distal end of the verumontanum
- When severe, may present *in utero* with severe oligohydramnios, hydroureteronephrosis or ascites
- Reflux occurs in up to 60% of cases

Imaging features

Micturating cystourethrogram
- 'Gold-standard' diagnostic study
- Abrupt transition from a dilated posterior urethra to a small bulbous urethra at the level of the valves
- The actual valve tissue may not be visible

Prune belly syndrome

- Triad of abdominal wall hypoplasia, cryptorchidism and dilatation of the urinary tract
- One in 40,000, not inherited
- Only boys are affected
- 20% of affected babies die in infancy
- Associations
  - Pulmonary hypoplasia
  - Polydactyly or syndactyly
  - Malrotation
  - Scoliosis
  - Congenital heart disease
  - Pneumothorax
  - Microcephaly
  - Imperforate anus

Imaging features

- Hypertrophied bladder with severe vesicoureteral reflux
- Tortuous ureters and renal dysplasia

Tumours of the renal tract

Wilms' tumour

- Commonest renal tumour of childhood
- Genetic mutations have been identified
- Male and females equally affected
- Median age at presentation is 3 years
- Bilateral in 5% of causes
- Usually synchronous when bilateral
- 5-year survival rates can be up to 95% in children with favourable histology
- Associations
  - WAGR (Wilms' tumour, Aniridia, Genitourinary anomalies and mental Retardation)
  - Denys–Drash syndrome
  - Beckwith–Wiedemann syndrome
  - Perlman syndrome
  - Hemihypertrophy

Imaging features

Plain X-ray
- Mass predominantly in the flank with displacement of bowel gas

Ultrasound
- Heterogeneous mass with IVC invasion. Doppler ultrasound is better than MRI for assessing venous involvement

CT
- Calcification is seen in 10% of cases
- Enhances poorly post-contrast

Neuroblastoma

- Tumours arising from the neural crest along the sympathetic chain, or adrenal medulla
- Commonest solid neoplasm in children and infants, and the third commonest malignant disease in children overall
- Location is unknown in 10% of cases
- Almost always bilateral
- Boys and girls are equally affected
- Median age at presentation is 2 years
- Metastases are found at time of presentation in up to 60% of cases
- Spreads via lymphatic and haematogenous routes to bone marrow and skeleton
- Better prognosis when the child is < 1 year old

Staging of neuroblastoma

- Stage 1: localised, with complete gross excision
- Stage 2a: localised, with incomplete gross excision
- Stage 2b: localised, with ipsilateral nodes positive for metastases
- Stage 3: unresectable unilateral or localised unilateral disease with contralateral nodes, or in the midline with bilateral extension
- Stage 4: any primary tumour with dissemination to distant nodes
- Stage 4s: 's' for special dissemination to skin, liver or bone marrow (limited to infants < 1 year old)

Imaging features

Plain X-ray
- Mass in abdomen
- Shows mass in the lungs in cases of extension, and metastases

Ultrasound
- Solid tumour with echogenic foci of calcification
- Echo-poor areas indicate haemorrhage or necrosis
- Encasement of vessels

CT and MRI
- For full assessment of extension and spread

Methylene diphosphonate (MDP) or metaiodobenzylguanidine (MIBG) scintigram
- Assesses for bone metastases

Disorders of sexual development

Ambiguous genitalia

True hermaphroditism
- 46XX mosaic or 46XY
- Both testes and ovaries are present in the fetus
- Rare

Female pseudohermaphroditism
- 46XX
- Fetus has two ovaries

Male pseudohermaphroditism
- 46XY
- Causes include androgen insensitivity and decreased synthesis of testosterone
- Testes present, but no müllerian structures
- Bilateral cryptorchidism
- Presents in adolescence with 'amenorrhoea'

- 'Streak gonads' should be removed promptly (because of the risk of gonadoblastoma)
- Calcification suggests malignancy
- Increased risk of Wilms' tumour in true gonadal dysgenesis

Cryptorchidism
- Undescended testis
- Prevalence is 3.5% at birth, which decreases to 0.8% by 1 year
- Commoner in premature children
- Familial predisposition
- 70% of cases are right-sided; most of the rest are bilateral
- Locations
  - In the inguinal canal (in 70% of cases)
  - Prescrotal in (15% of cases)
  - Intra-abdominal in (15% of cases)
- Associations include prune belly, Prader–Willi syndrome, Beckwith–Weidemann syndrome, Noonan's syndrome and Laurence–Moon–Biedl syndrome
- High incidence of malignancy and infertility
- Ultrasound confirms the diagnosis

Overview

Neonatal chest conditions

Diffuse conditions

- Low lung volumes with streaky perihilar densities
    - Hyaline membrane disease
    - Oxygen therapy and complication
- Large lung volumes with streaky perihilar densities
    - Meconium aspiration syndrome
    - Transient tachypnoea of the newborn
    - Neonatal pneumonia

Focal conditions

- Congenital cystic adenomatoid malformation
- Congenital lobar emphysema
- Pulmonary interstitial emphysema
- Congenital diaphragmatic hernia
- Pulmonary hypoplasia
- Sequestration
- Bronchogenic cyst

Upper airway problems in children

- Laryngomalacia
- Tracheomalacia
- Tracheal stenosis
- Epiglottitis
- Laryngeal papillomatosis
- Croup
- Foreign body aspiration
- Juvenile angiofibroma

Childhood chest conditions

- Pneumonia
- Chest in drowning
- Tuberculosis
- Cystic fibrosis
- HIV infection
- Immunodeficiency syndromes
- Chronic granulomatous disease

Neonatal chest conditions

Hyaline membrane disease

- Surfactant deficiency leading to collapse of the alveoli
- Respiratory distress within 2 hours of life; distress beginning after 8 hours is unlikely to be due to hyaline membrane disease
- Predisposing factors
    - Prematurity
    - Term infants of diabetic mothers
    - Second twins
    - Infants delivered by Caesarean section
- Treatment is with ventilation and exogenous surfactant
- Antenatal corticosteroids given to the mother have been shown to reduce the incidence
- Postnatal exogenous surfactant via endotracheal tube has been shown to reduce mortality (one of its complications, however, is pulmonary haemorrhage)

Imaging features

- Any opacity on plain X-ray in this age group should be considered as hyaline membrane disease unless proven otherwise
- Small-volume chest
- Ground-glass appearance in the lungs with fine reticulonodular markings
- Bell-shaped thorax in the unintubated baby
- Air bronchograms may be present and may extend to the periphery
- Consolidation and pleural effusion are very rarely seen

Complications 'due to oxygen therapy'

- Pulmonary interstitial emphysema occurs after 2–3 days
    - Presence of air in the lymphatic parenchymal tissues causing overdistension and subsequent rupture

- Usually seen as bilateral curvilinear lucencies on plain X-ray
- However, it may occur unilaterally if the endotracheal tube selectively enters one bronchus during intubation
- Acquired lobar emphysema
- Interstitial fibrosis occurs after 28 days; also known as bronchopulmonary dysplasia

Evolution of bronchopulmonary dysplasia

- < 4 days: mucosal necrosis
- 1 week: oedema with exudates
- 2 weeks: bronchial metaplasia
- 1 month: fibrosis (mortality 40–50%)
- In infants who survive, improvement in the appearance of the chest radiographs is seen, even progression to a normal radiograph at 3–5 years in about 10% of cases

Meconium aspiration syndrome

- Meconium-filled amniotic fluid breathed into the infant's lungs during delivery
- Significant only if aspirated to below the level of vocal cords
- Occurs in 1% of all full-term neonates
- Usually clears in 3–5 days
- Complications include persistent fetal circulation and pulmonary hypertension

Imaging features

CXR
- Hyperinflated lungs
- Atelectasis with patchy bilateral opacities
- Pneumothorax or pneumomediastinum in 25% of cases
- CXR returns to normal by 1 year of age

Transient tachypnoea of the newborn

- Delayed clearance of intrauterine pulmonary liquids ('wet lungs')
- Occurs in 5% of full-term infants

- Main differential diagnoses are group B streptococcal sepsis and total anomalous pulmonary venous drainage
- May lead to persistent fetal circulation
- Predisposing factors
  - Elective Caesarean section (transient tachypnoea seen in 9% of cases)
  - Maternal diabetes
  - Maternal sedation
  - Hypoproteinaemia
  - Hypervolaemia
  - Male sex

Imaging features

CXR
- Interstitial oedema (caused by fluid overload)
- Lungs clear in 48–72 hours as a rule

Neonatal pneumonia

- 1 in 200 live births
- Risk factors include prolonged labour, premature rupture of membranes and placental infection
- Group B streptococcus is the most common causative organism (acquired in the birth canal)
- Others causative organisms include *Pseudomonas, Enterobacter, Staphylococcus* and *Klebsiella* species
- Empyema can develop as a complication, mostly due to staphylococcus or *Klebsiella*, rarely streptococci

Imaging features

- Patchy, asymmetric bilateral infiltrates
- Pleural effusions

Infants

Congenital cystic adenomatoid malformation

- Anomalous development of terminal respiratory structures resulting in polypoid glandular lung tissue without normal alveolar differentiation
- Communicates with the bronchial tree
- Respiratory distress within first few days of life, but may present up to 1 year of age

- Usually confined to one lobe; equally common in all lobes
- Rarely undergoes sarcomatous degeneration
- Can cause pulmonary hypoplasia if large
- Associations
  - Pectus excavatum (in 25% of cases)
  - Cardiac malformations
  - Renal agenesis
  - Prune belly syndrome
  - Jejunal atresia
  - Bronchopulmonary sequestration

Imaging features

Antenatal ultrasound
- Echo-bright cysts
- Fetal ascites

CXR
- Unilateral cystic mass
- Multiple fluid levels (even in the absence of infection)
- Contralateral mediastinal shift
- Spontaneous pneumothorax

CT
- Complex cystic structure with surrounding air trapping

Causes of an echo-bright intrathoracic mass on antenatal ultrasound

- Congenital diaphragmatic hernia
- Congenital cystic adenomatoid malformation
- Intralobar pulmonary sequestration

Congenital lobar emphysema

- Progressive lobar over-distension, caused by narrowing of a bronchial segment
- Bronchial cartilage dysplasia or immaturity is the usual culprit
- Vascular compression or extrinsic mass lesions can also lead to lobar emphysema
- Presents in the first 6 months of life
- Males more commonly affected than females
- Idiopathic in 50% of cases

- Sites: Left upper lobe in 40% of cases, right middle lobe in 30%, right lower lobe in 20%; bilateral in 5%
- Congenital heart defects are seen in 10% of cases, e.g. patent ductus arteriosus, ventral septal defect
- Can cause pulmonary hypoplasia

Imaging features

CXR
- Expanded hyperlucent lobe
- Variable degrees of atelectasis of the adjacent lung
- Contralateral mediastinal shift

CT
- Hyperlucent, expanded lobe with reduced vascularity and midline substernal lobar herniation
- Usually the mediastinum is shifter to the opposite side

Congenital diaphragmatic hernia

- Failure of closure of the pleuroperitoneal membrane
- Males more commonly affected than females
- One in 2500 live births
- The left side is more commonly than the right; bilateral in 5% of cases
- Present later than 1 year of age in 10% of cases
- Delayed onset of this condition is related to group B streptococcal infection
- Complications include pulmonary hypoplasia and persistent fetal circulation
- Neonatal death occurs in 35% of cases, still birth in 35–50%
- Multiple associations
  - CNS abnormalities: spina bifida (with neural tube defect in 30% of cases), encephalocele and anencephaly
  - Pulmonary hypoplasia
  - Intestinal malrotation (in 95% of cases)
  - Trisomy 13, trisomy 18
  - Infections: cytomegalovirus and rubella
  - Cardiovascular anomalies (in 20% of cases)

Bochdalek's hernia versus Morgagni's hernia

- Bochdalek's hernia accounts for 90% of cases; Morgagni's hernia accounts for 10% of cases
- Bochdalek's hernia is located posteriorly; Morgagni's hernia is located anteriorly
- Bochdalek's hernia is commoner on the left; Morgagni's hernia is commoner on the right

Imaging features

Antenatal ultrasound
- Echo-bright solid or cystic mass positioned behind the left atrium and ventricle in the thorax
- Contralateral mediastinal shift
- Polyhydramnios
- Absent stomach in the abdomen

CXR
- Bowel loops in the chest

Oral contrast study
- Used to confirm the anatomy

Pulmonary hypoplasia

- Underdevelopment of lung parenchyma and vasculature
- Hypoplastic lung is supplied by the aorta and drained by the IVC or portal vein
- Almost always right-sided (commonest site is the right middle lobe)
- Associations
  - Diaphragmatic hernia or accessory diaphragm
  - Congenital tracheal stenosis
  - Bronchiectasis
  - Congenital heart disease, e.g. atrial septal defect, ventricular septal defect, patent ductus arteriosus, tetralogy of Fallot
  - Skeletal problems, e.g. osteogenesis imperfecta, hemivertebra, hypoplastic ribs with or without notching, early-onset scoliosis

Types of pulmonary hypoplasia: primary and secondary

- Primary idiopathic pulmonary hypoplasia
- Secondary bilateral or unilateral pulmonary hypoplasia
- Bilateral pulmonary hypoplasia secondary to oligohydramnios or a restricted chest cage (resulting from skeletal dysplasias)
- Unilateral pulmonary hypoplasia secondary to congenital diaphragmatic hernia, hydrothorax or Swyer–James (McLeod) syndrome
- Acquired pulmonary hypoplasia secondary to infection

Imaging features

Antenatal ultrasound
- Small thorax
- Oligohydramnios

CXR
- Small hyperlucent lung
- Diffuse pattern of scarring

Fluoroscopy
- Little change in volume with respiration

CT
- Pruned appearance with mosaic pattern of air trapping

Scimitar syndrome (pulmonary venolobar syndrome)

- Aplasia or hypoplasia of one or more lobes of the right lung with partial or complete anomalous pulmonary venous return
- Absent or small pulmonary artery
- Males more commonly affected than females
- Associations include atrial septal defect, tetralogy of Fallot, hemivertebra and rib anomalies

Imaging features

CXR

- Classic finding is of a 'scimitar' vein (shaped like a Turkish sword), seen medial and inferior to the IVC

Pulmonary sequestration

- Congenital mass of aberrant pulmonary tissue that has no connection with the bronchial tree or the pulmonary arterial system
- Typically in posteromedial segments of the lower lobes
- Two types: extralobar and intralobar
- Extralobar pulmonary sequestration
  - Presents with respiratory distress in neonates
  - Aberrant lung tissue with its own pleural lining
  - Usually airless, unless it communicates with the bowel
  - Males more commonly affected than females
  - More commonly on the left side than the right, usually adjacent to the diaphragm
  - Arterial blood is supplied by the aorta (or, rarely, by the coeliac artery)
  - Venous drainage is by the IVC, the azygos system or the portal veins
  - Associations are common
- Intralobar pulmonary sequestration
  - Presents with chest infections in older children
  - No separate pleural lining
  - Airless or cystic lung mass
  - Arterial blood is supplied by the aorta
  - Venous drainage is by the pulmonary veins into the left atrium
  - Associations are uncommon (however, skeletal associations are more common)
- Associations
  - Pulmonary hypoplasia
  - Diaphragmatic defects
  - Bronchogenic cysts
  - Anomalous pulmonary venous circulation
  - Tracheo-oesphageal fistula

Imaging features

- *Antenatal US:* Echo-bright solid/cystic mass within chest cavity. Colour Doppler can be used to identify anomalous vessels
- *CXR:* Solid/cystic opacity near diaphragm. Air fluid levels with air bronchograms if infected
- *CT:* Bronchial mucus plugs
- Solid/cystic mass
- Hyperinflated lung
- Air-fluid levels if infected

Bronchogenic cyst

- Developmental cyst lined by respiratory epithelium caused by ectopic bronchial budding during embryogenesis
- *Site:* 85% occur in mediastinum when early in development. Posterior > middle > anterior
- Typically lower lobes when occurs late in development. Right> left

Imaging features

CXR

- Oval mass projecting from the mediastinum

CT

- Well-defined, fluid-filled or air-filled cyst in the medial third of the lung or mediastinum
- Cysts rarely calcify

MRI

- Fluid-filled cyst (low signal on T1WI, high signal on T2WI)

Upper airway pathologies

Choanal atresia

- Neonatal nasal obstruction due to failure of perforation of the oronasal membrane
- One in 5000 live births
- Bilateral disease is commoner than unilateral
- May be bony (in 90% of cases) or membranous (10%)
- Causes severe respiratory distress in the neonate (immediately after birth)

- Associations (75% are associated with other abnormalities)
  - Craniosynostosis
  - Congenital heart disease
  - Tracheo-oesophageal fistula
  - Intestinal malrotation
  - Polydactyly
  - Treacher–Collins syndrome, fetal alcohol syndrome, DiGeorge's syndrome

Imaging features

CT
- Axial CT is the investigation of choice
- Enlarged vomer
- Fusion of the bony aspects of the pterygoid process and the palatine bone
- Narrowing of the posterior choanae to < 3.4 mm

Congenital bronchial atresia

- Characterised by obliteration of the proximal lumen of a segmental bronchus with preservation of distal structures
- Pathogenesis unknown but proposed to be secondary to vascular insult
- Air enters the affected segment via collateral channels, producing over-inflation and air trapping
- Usually asymptomatic
- May present in older children with chest infections
- Commonest site is in apicoposterior aspect of the left upper lobe
- Associations
  - Congenital cystic adenomatoid malformation
  - Lobar emphysema (however, there is no mucus plug in this case)

Imaging features

Antenatal ultrasound
- Echo-bright mass with dilated bronchi

Plain X-ray
- Trapped air during expiration accompanied by a central 'mass' next

to the hilum, simulating collapse of the left upper lobe (corresponding to the mucocele)

Laryngomalacia (supraglottic hypermobility syndrome)

- Laryngeal collapse with inspiration secondary to infolding of the aryepiglottic folds
- Presents with inspiratory stridor in the first year of life
- Self-limiting condition
- Stridor improves with activity, prone positioning and neck extension
- Usually assessed by laryngoscopy

Tracheomalacia (soft trachea)

- Characterised by collapse of the trachea with expiration
- Can be focal or diffuse
- Focal disease is seen secondary to congenital abnormalities, e.g. a vascular ring
- Can be extrinsic (the commoner type) or intrinsic (caused by weakness of supporting structures)
- Can be primary (associated with chondromalacia, relapsing polychondritis and prematurity) or secondary (associated with vascular rings and mediastinal causes)
- Clinically produces expiratory or biphasic stridor
- Congenital diffuse tracheomalacia improves by age 6–12 months as the structural integrity of the trachea is gradually restored

Imaging features

- Fluoroscopy and oesophagography are diagnostic
- Fluoroscopy shows an exaggerated decrease in the calibre of the trachea during expiration

Associations of tracheal compression

- Aberrant origin of the innominate artery (left of the trachea in 30% of cases)
- Double aortic arch (posterior indentation from the right-sided arch more prominent)
- Right aortic arch
- Pulmonary 'sling' (left pulmonary artery from the right pulmonary artery crossing between the trachea and oesophagus)
- High cervical aortic arch

Tracheal stenosis

- Can be primary or secondary
- Primary tracheal stenosis
  - Intact tracheal rings
  - Associated with vascular ring, pulmonary sling and H-type tracheo-oesophageal fistulae
- Secondary tracheal stenosis is seen with a subglottic haemangioma (soft tissue mass causing compression)
- Present during the first year of life in 90% of cases, often with biphasic stridor
- Frontal and lateral high-voltage, filtered radiographs are used to give a clear visualisation of the stenosed segment

Acute epiglottitis

- Life-threatening condition
- Presents with expiratory stridor and dysphagia
- Caused by infection with *Haemophilus influenzae* type B
- Commonest age is 3–6 years

Imaging features

CXR
- Lateral film shows thickened aryepiglottic folds
- Thickened epiglottis ('thumb' sign)

- Subglottic narrowing secondary to oedema
- Distended hypopharynx and pyriform sinuses
- Caution: complete obstruction of the epiglottis can be precipitated by handling the neck of the child during radiographic positioning

Croup (laryngotracheobronchitis)

- Subglottic location
- Caused by infection with parainfluenza virus, respiratory syncytial virus or bacteria such as staphylococci and *Clostridium diphtheriae*
- Affects children aged 6 months to 3 years

Imaging features

CXR
- Subglottic narrowing on anteroposterior view ('steeple' sign)
- Loss of subglottic shoulder
- Anteroposterior film cannot distinguish between croup and epiglottitis, and a lateral view is required to exclude epiglottitis

Fluoroscopy
- Shows that the narrowing is most obvious on inspiration

Foreign body

- Typical age of presentation is 6 months to 4 years
- Most commonly lodged in the right bronchus, followed by the left bronchus and then the larynx and trachea

Imaging features

- Unilateral air trapping, which indicates a bronchial foreign body unless proven otherwise
- Only 10% of foreign bodies are radio-opaque

Juvenile angiofibroma

- Benign vascular, locally invasive tumour
- Occurs almost exclusively in adolescent boys

- Treatment is with embolisation followed by resection
- Recurrence occurs in up to 30% of cases

Imaging features

Plain X-ray
- Anterior bowing of the posterior wall of the maxillary sinus
- Large mass in the nasopharynx with or without bony erosion

CT
- Best for showing bony involvement

MRI
- Best for showing sinus extension

Childhood chest conditions

Childhood pneumonia

- Mycoplasmal in 30% of cases, with segmental, subsegmental or reticulonodular interstitial infiltrates, lobar involvement in the lower lobes and effusions in 20%
- Viral in 65% of cases, with peribronchial thickening, hyperinflation and scattered atelectasis
- Bacterial in 5% of cases, caused by infection with the pneumococcus, *Staphylococcus aureus* or *Haemophilus influenzae*
- Fungal pneumonia is associated with mycetoma or allergic bronchopulmonary aspergillosis (seen in asthma and cystic fibrosis, with mucus plugs in the bronchi, outlined by collateral air drift, which appears like a gloved finger)
- Round pneumonias respond rapidly to treatment

Swyer–James (MacLeod) syndrome (bronchiolitis obliterans)

- Acquired pulmonary hypoplasia
- Seen as a small hyperlucent lung with diminished vessels (focal emphysema) following a viral respiratory tract infection

Childhood tuberculosis

- In children most tuberculosis is primary
- Miliary tuberculosis is due to haematogenous spread and is more common in post-primary tuberculosis

Imaging features

- Primary tuberculosis
  - Ill-defined consolidation, which may be subsegmental or lobar, involving any lobe
  - Typically unilateral hilar or paratracheal lymphadenopathy
  - Pleural effusions are uncommon
- Miliary tuberculosis
  - Multiple 'millet'-like nodules (1–2 mm in diameter) diffusely spread throughout both lungs

Chest in drowning

- Pulmonary oedema with a normal-sized heart
- Changes resolve over 5–10 days
- Admission X-ray may be normal, and a repeat X-ray after 24 hours is mandatory
- Can lead to acute respiratory distress syndrome (ARDS) in severe cases
- Pneumomediastinum and pneumothorax are recognised complications

Cystic fibrosis

- Autosomal-recessive inheritance
- Abnormality on chromosome 7
- Commoner in Caucasians
- Affects exocrine glands (in the skin, pancreas, chest and paranasal sinuses)
- In the lungs, the upper lobes are most severely affected
- Early pathogens are *Staphylococcus aureus* and *Haemophilus influenzae*
- Late pathogens are *Pseudomonas aeruginosa* and *Burkholderia cepacia*
- The earliest presentation is with a bronchiolitis-like illness, reflecting small airway obstruction

Imaging features

CXR
- Overinflated lungs with or without air space shadowing

- Used for severity scoring
- Portacath tip should be in the superior vena cava (SVC)

AIDs in children

- *Pneumocystis carinii*, cytomegalovirus and *Aspergillus* are the commonest chest pathogens
- CXR in *Pneumocystis carinii* pneumonia shows perihilar haze, which is progressive with air bronchograms and hyperinflation; pneumatocoeles, pneumothoraces may develop later
- Cytomegalovirus causes a more prominent reticulonodular pattern in the outer third of the lung
- Lymphocytic interstitial pneumonia may be the presentation of AIDS, with ground-glass attenuation, poorly defined centrilobular nodules, and thickening of the interstitium along the lymphatic vessels with lymphadenopathy
- Biopsy is ultimately required to establish the diagnosis

Chronic granulomatous disease

- X-linked or autosomal-recessive condition in which phagocytes can engulf but not kill organisms
- Boys are affected
- Pathogens include *Staphylococcus aureus*, *Staphylococcus epidermidis*, *Escherichia coli*, *Klebsiella* species, *Salmonella* species and fungi
- Normal antibodies, normal cell-mediated immunity

Imaging features

- Lymphadenopathy, abscesses, fibrosis, effusions and parenchymal or nodal calcification

DiGeorge's syndrome

- Congenital thymic aplasia
- Absent parathyroid glands
- Associated with congenital heart defects, oesophageal atresia and mandibular hypoplasia
- Patients have deficient T-cell function

Thymus and mediastinal masses

Thymus

- Usual extent is from the level of left brachiocephalic veins up to the level of the pulmonary arteries
- However, in young infants it may extend into the neck and down to the level of the diaphragm
- Starts involuting at 3–4 years of age
- Temporary involution seen during acute illnesses

Imaging features

CXR

- Thymus is normally prominent on CXR during the first few years of life
- Normal gland is not radio-opaque, and bronchial markings can be seen through it
- In the presence of a pneumomediastinum, thymic lobes may be elevated and well demarcated, owing to air outlining their inferior margins
- A normal thymus never compresses the trachea

Ultrasound

- Echotexture similar to that of the liver: generally hypoechoic with linear or punctuate echoes
- In children < 5 years of age, seen as quadrilateral with convex lateral borders
- In children > 5 years of age, seen as triangular with concave or straight margins
- Nodularity is not a normal finding at any age
- Heterogeneity seen only in children > 10 years of age, when fatty tissue starts replacing the normal gland
- Heterogeneity, calcification and cystic changes are abnormal in children

MRI

- In children < 10 years of age, thymus seen as an intermediate signal on T1WI (similar to muscle and liver)
- Seen as homogeneous mild hyperintensity on T2WI

Thymomas

- Rare in childhood (< 5% of mediastinal tumours)
- Usually occur in isolation, i.e. not with myasthenia gravis
- Calcification is uncommon

Mediastinal masses

- Causes of anterosuperior mediastinal masses
  - Goitre
  - Aneurysm
  - Parathyroid tumour
  - Oesophageal tumour
  - Angiomatous tumour
  - Teratoma
  - Thymoma
  - Pericardial cyst
  - Lymphoma
  - Morgagni's hernia
  - Lipoma
  - Bronchogenic cyst
- Causes of middle mediastinal masses
  - Lymphoma
  - Lymph node hyperplasia
  - Bronchogenic tumour
  - Bronchogenic cyst
- Causes of posterior mediastinal masses
  - Neurogenic tumour
  - Aneurysm

  - Enteric cyst
  - Oesophageal tumour
  - Bronchogenic tumour
  - Bronchogenic cyst

Miscellaneous useful tables

Common causes of lung 'white out' and opaque hemithorax

- Congenital diaphragmatic hernia
- Agenesis of the lung
- Pleural effusion
- Empyema
- Atelectasis
- Consolidation and large tumours (rare)

Common causes of bubbly chest in infants

- Congenital cystic adenomatoid malformation
- Congenital diaphragmatic hernia
- Pneumatoceles
- Pulmonary interstitial emphysema (often bilateral)
- Congenital lung cysts
- Abscesses
- Bronchopulmonary dysplasia (often bilateral)

Fetal circulation

- Oxygenated blood leaves the placenta via a solitary umbilical vein
- It reaches the umbilicus in the umbilical cord and then runs in the falciform ligament to the porta hepatis
- Here it joins the intrahepatic left portal vein and most blood passes via the ductus venosus into the left hepatic vein and the IVC
- Blood entering the right atrium is directed by a valve towards the foramen ovale, through which it enters the left atrium
- Some blood enters the pulmonary artery, but resistance diverts most of it via the ductus arteriosus to the descending aorta
- Each internal iliac artery gives an umbilical artery, which passes deoxygenated blood back to the placenta in the umbilical cord

Pulmonary plethora without cyanosis

- Causes
  - Atrial septal defect (ASD)
  - Ventricular septal defect (VSD)
  - Patent ductus arteriosus (PDA)
- Left-to-right shunts increase pulmonary blood flow (pulmonary hypertension) if untreated
- Large high-pressure shunts, e.g. VSD, PDA, can cause pulmonary hypertension within the first few years of life, with plethora but no cyanosis
- Smaller low-pressure shunts, e.g. ASD, often do not present until adulthood
- When pulmonary resistance rises above systemic resistance, shunt reversal occurs with cyanosis (Eisenmenger's syndrome)

Cyanosis without pulmonary plethora

- Causes
  - Tetralogy of Fallot (TOF)
  - Ebstein's anomaly
  - Tricuspid atresia

Tetralogy of Fallot

- Four features of TOF
  - Pulmonary stenosis
  - Right ventricular hypertrophy
  - Large ventricular septal defect
  - Aortic valve overrides ventricular septum
- Pulmonary stenosis is usually progressive, with cyanosis developing at about 3 months of age
- Patients often adopt a squatting posture, which forces blood through the pulmonary stenosis
- Multiple associations, including coronary artery and valvular anomalies
- Treatment
  - Blalock–Taussig shunt (from the subclavian artery to the ipsilateral pulmonary artery)
  - Surgical closure of the VSD and relief of the pulmonary stenosis

Imaging feature

CXR
- Boot-shaped heart
- Elevated apex (caused by right ventricular hypertrophy)
- Small pulmonary trunk
- Right aortic arch in 25% of cases
- Pulmonary oligaemia

Ebstein's anomaly

- Displacement of the tricuspid valve deep into right ventricular cavity
- Proximal right ventricle is atrialised but contracts synchronously with the remainder of the ventricle
- Impaired ventricular function, with cyanosis and oligaemia
- Severe tricuspid regurgitation and massive right atrial dilatation
- Associated with other structural and conduction defects

- Wolf–Parkinson–White syndrome is a common cause of death
- Mortality is 50% in the first year of life

Imaging features

CXR
- Box-shaped heart
- Dilated azygous vein

Tricuspid atresia

- Complete agenesis of the tricuspid valve
- Fibrous tissue occupies the cleft between the right atrium and the right ventricle
- Obligatory right-to-left ASD or patent foramen ovale to sustain life
- Most also have a small VSD allowing some left-to-right flow through a hypoplastic right ventricle to the pulmonary artery
- Severe cyanosis at birth
- Rarely there can be pulmonary plethora (if the VSD is large)
- Surgical shunt procedures
  - Glenn's anastomosis (from the SVC to the pulmonary artery)
  - Fontaine's operation (from the right atrium to the pulmonary artery)

Imaging features

MRI and echocardiogram
- Large right atrium
- Hypoplastic ventricle

Cyanosis with pulmonary plethora

- Causes
  - Transposition of the great arteries
  - Total anomalous pulmonary venous connection
  - Truncus arteriosus
  - Tricuspid atresia with a large VSD

Transposition of the great arteries

- Systemic and pulmonary circulations are in parallel
- Aorta arises from the right ventricle, the pulmonary artery from the left ventricle
- Cyanosis at birth with pulmonary plethora
- Shunt-dependent, i.e. relies on ASD, VSD or PDA to sustain life
- Treated with prostaglandin E1 to stop

closure of the ductus arteriosus
- 90% mortality in first year of without surgical intervention

Imaging features

CXR
- 'Egg-on-a-string' sign
- Right ventricular hypertrophy
- Narrow vascular pedicle—pulmonary trunk lies posteriorly

Congenitally corrected transposition of the great arteries

- Ventricles are transposed
- The right ventricle is on the left side; it receives blood from the left atrium and empties into the pulmonary trunk
- The left ventricle is on the right side; it receives blood from the right atrium and empties into the aorta
- No cyanosis

Total anomalous pulmonary venous connection

- Pulmonary veins all drain to the systemic veins or the right atrium
- The SVC is the commonest site for the connection
- Complete left-to-right shunt: shunt-dependant (ASD or patent foramen ovale)
- Pulmonary vein may be obstructed, causing low cardiac output

Imaging features

CXR
- 'Figure-of-eight'-shaped heart

Scimitar syndrome

- Partial anomalous pulmonary venous connection
- Associated with a hypogenetic right lung
- Anomalous vein seen adjacent to the right side of the heart
- Most commonly drains to subdiaphragmatic IVC
- Occurs almost exclusively on the right side

Truncus arteriosus

- Failure of septation of the embryonic truncus arteriosus
- A single vessel drains both ventricles, supplying the systemic, pulmonary and coronary circulations
- Moderate cyanosis and pulmonary plethora

Imaging features

CXR
- Truncus is larger than a normal ascending aorta

Aortic arch anomalies

- Only 70% of the population have the classic aortic arch branch pattern
- Common variations
  - A 'bovine arch' (the commonest arch anomaly, seen in 22% of people), in which the left common carotid artery arises from the right brachiocephalic artery
  - Left arch with aberrant right subclavian artery
  - Left vertebral artery arising directly from arch (seen in 5% of people)
  - Common origin of left common carotid and subclavian arteries (seen in 2% of people)
  - Separate origin of the right common carotid and subclavian arteries (rare)

Aberrant right subclavian artery

- The right subclavian artery arises as the last branch of the aortic arch and ascends obliquely towards the right side of the body
- It traverses the mediastinum posterior to oesophagus in 80% of cases, between the oesophagus and the trachea in 15%, and anterior to the trachea in 5%
- Associated with congenital heart defects in 10–15% of cases
- Usually asymptomatic; rarely causes 'dysphagia lusoria'

Imaging features

CXR
- Right paratracheal opacity
- Opacity posterior to the trachea on lateral views

CT
- Seen as the last and most posterior vessel to come off the arch

> Persistence of the primitive right arch is referred to as Kommerell's diverticulum

Double aortic arch

- Forms a vascular ring around the trachea and oesophagus
- Presents in neonates and children with respiratory distress and/or stridor
- The descending aorta is left-sided in 75% of cases
- The ascending aorta divides into separate right and left arches, which pass on either side of trachea; the right arch is higher than the left
- Each arch gives a single subclavian and common carotid artery
- The subclavian arteries arise posterior to the carotid arteries
- The right arch crosses behind the oesophagus to join the left as the descending thoracic aorta

Imaging features

Axial CT and MRI
- Four vessels evenly spaced around trachea ('four artery' sign)

Contrast swallow
- Lateral view shows posterior indentation
- Frontal view shows bilateral indentations ('reverse S-shape')

Right-sided aortic arch

- Incidence is 1%
- 'Mirror' branching in two thirds of cases; in order of appearance, the left brachiocephalic artery, the right common carotid artery and the right subclavian artery; associated cyanotic congenital heart disease in 99% of cases

- Aberrant left subclavian artery in one third of cases; in order of appearance, the left common carotid artery, the right common carotid artery, the right subclavian artery and an aberrant left subclavian artery; commonly associated with slings and rings

Coarctation of the aorta

- Eccentric luminal narrowing caused by infolding of the aortic wall
- Most commonly a focal narrowing distal to the origin of the left subclavian artery
- Blood flow to the descending aorta is via intercostal collateral vessels
- Rarely, a long segment of tubular hypoplasia presenting in neonates with heart failure and congenital cardiac anomalies
- Associations
  - Bicuspid aortic valve
  - Turner syndrome (45XO)
  - Berry aneurysms

Imaging features

CXR
- 'Figure three' sign of pre- and post-stenotic dilatation
- Inferior rib notching (on third to ninth ribs), caused by dilated intercostal collateral vessels

- Unilateral right-sided rib notching if the coarctation is proximal to the left subclavian artery
- Unilateral left-sided rib notching if the coarctation is proximal to an aberrant right subclavian artery

MRI
- Modality of choice
- Clearly depicts extent of the coarctation and collateral vessels
- T1 spin echo imaging (black blood imaging) in a left anterior oblique position is suitable for measuring the aortic calibre before and after repair of the coarctation

Pseudocoarctation

- Elongation of the ascending aorta ('high aortic arch')
- Arch buckles at the insertion of the ligamentum arteriosum
- No pressure gradient across buckle
- Associated with trauma, hypertension, bicuspid aortic valve, PDA, VSD, aortic stenosis, single ventricle and ASD

Imaging features

- No rib notching
- Anteromedial deviation of the aorta and oesophagus on contrast studies

Injuries

Non-accidental injury

> **Skull fractures seen in non-accidental injury**
>
> - Complex patterns with fracture crossing sutures
> - Non-parietal fracture in infants
> - Bilateral fractures
> - Delayed presentation

Imaging features

CT
- Hyperacute blood may be hypodense
- Recent clotted blood is hyperdense, evolving to isodense in about 10 days and becoming hypodense 3–4 weeks after the trauma
- Extradural haematoma is infrequently associated with non-accidental injury; a subdural haematoma is typical

Limb and skeletal injuries

- Commonest fracture is diaphyseal
- Most specific fracture is metaphyseal
- High specificity injuries
  - Posterior rib
  - Multiple ribs
  - Acromion of the scapula
  - Pelvis
- Low specificity injuries:
  - Clavicle
  - Shaft fractures outside infancy
  - Parietal skull fractures outside infancy
- Typical abdominal injuries
  - Traumatic pancreatic pseudocyst
  - Liver laceration
  - Retroperitoneal haemorrhage
  - Splenic and renal injuries (though rare)
- Mimics of non-accidental injury
  - Normal variants, e.g. nutrient foramina
  - Birth trauma (in the middle one third of the clavicle)
  - Generalised osteoporosis and over-tubulation
  - Osteogenesis imperfecta
  - Rickets in an older child
  - Neuropathy

Periosteal reaction in children

- Physiological
  - Most commonly occurs in infants
  - Seen in long bones as smooth lines running parallel to the cortex. It remains confined to the diaphysis
- Osteomyelitis, which typically involves the metaphyses in infants
- Scurvy
  - Rare in children < 6 months of age
  - Osteoporosis and abnormal bleeding tendency follow
- Neuroblastoma or leukaemia
- Caffey's disease
  - Characteristically involves the mandible
  - Cause unknown cause
  - Clinically presents with spontaneous limb pain

Osteogenesis imperfecta

- Autosomal-dominant condition
- Normal mineralization but inadequate osteoid formation
- Thin osteoporotic fragile bones
- One in 40,000
- Males and females are equally often affected
- Associated with deafness and otosclerosis
- Predisposes to intracranial bleeds (reduced platelet count)
- Types of osteogenesis imperfecta
  - Type I: ages 2–6 years
  - Type II: congenital disease, and lethal
  - Type III: progressive limb and spine deformities
  - Type IV: mildest form with best prognosis

Imaging features

- Bowing
- Coxa valga or coxa vara
- Kyphoscoliosis
- Cortical thinning
- Fractures with extensive callus
- Wormian bones in the skull
- Vertebral scalloping in the spine
- Protrusio acetabuli in the pelvis

Salter-Harris injuries

- Salter-Harris described five types of growth plate fractures, and this classification should be used in describing fractures that affect the growth plates
- Salter-Harris type I
  - May be difficult to detect radiologically without stress views
- Salter-Harris type II
  - The fracture passes through much of the growth plate but includes a piece of metaphyseal bone on one side
  - The periosteum is intact on the side with the metaphyseal fragment, but is torn on the opposite side
- Salter-Harris type III
  - Includes a piece of the epiphysis
- Salter-Harris type IV
  - Includes the metaphysis and the epiphysis
  - Usually intra-articular, and the commonest fracture of the lateral condyle
- Salter-Harris type V
  - Crush injury of growth plate from axial loading
  - Exceedingly rare
  - May lead to progressive angular deformity if part of the growth plate is damaged
  - Growth cessation at the end of the limb may occur if the entire growth plate is involved
  - Injuries may not be recognised until cessation of growth is noticed

Osgood–Schlatter disease

- Males are more commonly affected than females
- Incidence 25%

- Painful irregularity of the tibial tuberosity secondary to trauma
- Typically bilateral
- Thickened patellar tendon
- Obliteration of the infrapatellar fat pad

Cervical spine

- Anterior subluxation of C2 on C3
- 25% of children under 8 years of age have up to 3 mm of C3 on C4
- Anterior wedging of C3 is also a normal variant
- Crying may increase soft tissue thickness anteriorly

The limping child

Perthes' disease

- Avascular necrosis of the femoral head in children
- Peak age is 4–8 years
- Bilateral in up to 10% of cases
- Males are five times more commonly affected than females
- Usually idiopathic, but may be secondary to trauma

Imaging features

Plain X-ray
- Smaller femoral epiphysis on the affected side, typically with sclerosis
- Widened joint space (secondary to thickened intra-articular cartilage, joint fluid or joint laxity)
- Later, a lucent subchondral fracture line appears, followed by fragmentation of the femoral head

CT
- Loss of asterisk in the centre of the femoral head ('asterisk' refers to the stellate pattern of crossing trabecula in the centre of a normal femoral head)

MRI
- Marrow signal from femoral epiphysis is low on T1WI and high on T2WI
- Double-line sign: sclerotic rim between viable and non-viable bone is edged by a high-signal rim of granulation tissue

Slipped upper femoral epiphysis

- Atraumatic fracture through the physeal plate
- Usually one-sided
- Associations
  - Trauma (Salter-Harris type I injury)
  - Growth spurt (commonly seen in boys aged 8–17 years)
  - Renal osteodystrophy and rickets
  - Childhood irradiation
  - Growth hormone or steroid treatment
  - Developmental dysplasia of the hip
  - Perthes' disease
  - Endocrine problems, e.g. hypothyroidism, hypoestrogenism, acromegaly, cryptorchidism, pituitary adenoma, parathyroid adenoma
- Complications
  - Avascular necrosis (seen in 10–15% of cases)
  - Coxa vara
  - Osteoarthritis (in 90% of cases)
  - Discrepancy in limb length

Imaging features
- Widened growth plate (prior to the slip)
- Posteromedial displacement of head during the slip
- Decrease in the neck–shaft angle
- If long-standing, then one sees sclerosis and irregularity with a widened physis

Childhood osteomyelitis

- Infection of the bone and bone marrow
- May occur from haematogenous spread (commonest cause in children), direct inoculation from trauma or spread from infection in adjacent soft tissue
- Usually affects a single bone
- Commonest sites are metaphyses of the proximal tibia, the distal femur, the wrist, the distal radius, the shoulder and the proximal humerus
- *Staphylococcus aureus* is the most commonly identified causative organism
- Others organisms include group B streptococci, other streptococci, *Escherichia coli* and *Kingella kingae*

- *Pseudomonas* is more typical of penetrating trauma and *Salmonella* is seen in patients with sickle cell anaemia

Imaging features
Bone scan
- Positive in 24 hours of symptoms developing

Plain X-ray
- Soft tissue swelling is seen initially
- Fat plane obliteration is seen after 3 days
- Periosteal reaction is seen after 5–7 days
- Involucrum formation is seen after 20 days
- Sequestrum is seen after 30 days; this is a specific sign of active infection in chronic osteomyelitis
- In chronic osteomyelitis, a Brodie's abscess may be seen as an elongated, radiolucent lesion in the long bone, with marked surrounding bony sclerosis
- Brodie's abscess is typically seen in the metaphysis of the tibia

MRI
- In the early stages, infected marrow is low in signal intensity on T1WI, with correlating high signals on T2WI and short inversion time inversion recovery (*STIR*) sequences
- Post-contrast enhancement is seen
- In chronic cases, the signal drops on T1WI and T2WI secondary to fibrosis, and no enhancement is seen after contrast

Nutritional diseases

Rickets
- Osteomalacia in the skeletally immature patient

Imaging features
- Widened and irregularly shaped metaphyses with flaring
- Cupping and fraying of the metaphyses is typical
- Metaphyseal spurs are also a feature
- Poorly mineralised epiphyseal centres with delayed appearance
- Periosteal reaction may be present
- Coarse trabeculation noted (a ground-glass appearance is not a feature)

- Soft bones with deformities, e.g. bowing
- Risk of Salter–Harris type I fractures in weight-bearing areas

Scurvy

- Caused by a long-term deficiency of vitamin C

Imaging features

- Ground-glass osteoporosis
- Increased density and widening of the zone of provisional calcification (white line of Frankl)
- Metaphyseal spurs or marginal fractures (Pelkan's sign)
- Transverse radiolucent band at the metaphysis subjacent to the zone of provisional calcification (scurvy line or Trummerfield's zone, which is a site of fractures and infarction)
- Parke corner sign: subepiphyseal infarction leading to cupping of the epiphysis
- Ring of increased density surrounding the epiphysis (Wimberger's sign)
- Periosteal elevation
- Sites of abnormalities include the distal end of femur, the proximal and distal ends of the tibia and fibula, the distal end of the radius and ulna, the proximal humerus, and the distal ends of the ribs

Developmental dysplasia of the hip

- One in 400
- Bilateral in 30% of cases
- Rare in Asians and Africans
- The left side is affected in 70% of cases
- Predisposing factors
  - Female sex
  - Breech delivery
  - First-born infants
  - Oligohydramnios
  - Positive family history
- Associations include sternomastoid tumour, torticollis, talipes, scoliosis and Down's syndrome
- Complications in untreated cases
  - Permanent dislocation or subluxation
  - Pseudoarthrosis
  - Shortening of the limb

- Early arthritis
- Avascular necrosis, though this is rare (commoner in treated cases)

Imaging features

Ultrasound
- At least 50% of the normal femoral head is covered by acetabulum; in developmental dysplasia of the hip, less than 50% is covered
- The acetabular cartilage is deformed
- The alpha angle is < 60°

Plain X-ray
- Puttis triad
  - Superolateral displacement of the proximal femur
  - Increased acetabular angle (normal angle is 15–30°)
  - Anteversion of the femoral neck

Juvenile rheumatoid arthritis and juvenile chronic arthritis

- Arthritis of unknown cause persisting for at least 6 weeks in a child under 16 years of age

Imaging features

Plain X-ray
- Periarticular soft tissue swelling
- Juxta-articular osteopenia
- Periosteal reaction is commonly seen in the metacarpals and metatarsals
- Advanced skeletal maturity, secondary to local hyperaemia
- Joint ankylosis in advanced cases

Down's syndrome (trisomy 21)

- Characteristic skeletal abnormalities
  - Short stature
  - Reduced bone mass
  - Atlantoaxial instability
  - 11 pairs of ribs
  - Ossification of the posterior longitudinal ligament
  - Two ossification centres in the manubrium
  - Flared iliac wings

Achondroplasia

- Autosomal-dominant, rhizomelic, short-limb dwarfism
- Normal intelligence and life span

Imaging features
- Lumbar kyphosis in infancy, progressing to exaggerated lordosis in adulthood
- Enlarged skull with narrowed cranial foramina and narrow foramen magnum leading to a communicating hydrocephalus
- Bullet-shaped vertebral bodies in infancy, vertebra plana in adulthood
- Squared iliac wings in the pelvis with 'champagne glass' inlet
- Long bones are short and wide
- Spinal and cranial stenosis, which are the major causes of morbidity

Congenital scoliosis

- Spinal curvature with vertebral anomalies
- Males and females are equally commonly affected
- Most commonly located in the thoracic spine
- Surgery is recommended for scoliotic curves that are progressing > 10° per year

Vertebral anomalies

- **Hemivertebra:** unilateral or anterior vertebral hypoplasia
- **Butterfly vertebra:** central vertebral cleft due to failure of central vertebral body development
- **Fused or block vertebra:** embryological failure of segmentation
- **Kippel–Feil syndrome:** multiple cervical segmentation anomalies

Miscellaneous pathologies

Scheuermann's disease
- Vertebral osteochondrosis
- Kyphosis > 35°
- Thoracic spine is affected in 75% of cases

Imaging features
- Progressive narrowing of disc spaces
- Anterior wedging
- More than three vertebral bodies affected
- Multiple Schmorl's nodes

Blount's disease
- Congenital tibia vara
- Abnormal enchondral ossification secondary to stress or compression
- Obese Afro–Carribean children presenting with painful bowed legs is a typical presentation

Imaging features
- Fragmented medial tibial epiphysis
- Irregular medial physeal line or bridging
- Tibial–femoral angle > 15°
- Metaphyseal–diaphyseal angle > 11°

Freiberg's disease
- Osteonecrosis of distal end of the second and third metatarsals
- Female preponderance
- Associated with hallux valgus and a short first metacarpal

Club foot (talipes equino varus)
- One in 1000
- Anteroposterior talocalcaneal angle < 20° (normal angle is 20–40°)
- Lateral talocalcaneal angle > 35° (normal angle is 35–50°)
- Adduction and varus deformity of the forefoot
- Talonavicular subluxation is an associated finding

Congenital vertical talus (rocker bottom feet)
- Dorsal dislocation of the navicular bone on the talus
- Associations include meningomyelocele, arthrogryposis and trisomies 13–18

Accelerated skeletal maturity
- Causes
  - Hyperthyroidism
  - Pseudohypoparathyroidism
  - Hypothalamic mass lesions

- McCune–Albright syndrome
- Idiopathic precocity
- Adrenal and gonadal tumours
- Acrodysostosis

Wormian bones (sutural bones)

- Causes
  - Cleidocranial dysostosis
  - Pyknodysostosis
  - Osteogenesis imperfecta
  - Hypothyroidism
  - Down's syndrome

Caffey's disease (infantile cortical hyperostosis)

- Seen in infants aged < 6 months
- Possible viral aetiology
- Multifocal, self-limited and benign condition

Imaging features

- New bone formation along the mandibles, clavicles and ulna bones

Coxa valga

- Neck shaft angle > 135°
- May be a normal variant
- Common causes of acquired form:
  - Juvenile rheumatoid arthritis
  - Poliomyelitis
  - Diaphyseal aclasis

Coxa vara

- Neck shaft angle < 120°
- Can be congenital (noted at birth and differentiable from congenital dislocation of the hips by MRI), developmental (autosomal dominant, progressive), or acquired (traumatic)

Imaging features

- Deformity in the subtrochanteric region
- An angle < 45° usually corrects itself, whereas an angle of > 60° (or a neck shaft angle < 110°) usually requires surgery

Chapter 6

Central nervous system, and head and neck

Supratentorial intra-axial tumours

Gliomas

Astrocytoma

- 80% of adult gliomas
- Primarily involve white matter
- Grades I and II: low grade, slow growing, younger patients
- Grades III and IV: high grade, aggressive, older patients
- 20% calcify, making astrocytoma the commonest overall cause of a calcified brain tumour

Glioblastoma multiforme (grade IV astrocytoma)

- Commonest primary brain tumour
- Worst prognosis (mean survival 12 months)
- Peak age: sixth decade
- Associated with neurofibromatosis type 1, Turcot's syndrome, Li–Fraumeni syndrome

Imaging features

CT and MRI
- Large, usually solitary mass within cerebral white matter
- Tendency to cross midline via corpus callosum ('butterfly' glioma)
- Extensive oedema and mass effect
- Thick irregular rim enhancement

Main differential diagnoses

- Cerebral abscess: typically thinner, uniform rim
- Metastases: typically multifocal
- CNS lymphoma: typically multifocal

Oligodendroglioma

- 15% of adult gliomas
- Slow growing, solid tumour
- Commonest location is frontal lobe white matter
- Typically presents with seizures

Imaging features

CT
- Low-attenuation mass
- 90% contain calcifications

Ependymoma

- 5% of adult gliomas, but much commoner in children
- Tumour arises from ependymal cells, which line the ventricles
- Slow growing (grade II) tumour
- 70% occur in the brain: commoner in children
- 30% occur in the spine: commoner in adults
- Commonest locations in the brain:
  - Children: within fourth ventricle
  - Adults: within lateral ventricles
  - Within parenchyma adjacent to ventricles (cell rests)

Supratentorial metastases

- Two thirds of all brain metastases
- Two thirds are multiple
- Two thirds of patients are symptomatic
- Commonest primaries: small cell carcinoma of the lung, breast carcinoma, melanoma
- Imaging cannot specify tissue of origin

Haemorrhagic metastases: common primary tumours

- Small cell carcinoma of the lung
- Melanoma
- Thyroid carcinoma
- Renal carcinoma
- Choriocarcinoma

Calcified metastases (rare): common primary tumours

- Gastrointestinal tumour (mucinous adenocarcinoma)
- Breast carcinoma
- Sarcoma
- After chemotherapy or radiotherapy, e.g. lymphoma
- Squamous or adenocarcinoma of lung

High-attenuation metastases on non-contrast CT: common primary tumours

- Lymphoma
- Haemorrhagic metastases
- Calcified metastases

Imaging features

CT
- Small spherical lesions at grey–white matter junction with extensive (disproportionate) surrounding oedema
- Most are of low attenuation on non-contrast scans
- Double-dose contrast with delayed imaging is most sensitive modality
- Small lesions display homogeneous enhancement
- Large lesions display rim enhancement (because of central necrosis)

MRI
- Most sensitive modality (especially for posterior fossa lesions)
- Small foci of high T2 signal with extensive surrounding oedema
- Display homogeneous or rim enhancement
- Delayed scans do not improve sensitivity

Melanoma metastases

Imaging features

MRI
- High signal on T1-weighted image (TIWI)
- Low signal on T1-weighted image (T2WI)
- Paramagnetic effects shorten T1 and T2 relaxation times

CNS lymphoma

Primary tumours

- 90% of CNS lymphomas
- Most are non-Hodgkin's B-cell lymphoma
- Most patients are immunocompromised, although it can occur in immunocompetent patients

Secondary tumours

- 10% of CNS lymphomas
- Occurs as part of a systemic non-Hodgkin's lymphoma

- Most are supratentorial
- Commonest site is periventricular, contacting the ependymal lining
- Symptoms are caused by mass effect: headaches, confusion, seizures
- Prognosis is very poor, with mean survival of only a few months

Imaging features if immunocompromised

Non-contrast CT
- Multiple high-attenuating lesions of variable size

MRI
- Lesions isointense on T1WI
- Central high-signal necrotic areas on T2WI
- Extensive surrounding oedema and rim enhancement
- Ependymal enhancement along adjacent ventricular wall

Imaging features if immunocompetent

CT and MRI
- Unifocal lesion
- Minimal surrounding oedema
- Absence of central necrosis
- Homogeneous enhancement

Lymphoma versus toxoplasmosis

- Lymphoma more likely if lesion is solitary
- Lymphoma shows subependymal enhancement
- Lymphoma shows more uptake of thallium-201
- Lymphoma shows meningeal enhancement (a late feature)

Supratentorial extra-axial tumours

Meningioma

- Commonest extra-axial tumour
- Second commonest primary brain tumour (the commonest being glioma)
- 20% of all brain tumours, more common in females than in males
- Arise from arachnoid cell rests ('cap cells')
- Risk factors are radiation (up to 30 years lag) and neurofibromatosis type 2

- Vast majority are benign and exert symptoms via pressure effects
- Parasagittal meningiomas often cause contralateral leg weakness
- 2% are malignant, with parenchymal invasion and distant metastases
- Skull-base meningiomas are often unresectable

Types

- Globular (the majority): flat, dural-based lesion with a lobulated outer margin
- En-plaque: sheet-like, poorly vascular lesion

Common sites

- 90% are supratentorial
- Parasagittal: often occlude the superior sagittal sinus
- Cerebral convexities
- Sphenoid wing

Uncommon sites

- Suprasellar, cerebellopontine angle, optic nerve sheath, spinal, intraventricular, intraosseous
- 1% arise outside CNS, e.g. in the paranasal sinuses, mediastinum, lung

Imaging features

Plain skull X-ray

- Usually normal
- May see a focal area of hyperostosis or calcifications
- May see an enlarged foramen spinosum, which represents an enlarged middle meningeal artery supplying these hypervascular tumours

Causes of focal skull vault hyperostosis

- Meningioma
- Paget's disease
- Fibrous dysplasia

CT

- Well-circumscribed, high-attenuating, broad-based extra-axial mass

- 20% are isoattenuating to brain parenchyma
- 20% show calcifications
- 20% show focal hyperostosis, which is reactive and not a sign of invasion
- Variable degree of adjacent parenchymal brain oedema
- Display uniform and intense enhancement

MRI

- Isointense on T1WI and mildly hyperintense on T2WI
- 'Cleft sign': thin CSF space between lesion and underlying brain
- Perilesional flow voids
- Avid, intense uniform enhancement
- 70% display dural tail enhancement

Causes of dural tail sign

- Meningioma
- Schwannoma
- Dural metastases
- Lymphoma
- Tuberculoma
- Sarcoidosis
- Glioma

MR spectroscopy

- Characteristic alanine peak

Catheter angiography

- Highly vascular lesion (except en-plaque type)
- Supplied by meningeal branches of the external carotid artery
- Early tumour blush and delayed washout

Recognised atypical imaging features

- Intralesional cysts
- Ring enhancement
- Focal areas of non-enhancement

Leptomeningeal metastases

- Metastasises to pia and arachnoid mater
- Seen in late-stage, disseminated malignancy
- Commoner than dural metastases

- Commonest primary tumours are breast, lung and melanoma

Imaging features

MRI
- Best sequences are FLAIR and T1 post-contrast
- Nodular surface enhancement that follows the gyral contours
- Commonest locations are cerebral convexities and basal cisterns
- Main differentials are bacterial or fungal meningitis and sarcoidosis

> **Detection rates for leptomeningeal metastases**
>
> - 25% with MRI
> - 50% with single lumbar puncture
> - 95% with serial lumbar punctures

Diploic space metastases

- Common: seen in 10% of patients with brain metastases

Imaging features

CT
- Focal destructive bone lesion

MRI
- Low signal tumour within high signal fatty marrow on T1WI

Infratentorial intra-axial tumours

Infratentorial metastases

- One third of all brain metastases
- In two thirds of cases there are multiple metastases
- Commonest infratentorial tumour in adults
- Commonest location is the cerebellar hemispheres
- Most common primary tumours are small cell carcinoma of the lung, carcinoma of the breast, melanoma

Imaging features

MRI
- Contrast-enhanced MRI is most sensitive technique
- Low signal intensity on T1WI
- Variable signal intensity on T2WI
- Extensive surrounding oedema

Cerebellar haemangioblastoma

- Benign vascular tumour of young adults
- 20% associated with von Hippel–Lindau disease
- Cerebellar signs are common
- 40% are associated with polycythaemia because of erythropoietin secretion
- Surgical resection is of nodule alone as cyst is non-neoplastic
- Juvenile pilocytic astrocytoma has similar imaging features

Imaging features

CT and MRI
- Large cystic mass with an enhancing mural nodule
- Prominent flow voids from vessels feeding the nodule
- No calcifications

Haemangioblastoma versus pilocytic astrocytoma

- Haemangioblastomas occur in an older age group (30–40 years versus 5–15 years)
- Haemangioblastoma nodules are hypervascular whereas pilocytic astrocytomas are hypovascular
- History of von Hippel–Lindau disease suggests haemangioblastoma

Radiation- or chemotherapy-induced brain damage

Transient white matter oedema

- Occurs early, often within weeks of treatment
- Common asymptomatic incidental finding
- Resolves spontaneously
- Diffuse white-matter high signal on T2WI

Focal radiation necrosis

- Occurs late, > 6 months after treatment
- Coagulative destruction of white matter
- Occurs adjacent to resected tumour bed
- Mimics tumour recurrence

Imaging features

MRI
- Conventional sequences are non-specific
- Focal high signal area on T2WI with central or ring enhancement

Radiation necrosis versus tumour recurrence

- Choline:creatine ratio > 3 with MR spectroscopy in tumour recurrence

- Increased uptake with F-18-DG PET scanning in tumour recurrence

Necrotising leukoencephalopathy

- Severe diffuse form of radiation injury
- Complication of chemotherapy (intrathecal or intravenous)
- Increased risk if combined with radiotherapy
- Diffuse bilateral white-matter high signal on T2WI

Other late effects of radiation

- Cerebral and cerebellar atrophy
- Radiation induced tumours, e.g. meningioma, gliomas, sarcomas

Medulloblastoma

- Commonest posterior fossa tumour in children
- A primitive neuroectodermal tumour
- Fast growing, aggressive tumour
- Two age peaks:
  - – First decade (75%): midline (vermis, roof of fourth ventricle)
  - – Third decade (25%): parasagittal (cerebellar hemispheres)
- 40% have leptomeningeal 'drop' metastases at time of diagnosis, which can seed anywhere along the neuroaxis but are most common over the cerebral convexities and lumbosacral region
- 5% have bone metastases (osteoblastic) at time of diagnosis
- Treatment is with surgical resection and full neuroaxis irradiation

Imaging features

CT
- Large hyperdense midline mass with homogeneous enhancement
- 90% have hydrocephalus secondary to ventricular obstruction
- Atypical features:
  - – Calcified (10%)
  - – Haemorrhagic components (10%)
  - – Cystic components (10%)
  - – Non-enhancing

MRI
- Typically low T1 and high T2 signal
- FLAIR and T1 post-contrast are best sequences for drop metastases
- Seen as nodular surface enhancement following gyral contours

Other paediatric causes of 'drop' metastases

- Medulloblastima
- Ependymoma
- Germinoma
- Pineoblastoma

Juvenile pilocytic astrocytoma

- Second commonest posterior fossa tumour in children
- Peak age 10 years, associated with neurofibromatosis type 1
- Commonest location is in cerebellar hemispheres
- Slow growing
- Present with progressive headache, ataxia
- Rarely occur in optic nerves or hypothalamus

Imaging features

CT
- Well-defined cystic mass with an avidly enhancing mural nodule
- Very similar appearance to that of cerebellar haemangioblastoma
- 10% calcify

MRI
- Cyst is of low T1 and high T2 signal
- Mural nodule displays prominent enhancement

Ependymoma

- Slow growing tumour arising from ependymal lining of ventricles
- 70% occur in the brain: commoner in children
- 30% occur in the spine: commoner in adults
- Commonest locations in children is within the fourth ventricle
- Fourth ventricle tumours typically extend through foramina of Luschka and Magendie, and do not invade through ventricular walls

Imaging features

CT
- Large low-attenuation midline tumour obliterating the fourth ventricle
- Non-communicating hydrocephalus
- 50% contain calcifications, 50% contain cystic elements

CT features: ependymoma versus medulloblastoma

- Ependymoma is a high-attenuation lesion, rarely calcified and rarely cystic
- Medulloblastoma is a low-attenuation lesion, commonly calcified and commonly cystic

MRI
- Heterogeneous signal on T1WI and T2WI
- Solid components enhance

Brainstem glioma

- High-grade, aggressive tumour with a poor prognosis
- Commonest location is the pons
- Present early with cranial nerve palsies
- Hydrocephalus uncommon at time of diagnosis

Imaging features

CT and MRI
- Asymmetric expansion of pons and medulla
- Effacement of pre-pontine cistern
- Posterior displacement of fourth ventricle

Arnold–Chiari malformation

Arnold–Chiari malformation type 1

- Presents in adulthood

Imaging features

- Small posterior fossa
- Normal-sized foramen magnum
- Tonsillar herniation > 5 mm
- Elongated fourth ventricle in a normal position
- Obliterated cisterna magna
- Associations:
  - Syringomyelia (25%)
  - Hydrocephalus (25%)
  - Fused cervical vertebrae (Klippel–Feil syndrome)
  - Fused atlanto-occipital junction
  - Platybasia
- No myelomeningocele, no supratentorial abnormalities

Arnold–Chiari malformation type 2

- Presents with respiratory disease in newborns

Imaging features

- Small posterior fossa
- Wide foramen magnum with variable herniation of tonsils, vermis, medulla or pons
- Scalloped clivus and petrous ridges
- Dysplasia of membranous skull, which disappears by 6 months of age
- Elongated or obliterated low-lying fourth ventricle
- Obliterated cisterna magna
- Associations:
  - Myelomeningocele (95%)
  - Non-communicating hydrocephalus (95%)
  - Syringomyelia
  - Tethered cord

- Supratentorial anomalies
  - Thinning of tentorium, wide incisura
  - Upward herniation of cerebellum
  - Dysgenesis of corpus callosum
  - Large massa intermedia with small third ventricle
  - Small gyri

Dandy–Walker malformation

- Sporadic condition
- 50% mortality in first year of life
- Dysembryogenesis of the fourth ventricle
- Risk in subsequent pregnancies < 5%
- Associated anomalies (in 90% of cases):
  - Lipoma or agenesis of corpus callosum
  - Holoprosencephaly
  - Gyral malformations
  - Klippel–Feil syndrome

Imaging features

CT and MRI

- Large posterior fossa
- Large posterior fossa cyst connected to fourth ventricle
- Elevated tentorium cerebelli
- Key feature is agenesis of cerebellar vermis
- Small and widely separated cerebellar hemispheres
- 75% have non-communicating hydrocephalus

Corpus callosum anomalies

Lipoma of the corpus callosum

- Congenital pericallosal malformation (not a tumour)
- Caused by abnormal resorption of the primitive meninges
- Always associated with hypoplasia or agenesis of corpus callosum
- Asymptomatic incidental finding in 50%
- 50% have seizures, mental retardation
- Other associations are midline frontal lipoma and encephalocele

Imaging features

CT
- Midline area of low attenuation (fat)
- Often contains areas of calcification

MRI
- Sagittal T1 is best sequence
- Complete or partial absence of corpus callosum
- High signal intensity
- Chemical shift artefact seen at lipoma–tissue interface in the frequency encoding direction

Hypoplasia or agenesis of the corpus callosum

- Normal sequence of formation is genu, anterior body, posterior body, splenium, rostrum
- Hypoplasia (partial absence)
  - Typically the last three sections to form are absent
  - Associated with lipoma of the corpus callosum, fetal alcohol syndrome
- Agenesis (complete absence)
  - Multiple associations, including Dandy–Walker malformation, holoprosencephaly and lipoma of the corpus callosum

Imaging features

MRI and cranial ultrasound
- High riding third ventricle (between lateral ventricles)
- Parallel lateral ventricles
- Colpocephaly (dilated occipital horns)
- Absent corpus callosum
- Medial sulci have a radial configuration towards the midline

Phakomatoses

Sturge–Weber syndrome

- Rare sporadic disease (1 in 50,000)
- Contralateral hemiparesis, hemiatrophy, hemianopia, seizures
- Ipsilateral leptomeningeal angioma
- Ipsilateral choroidal haemangioma
- Ipsilateral facial port wine stain:
  - Maxillary distribution: parietal lobe angioma (commonest)

- Ophthalmic distribution: occipital lobe angioma
- Mandibular distribution: frontal lobe angioma
- Leptomeningeal angioma:
  - Underlying cortical hemiatrophy
  - Age-related gyral 'tramtrack' calcifications
  - Overlying skull vault thickening
  - Ipsilateral choroid plexus hypertrophy
  - Ipsilateral dilated subependymal veins
  - Bleeding (rare)

Causes of gyral calcification

- Old infarct
- Meningoencephalitis
- Intrathecal chemotherapy
- Sturge–Weber syndrome

Tuberous sclerosis

- Autosomal-dominant (70% are new mutations)
- Epilepsy and mental retardation
- Skin abnormalities:
  - Adenoma sebaceum
  - Shagreen patches
  - Ash leaf macules
  - Periungual fibromas
  - Café au lait spots
- Renal abnormalities
  - Angiomyolipoma
  - Renal cysts
  - Renal cell carcinoma
- CNS abnormalities
  - Multiple cortical hamartoma (90%)
  - Multiple subependymal hamartoma (90%)
  - Heterotopic grey-matter islands (90%)
  - Giant cell astrocytoma (15%)
  - Subependymal tumour located near foramen of Munro
  - Enlargement, causing obstructive hydrocephalus
  - Transformation into high-grade astrocytoma
- Other abnormalities
  - Cardiac rhabdomyoma
  - Bone cyst
  - Retinal hamartoma, which can calcify

Neurofibromatosis

Neurofibromatosis type 1

- Autosomal dominant, chromosome 17
- One case per 3000 births
- Intracranial abnormalities
  - Optic nerve glioma (20%)
  - Cerebral gliomas
  - CNS hamartomas (pons, globus pallidus, thalamus)
  - Cranial nerve neurofibromas (VIII and V commonest)
  - Hydrocephalus (aqueductal stenosis)
  - Craniofacial plexiform neurofibroma
  - Not associated with meningioma or acoustic schwannomas
- Bony abnormalities
  - Multiple non-ossifying fibromas
  - Bowing of tibia and pseudarthrosis
  - Ribbon ribs
  - Scoliosis (with a sharp, angular, high thoracic curve) in 40%
  - Dural ectasia (posterior scalloping)
  - Widened neural foramina
- Vascular abnormalities
  - Coarctation of the aorta
  - Stenoses of major vessels, e.g. the carotid arteries
  - Hypertension (renal artery stenosis and phaeochromocytomas)
- Lung abnormalities
  - Lower zone fibrosis
  - Intercostal neurofibromas
- Gastrointestinal
  - Intussusception (submucosal neurofibromas)
  - Increased incidence of carcinoid and gastrointestinal stromal tumours

Neurofibromatosis type 2

- Autosomal dominant, chromosome 22
- One case per 50,000 births

Neuroibromatosis type 2 versus neurofibromatosis type 1

- Cutaneous signs are much less common
- Not associated with learning difficulties
- Not associated with optic nerve glioma
- Associated with meningiomas and acoustic schwannomas

---

von Hippel–Lindau disease

- Autosomal dominant, chromosome 3
- One per 40,000 births
- Absence of cutaneous signs
- Haemangioblastomas develop in 50%
  - 50% of patients with von Hippel–Lindau disease develop them
  - 20% of all haemangioblastomas are associated with von Hippel–Lindau disease
  - Benign slow growing vascular tumours
  - Cerebellum is commonest site followed by spinal cord
  - Occasionally they secrete EPO causing polycythaemia
  - Large cystic lesion with an avidly enhancing mural nodule
- Retinal angiomas develop in 70% and are commonly multiple and bilateral
- Multiple visceral organ neoplasms include:
  - Renal cell carcinoma (and cysts)
  - Phaeochromocytoma
  - Pancreatic cystadenocarcinoma and islet cell tumours
  - Endolymphatic sac tumour (causing sensorineural deafness)
  - Cystadenocarcinoma of epididymis

Diagnostic criteria for von Hippel–Lindau disease

- More than one CNS haemangioblastoma or
- One CNS haemangioblastoma and visceral manifestations or
- Any manifestation and family history of VHL

Arachnoid cyst

- Benign congenital intra-arachnoid cyst filled with cerebrospinal fluid (CSF)
- Caused by a focal splitting of the arachnoid membrane
- Commonest location is the anterior aspect of middle cranial fossa
- 10% occur at the cerebellopontine angle
- Often an asymptomatic incidental finding but slow expansion with pressure

effects can cause headaches, seizures or hydrocephalus

Recognised complications

- Intracystic haemorrhage (neurosurgical emergency)
- Adjacent subdural haematoma

Imaging features

CT

- Well-defined, low-attenuating lesion
- No calcifications, no enhancement
- Thinning of overlying calvarium, which displaces adjacent structures

MRI

- Isointense to CSF on all sequences including FLAIR
- Hypogenesis of adjacent structures, e.g. temporal lobe

Arachnoid cyst versus epidermoid

- Cyst displaces structures; epidermoid encases structures
- Cyst is dark on FLAIR; epidermoid is bright
- Cyst is dark on diffusion-weighted imaging (DWI); epidermoid is bright

Spinal dysraphism

- Incomplete midline fusion of the bony spine

Spina bifida occulta

- 15% of spinal dysraphisms
- Bony defect is covered by skin
- Usually at the L5 or S1 levels
- Common incidental plain film finding
- Majority have no neurological deficit
- Majority have a midline cutaneous lesion marking level of defect
- Can be associated with other cord lesions, e.g. diastematomyelia

Spina bifida aperta

- 85% of spinal dsyraphisms
- Bony defect not covered by skin

- Spinal contents are exposed
- Commonest subtype is myelomeningocele
- Commonest location is lumbosacral
- Risk factors:
  - mother aged > 35 years
  - Lack of folic acid
  - Positive family history
- 95% have a neurological deficit
- Common associations:
  - Scoliosis
  - Hydrocephalus
  - Arnold–Chiari malformation type 2
  - Tethered cord
  - Diastematomyelia
  - Syringomyelia

Other associations of myelomeningocele

- Rockerbottom and club foot
- Valgus deformity of hip
- Exuberant callus formation
- Metaphyseal fractures

Diastematomyelia

- Congenital sagittal cleft through cord splitting it into two 'hemicords'
- Each hemicord has its own central canal
- The hemicords often reunite distally
- Subtypes
  - Type I: both hemicords contained within a single dural sheath with no bony or fibrous septum between them
  - Type II : both hemicords have their own dural sheath and are separated by a bony or fibrous septum
- Commonest location is thoracolumbar junction region
- Site of the split is often marked by an overlying cutaneous lesion
- Presents in teenage years with progressive lower limb neurological problems
- Association:
  - Tethered cord (>50%), s
  - Scoliosis (>50%)
  - Dysraphism
  - Syringomyelia

Tethered cord

- Abnormal dorsal fixation of the filum terminale
- Caused by a fibrous band, lipoma or intrathecal dermoid
- Cord unable to ascend during growth spurt becomes 'stretched'
- Progressive lower limb weakness and bowel and bladder dysfunction

Imaging features

MRI
- Thickened filum (> 2 mm)
- Low-lying conus (below L2 level)
- Dorsal fixation of cord,
- Lipoma (in the filum or cutaneous)
- Dysraphism

Syringomyelia

- Fluid filled cavity within the spinal cord, which slowly expands, compressing nerve fibres

Congenital syringomelia

- Commonest type
- Dilatation of central canal

- Lower cervical cord
- Associations
  - Arnold–Chiari malformation type 1 (>50%)
  - Dysraphism
  - Diastematomyelia
  - Scoliosis
  - Tethered cord
- Clinical features
  - Horner's syndrome
  - Loss of pain and temperature sensation over the shoulder (leading to a Charcot joint)
  - Upper motor neurone signs in legs, lower motor neurone signs in arms

Acquired syringomeylia

- Fluid-filled cavity within cord parenchyma
- Thoracic cord
- Associations
  - Cord tumours
  - Trauma
  - Infection

Imaging features

MRI
- Cord expansion with low T1 and high T2 signal in cavity

Bacterial meningitis

- Inflammation of the leptomeninges (pia and arachnoid) with development of a subarachnoid exudate
- Unenhanced CT and MRI usually normal
- Post contrast may see leptomeningeal enhancement
- Lumbar puncture is needed to establish the diagnosis

Complications

- Arterial thrombosis with infarction
- Venous sinus thrombosis with infarction
- Cerebritis leading to abscess formation
- Ventriculitis (ependymal enhancement)
- Hydrocephalus caused by exudative adhesions
- Subdural empyema

Causes of leptomeningeal enhancement
• Bacterial meningitis
• Tuberculous or fungal meningitis
• Carcinomatosis
• Lymphoma
• Subarachnoid haemorrhage
• Sarcoidosis

Subdural empyema

- Purulent fluid collection in the subdural space
- Neurosurgical emergency with mortality around 20%
- Rapid neurological deterioration (seizures, focal signs, coma)
- Causes
  - Sinusitis (frontal sinuses most commonly involved)
  - Mastoiditis
  - Meningitis
  - Trauma (penetrating injury)

Imaging features

MRI
- Much more sensitive than CT

- Commonest over cerebral convexities (especially frontal lobe)
- Proteinaceous fluid is of intermediate signal on T1WI and T2WI
- Peripheral enhancement around collection
- Underlying sulcal effacement and cerebritis

Brain abscess

- Streptococcus milleri is the commonest organism
- Begins as an area of cerebritis which develops a capsule
- Fever, raised WCC, seizures, focal neurology
- Neurosurgical emergency requiring drainage and antibiotics

Causes
Direct spread
• Sinusitis (frontal lobe abscess)
• Mastoiditis (temporal lobe abscess)
• Meningitis
Haematogenous spread
• Immunocompromise
• Endocarditis
• Intravenous drug use
• Right-to-left cardiac shunts
• Pulmonary arteriovenous malformation

Imaging features

CT and MRI
- Typically a solitary lesion in a subcortical location
- Extensive surrounding oedema and 'mass effect'
- Classically displays a uniform thin rim of enhancement
- Steroids reduce the degree of enhancement
- Restricted diffusion on DWI (unlike a tumour, which displays normal diffusion)

Solitary rim-enhancing lesion

- High grade glioma
- Metastasis
- Cerebral infarct
- Resolving haematoma
- MS plaque in acute stage
- Lymphoma (in immunocompromised)
- Tuberculoma
- Radiation necrosis
- Arteriovenous malformation
- Thrombosed aneurysm

Multiple rim-enhancing lesions

- Metastases
- Septic emboli
- Bacterial endocarditis
- Intravenous drug use
- Toxoplasmosis
- CNS lymphoma
- Fungal infection
- Neurocysticerosis

Herpes simplex encephalitis

- In adults caused by herpes simplex virus (HSV)-1
- In neonates caused by HSV-2
- Virus lies dormant in cranial nerve ganglia
- Rapid deterioration, with behavioural changes, seizures and coma
- Mortality approximately 50%
- Empirical antiviral treatment should be given if there is a clinical suspicion

Imaging features

CT
- Findings often normal in first 5 days

MRI
- Findings usually apparent within first 2 days
- FLAIR is the best sequence
- Unilateral diffuse high T2 signal in frontal and temporal lobes
- Progresses to bilateral disease and parietal lobe involvement*

- Key features
  - Sparing of lentiform nucleus
  - Streaky contrast enhancement around sylvian fissure
  - Petechial haemorrhages
- Diffuse brain involvement is seen in AIDS patients

Tuberculosis

- Immunocompromised are most at risk

Tuberculous meningitis

- Commonest manifestation of cranial tuberculosis
- Leptomeningeal enhancement
- Hydrocephalus caused by exudative adhesions

Tuberculoma

- Develops in 25% of patients
- Usually solitary lesion in the posterior fossa

Imaging features

CT
- Isoattenuating lesion with surrounding oedema
- Central focus of calcification in 25%

MRI
- Low T1, high T2 signal and ring enhancement

AIDS-related CNS infections

- MRI is the modality of choice in all these conditions

Incidence of AIDS-related CNS infections

- HIV encephalitis: 60%
- Toxoplasmosis (opportunistic infection): 30%
- Cryptococcus (opportunistic infection): 5%
- Progressive multifocalleukoencephalopathy: 3%
- Cytomegalovirus encephalitis, tuberculoisis: 2%

HIV encephalitis

- Caused by HIV virus directly
- Dementia-like picture
- Slowly progressive, diffuse high T2 signal in centrum semiovale and periventricular white matter
- No enhancement or mass effect
- Diffuse cerebral, cerebellar and brainstem atrophy

Toxoplasmosis

- Commonest opportunistic CNS infection in AIDS
- Reactivation of prior infection with Toxoplasma gondii (from cat faeces)
- Usually multiple small abscesses with surrounding oedema
- Main differential diagnosis is CNS lymphoma

Imaging features

MRI

- Predilection for basal ganglia and grey–white matter junction
- Homogeneous or thin rim of enhancement
- Most lesions resolve within a few weeks of treatment
- Some remain visible on imaging for years

Cryptococcus neoformans infection

- Second commonest opportunistic infection of the CNS
- Causes an insidious onset of meningitis
- Imaging features are usually normal, though may see subtle meningeal enhancement on post-contrast MRI

- Lumbar puncture needed to establish diagnosis (India ink stain)
- 25% will develop cryptococcomas

Cryptococcoma

- Pseudocysts fill dilated Virchow–Robin spaces
- Common in basal ganglia, thalamus and brainstem
- Multiple well-defined high T2 signal lesions
- No surrounding oedema or enhancement

Progressive multifocal leukoencephalopathy

- Progressive, fatal demyelinating disease
- Reactivation of JC virus, which destroys oligodendrocytes
- Focal neurological signs, e.g. limb weakness

Imaging features

MRI

- Diffuse bilateral white matter high signal (on T2WI and FLAIR)
- Commonest site is posterior centrum semiovale
- No enhancement or mass effect
- Extension into the gyri, following the outline of the overlying grey matter; this distinguishes it from HIV encephalitis

Cytomegalovirus encephalitis

- Imaging features indistinguishable from HIV encephalitis
- Diagnosis via PCR analysis of CSF
- Tendency to cause post-inflammatory parenchymal calcifications

Relevant vascular anatomy

Arterial supply of the central nervous system is via the paired internal carotid arteries and the paired vertebral arteries.

Internal carotid artery (ICA)

Course

The ICA enters the skull base through the carotid canal (in the petrous temporal bone). It exits through the foramen lacerum to enter the middle cranial fossa. It then enters the posterior part of the cavernous sinus and runs forward in the sinus before turning upwards to pierce its roof medial to the anterior clinoid process. Here it gives off the ophthalmic artery (which enters the orbit through the optic canal with the optic nerve). The ICA then turns backwards, curving over the roof of the sinus. It terminates by dividing into the anterior cerebral artery (ACA), the middle cerebral artery (MCA), which runs in the sylvian fissure, and the posterior communicating artery (PCOM).

Circle of Willis

The circle of Willis forms an anastomosis between the ICA and the vertebrobasilar system and lies in the interpeduncular fossa on the ventral surface of the brain. It comprises:

- The two PCOMs connecting the MCAs with the posterior cerebral arteries (terminal branches of the basilar artery)
- The anterior communicating artery (ACOM) uniting the two ACAs

Important branches of the ACA and MCA

ACA
- A1 segment (pre-ACOM): recurrent artery of Heubner, which supplies the anterior limb of the internal capsule and adjacent structures
- A2 segment (post-ACOM): this passes posterosuperiorly over the corpus callosum giving off the orbitofrontal, frontopolar, callosomarginal and pericallosal branches. These branches supply the frontal lobe and the medial aspect of the parietal lobe

MCA
- M1 segment (pre-MCA bifurcation): lenticulostriate perforating arteries, which supply the basal ganglia and adjacent deep structures
- M2 segment (post-MCA bifurcation): insular and cortical branches, which supply the insula and lateral surface of the cerebral hemispheres

Vertebral artery (VA)

Course

The VA is the first branch of the subclavian artery. It enters the C6 foramen transversarium (the vertebral vein exits at C7). It exits at the C1 foramen, running posterior to the lateral mass. It then enters the skull through the foramen magnum, and it unites with the other vertebral artery in the pre-pontine cistern to form the basilar artery.

Important branches of the vertebral arteries

- Paired anterior spinal arteries which unite and descend in the anterior sulcus of the cord
- Paired posterior inferior cerebellar arteries (PICAs) which supply the lateral medulla and posterior inferior cerebellum. The PICAs give off the posterior spinal arteries

Important branches of the basilar artery
- Paired anterior inferior cerebellar arteries (AICAs) supply the anterior aspect of the inferior cerebellum
- Perforator arteries supply the pons
- Paired superior cerebellar arteries supply the superior aspect of the cerebellum
- Basilar artery terminates as paired posterior cerebral arteries, which supply the occipital lobes

Venous sinus anatomy

- Paired internal cerebral veins run posteriorly in the roof of the third ventricle
- Paired basal veins of Rosenthal run posteriorly around both sides of the midbrain (between the posterior cerebral and superior cerebellar arteries)
- The internal cerebral and basal veins unite under the splenium of the corpus callosum to become the great cerebral vein of Galen
- The single inferior sagittal sinus runs posteriorly in the lower free edge of the falx cerebri; it joins the great cerebral vein to become the straight sinus
- The straight sinus runs posteriorly in the midline along the tentorium cerebelli
- The single superior sagittal sinus runs posteriorly in the upper aspect of the falx cerebri, joining the straight sinus at the venous confluence at the internal occipital protuberance
- The confluence divides into two transverse sinuses, which are asymmetrical and which run laterally
- The transverse sinuses become the sigmoid sinuses before entering the jugular foramina to become the internal jugular veins

Stroke

Definition

- An acute neurological deficit of presumed vascular origin lasting more than 24 hours

Classification

Thromboembolic (70% of strokes)

- In situ atherothrombosis
- Embolic
  - Carotid artery plaque
  - Left heart mural thrombus (AF, LV aneurysm)
  - Valve vegetations (endocarditis)
  - Paradoxical embolism (patent foramen ovale)
  - Pulmonary arteriovenous malformation

Primary cerebral haemorrhage (15% of strokes)

- Hypertensive bleed
- Amyloid angiopathy

Other causes (15% of strokes)

- Carotid or vertebral artery dissection
- Vasculitis (e.g. systemic lupus erythematosus)
- Arterial spasm (aneurysm rupture)
- Venous sinus thrombosis
- Cocaine use
- Acute hypotension (watershed infarct)
- Hypoglycaemia (occipital lobe infarct)
- Carbon monoxide poisoning (globus pallidus infarct)
- Periventricular leukomalacia (perinatal hypoxic or ischaemic insult)

Thromboembolic stroke

Pathophysiology

- 0–2 hours: reduced perfusion
- 2–6 hours: intracellular neuronal grey matter swelling (cytotoxic oedema)
- > 6 hours: vasogenic white matter oedema (blood–brain barrier breakdown)

Territorial involvement

- 50%: MCA
- 20%: lacunar
- 20%: vertebrobasilar system
- 10%: anterior cranial artery

Intravenous thrombolysis

Intravenous thrombolysis can be administered within 3 hours of onset provided intracerebral haemorrhage has been ruled out and strict clinical criteria have been met

MCA infarction

Imaging features in acute infarction

- There will be early signs of MCA territory thromboembolic stroke in the first 6 hours

CT (non-contrast)
- Hyperdense MCA sign (intraluminal thrombus)
- Loss of definition of lentiform nucleus
- Loss of definition of insular cortex
- Loss of grey-white matter differentiation

MRI (T1WI and T2WI)
- Normal or non-specific changes in the early stages.
- Absent flow void in a major occluded vessel is sometimes seen

MRI (DWI)
- Most accurate test for ischaemia in the first 6 hours
- Produces an MR image sensitised to the microscopic Brownian motion of water molecules
- Acute stroke appears bright on DWI (restricted diffusion of water)
- Acute stroke appears dark on the corresponding apparent diffusion coefficients (ADC) map image
- High DWI signal persists for around 5 days

MR spectroscopy
- Low N-acetyl aspartate
- High lactate peak

Imaging features in established infarction

CT
- Vasogenic white matter oedema develops
- Infarct becomes better defined and exerts mass effect
- Haemorrhagic transformation occurs in around 10% of cases

MRI
- High signal on T2WI
- Small petechial haemorrhages are commonly seen
- Contrast enhancement is typical beyond 48 hours (owing to opening of collateral vessels) in the cortex and overlying leptomeninges
- Enhancement may persist for up to 12 months

Imaging features in chronic stroke
- Well-defined area of brain atrophy with enlargement of adjacent CSF spaces

- Two phenomena, resulting from reduced cortical neuronal input, are recognised
  - Wallerian degeneration, with atrophy of ipsilateral corticospinal tracts
  - Crossed cerebellar diaschisis, with atrophy of the contralateral cerebellar hemisphere

Lacunar infarction
- Caused by occlusion of small deep penetrating end arteries, e.g. lenticulostriate branches of MCA or pontine perforators of the basilar artery
- Small (< 1 cm^2) areas of infarction in deep structures, e.g. basal ganglia, internal capsule, thalamus, pons, deep white matter
- Common in patients with diabetes or hypertension
- In the pons the infarcts never cross the midline, except following occlusion of a rare anatomical variant, the artery of Percheron

Imaging features

CT
- Small, well-defined areas of low attenuation

MRI
- Small areas of high signal on T2WI
- Small bright areas in the acute stages on DWI

ACA infarction
- Uncommon pattern of thromboembolic infarction
- Most often occurs secondary to vasospasm following subarachnoid haemorrhage

Imaging features

CT and MRI
- Infarct involving medial portion of the frontal lobe

Vertebrobasilar infarction
- Clinically presents with cerebellar signs, cranial nerve palsies, vertigo, lateral medullary syndrome (occlusion of PICA)

Cerebellar signs

- Nystagmus
- Slurred speech
- Intention tremor
- Past pointing
- Rebound
- Hypotonia
- Truncal ataxia
- Dysdiachokinesia
- Pendular knee jerk
- Drunken gait

Hint: Not Romberg's sign, which is caused by loss of joint position sense

Imaging features

CT and MRI
- Infarcts correspond to the vascular territory supplied by the occluded vessel
- Specific imaging features are the same as for the anterior circulation

Basilar artery thrombosis

- A rare but important variant of vertebrobasilar infarction
- Bilateral occipital lobe and thalamic infarcts
- Clinically causes occulomotor palsies, locked-in syndrome
- 90% mortality if untreated
- Treated with systemic thrombolysis (within 3 hours)
- Intra-arterial catheter-directed thrombolysis can improve the dismal prognosis in this condition

Imaging features

CT (non-contrast)
- May show hyperdense clot in the basilar artery

Primary cerebral haemorrhage

Main causes

- Hypertensive bleed
  - Elderly patients
    - Rupture of Charcot–Bouchard microaneurysms.
    - Solitary deep bleed in basal ganglia, thalami, pons
- Amyloid angiopathy
  - Normotensive elderly patients
  - Multifocal peripheral bleeds

Other causes

- Vascular malformations
- Cocaine use
- Brain tumours
- Coagulopathy
- Vasculitis
- Venous infarction
- Trauma

Imaging features

CT
- Focal area of high attenuation (60–80 HU) in the acute stage, which slowly decreases in size over several weeks becoming isodense with brain parenchyma
- Typically displays rim enhancement during this phase, eventually becoming a low-density area of encephalomalacia

MRI
- T2 gradient echo is the most sensitive sequence for blood breakdown products
- 0–2 days: low T1, low T2, deoxyhaemoglobin
- 3–7 days: high T1, low T2, methaemoglobin (intracellular)
- 7–14 days: high T1, high T2, methaemoglobin (extracellular)
- Chronic: low T1, low T2, haemosiderin

Special causes of stroke

Carotid dissection

- Accounts for 10–25% of strokes in young adults (< 45 years of age)
- Increased risk with fibromuscular dysplasia, Ehlers–Danlos syndrome, Marfan's syndrome or homocystinuria
- Most commonly occurs spontaneously or following minor, unrecalled trauma. Less commonly caused by major trauma or penetrating injuries
- Presents with headache, stroke or painful Horner's syndrome (in 50% of cases)

Imaging features

MRI
- Axial T1WI is the best sequence)
- Intimal flap (only seen in one third of cases).
- Narrowed true lumen.
- False lumen containing high signal thrombus.

MR angiography, CT angiography or catheter angiography
- Commonest location is cervical ICA at C1–C2 level
- Tapered narrowing of vessel over a few centimetres
- Lumen typically reconstitutes within the bony carotid canal

Watershed infarct

- Caused by an episode of profound hypotension, e.g. from cardiac arrest
- Affects regions of the brain located between major vascular territories, e.g. between ACA and MCA (anterior watershed) or between MCA and PCA (posterior watershed)
- Causes symmetrical deep cerebral white matter infarcts

Venous infarction

- Accounts for 1–2% of all strokes
- Commonest in children and young adults
- Non-specific symptoms (headache) evolving over several days
- Thrombotic occlusion of a dural venous sinus
- The bridging and cortical veins become occluded, causing regional ischaemia, cortical venous infarction and petechial haemorrhages
- Superior sagittal sinus is commonest sinus affected, followed by transverse sinus and sigmoid sinus

Causes

- Idiopathic in 25%
- Dehydration (in neonates)
- Adjacent infection, e.g. mastoiditis, subdural empyema
- Pregnancy

- Oral contraceptive pill
- Malignancy
- Vasculitis (lupus anticoagulant)
- Sagittal meningioma
- Paroxysmal nocturnal haemoglobinuria
- Congenital coagulation defects (deficiency of protein S, protein C or antithrombin III)

Imaging features

Non-contrast CT
- Hyperdense thrombus in a dural sinus: 'delta' sign, seen in about 25% of cases
- Haemorrhagic infarction at underlying grey–white matter junction
- Extensive thrombosis, which typically causes multifocal areas of haemorrhagic infarction that do not correspond to an arterial distribution and often occur some distance from occluded sinus

'Pseudodelta' sign: false positives

- Raised haematocrit (neonates)
- Subdural blood
- Subarachnoid blood

Contrast-enhanced CT or CT venography
- Modality of choice
- Collateral venous channels enhance peripherally around a non-enhancing thrombosed sinus: 'empty delta' sign, seen in about 30% of cases
- In chronic cases the falx and tentorium appear thickened, owing to the development of prominent collateral venous channels

MR venography
- Loss of normal flow void in the occluded sinus
- Direct visualisation of clot within the sinus
- Signal characteristics of clot vary with time, e.g. subacute thrombus is high signal on T1WI
- Adjacent subcortical cerebral oedema or infarction appears high signal on T2WI
- Low signal areas within this represent haemorrhage

Magnetic resonance venography (MRV)
- Provides complimentary information
- Sinus thrombosis appears as a segment of signal loss

Pitfalls of MRI
• Slow flowing blood gives high signal on T1WI and can mimic thrombus • Thrombus in the early stages gives low signal and can mimic a normal flow void

Deep cerebral venous thrombosis

- Devastating clinical event
- Occlusion of straight sinus, vein of Galen or internal cerebral veins
- Bilateral infarction of thalamus, basal ganglia and brainstem

Carotid artery imaging

Anatomy

- The common carotid artery (CCA) bifurcates at the C4 level into the ICA and ECA
- The ICA has no branches in the neck

Branches of the ECA
• Superior thyroid artery • Ascending pharyngeal artery • Lingual artery • Facial artery • Occipital artery • Posterior auricular artery • Temporal artery • Maxillary artery (the first branch is the middle meningeal artery; the terminal branch is the sphenopalatine artery)

ICA stenosis

- ICA stenosis of 70–99% has been shown to benefit from endarterectomy surgery (NASCET study)

- Methods of assessing ICA stenosis include Doppler ultrasound, MR angiography and catheter angiography

Doppler ultrasound of the carotids

Features of the normal ECA waveform

- ECA arises anteromedial to the ICA
- Side branches in the neck
- Demonstrates the 'temporal tapping' phenomenon
- Has a high resistance waveform, i.e. low end-diastolic flow
- Waveform has a characteristic notch and may dip below the baseline

Features of the normal ICA waveform

- No side branches in the neck
- No 'temporal tapping' phenomenon
- Has a low resistance waveform, i.e. high end-diastolic flow

Features of the normal CCA waveform

- Intima-media thickness, measured just proximal to carotid bulb is normally < 0.8 mm
- Thickening is recognised as an independent risk factor for cardiovascular events
- CCA waveform is higher resistance than ICA but lower than ECA
- Can normally dip below the baseline

Criteria for diagnosing ICA stenosis

- Direct signs
  - Peak systolic velocity in the ICA > 230 cm/second
  - ICA and CCA peak systolic velocity gradient > 4
- Indirect signs
  - Spectral broadening of ICA waveform - 'filling in' under curve
  - ECA waveform shows increased diastolic flow - 'ICA like'
- Atherosclerotic plaques
  - Echo-poor: unstable with a high risk of rupture
  - Calcified: stable with low risk of rupture

Limitations of ultrasound

- Calcified plaques interfere with Doppler interrogation
- Inability to visualise ICA lesions near the skull base
- Inability to image the origins of the neck vessels
- Difficult to distinguish high-grade stenosis from occlusion

MR angiography

- Contrast enhanced MR angiography is the technique of choice
- The most accurate non-invasive technique for evaluating the extracranial carotid vessels
- Can image the origins of the carotid arteries at the aortic arch
- Has a tendency to overestimate the degree of stenoses

Residual 'trickle' flow in high grade stenosis

- Residual flow: suitable for surgery
- Absent flow: unsuitable for surgery

Catheter angiography

- Definitive imaging test for distinguishing between high-grade stenosis and occlusion of the ICA
- Carries an approximate 1% risk of stroke

Carotid stenting

- Endovascular procedure as an alternative to endarterectomy
- Especially suited for patients with significant medical co-morbidities who are considered too high an anaesthetic risk
- Shortened hospitalisation and convalescence times
- Similar 30-day stroke risk to endarterectomy (approximately 5%)
- Distal embolic protection devices (filters) have been developed to reduce further the risk of stroke
- Can also be used to treat carotid dissection

Subclavian steal syndrome

- Narrowing (partial steal) or occlusion (complete steal) of the proximal subclavian (or brachiocephalic) artery. Blood flows in a retrograde direction down the same side vertebral artery to supply the distal subclavian artery
- This diverts blood flow away from the vertebrobasilar circulation causing syncopal episodes, vertigo and ataxia, classically induced by exercising the arm on the affected side.

Imaging features

Ultrasound
- Partial steal: antegrade flow during diastole and retrograde flow during systole
- Complete steal: retrograde flow during diastole and systole

Anatomy and physiology

- The pituitary fossa (sella turcica) houses the pituitary gland, which is connected to the hypothalamus via the infundibulum
- Composed of a large anterior lobe and smaller posterior lobe
- Anterior lobe produces prolactin, growth hormone (GH), thyroid stimulating hormone (TSH), adrenocorticotropic hormone (ACTH), luteinising hormone (LH) and follicle stimulating hormone (FSH)
- These hormones are secreted in response to releasing factors, which are carried by hypophyseal veins in the infundibulum (the exception being prolactin, which is inhibited by dopamine release)
- Posterior lobe produces antidiuretic hormone (ADH) and oxytocin
- These hormones are secreted in response to neuronal impulses travelling down the infundibulum

Relations of the pituitary gland

- Superior: diaphragm sella and suprasellar cistern
- Inferior: lamina dura and sphenoid sinus
- Lateral: cavernous sinuses
- Anterior: tuberculum sella
- Posterior: dorsum sella

The pituitary fossa is bordered by two anterior and two posterior bony projections, the clinoid processes.

Hypothalamus

- Forms roof of the suprasellar cistern and floor of the third ventricle
- Infundibulum arises from the tuber cinereum and projects down through the suprasellar cistern. It passes through a hole in the diaphragma sella to attach to the pituitary gland

Components of the hypothalamus

- Optic chiasma
- Tuber cinerum
- Infundibulum
- Mamillary bodies
- Posterior perforated substance

Normal MRI appearances of the pituitary

- T1WI: posterior lobe is high signal, anterior lobe is isointense
- T2WI: anterior and posterior lobes are isointense to white matter
- Post-contrast: homogenous enhancement of the whole gland; adjacent cavernous sinuses enhance more brightly than the pituitary

Pituitary disorders

Hypopituitarism

- Presents with lethargy, hypotension and impotence

Causes of hypopituitarism

- Macroadenoma
- Craniopharyngioma
- Radiation therapy
- Suprasellar meningioma
- Lymphocytic hypophysitis
- Trauma
- Haemochromatosis
- Sheehan's syndrome

Lymphocytic hypophysitis

- Autoimmune disease: lymphocytic infiltration of pituitary

- 90% of cases occur in women
- Often arises in late pregnancy
- Causes headaches, visual symptoms and hypopituitarism

Imaging features

MRI
- Swollen gland and infundibulum, which are of high T2 signal

Hyperprolactinaemia

- Presents with galactorrhoea, amenorrhoea, loss of libido and impotence

Causes of hyperprolactinaemia

- Prolactinoma
- Stalk compression by any suprasellar mass (inhibiting dopamine release)
- Anti-dopaminergic drugs, e.g. phenothiazines
- Lactation and pregnancy
- Hypothyroidism (TRH stimulates release)

Empty sella syndrome

- Herniation of CSF-filled subarachnoid space through the diaphragma sella
- Primary empty sella syndrome is the commonest type
  - Usually an incidental imaging finding
  - Caused by a congenital defect in the diaphragma sella
  - More common in females
  - Associated with hypertension, obesity and benign intracranial hypertension
  - Majority have normal endocrine function
  - Associated with spontaneous CSF rhinorrhoea
- Secondary empty sella syndrome
  - Occurs following destruction of pituitary gland
  - Causes include Sheehan's syndrome and radiotherapy
  - More marked degree of CSF herniation than in the primary type
  - Headaches and visual disturbance are common

Imaging features

Plain X-ray
- Enlarged sella turcica

CT and MRI
- Pituitary tissue is pushed posteroinferiorly within the sella
- Remainder of sella is filled with CSF
- Infundibulum extends to sella floor

Causes of a large sella turcica

Tumours
- Macroadenoma, e.g. acromegaly
- Craniopharyngioma
- Meningioma

Others
- Pituitary hyperplasia
- Hypothyroidism
- Nelson's syndrome following adrenalectomy
- Raised intracranial pressure
- Benign intracranial hypertension
- Empty sella syndrome

Causes of a small sella turcica

- Normal variant
- Low intracranial pressure
- Fibrous dysplasia
- Childhood irradiation
- Dystrophica myotonia
- Hypoptuitarism

Pituitary tumours

Microadenoma

- Very common in autopsy series
- Accounts for one third of pituitary adenomas presenting clinically
- Benign tumours < 1 cm in diameter
- Arise from the anterior lobe
- 75% secrete hormones (the other 25% are 'incidentalomas')
- Commonest hormone secreted is prolactin
- Less commonly GH is secreted (causing acromegaly)
- Rarely ACTH, TSH or FSH are secreted

Imaging features

MRI (modality of choice)
- Modality of choice
- Subtle low signal area on T1WI, subtle high signal area on T2WI
- Commonly off midline
- Adenoma is non-enhancing post contrast
- Non-specific signs
  - Depression of sella floor
  - Contralateral deviation of infundibulum
  - Convex diaphragma sella (normally seen with gland hypertrophy caused by pregnancy or hypothyroidism)

Differential diagnoses

Rathke cleft cyst
- Arises from Rathke pouch remnants
- Small non-enhancing benign intrapituitary cyst
- Majority are incidental findings
- If large can extend into the suprasellar region

Pituitary metastases
- Very rare

Macroadenoma

- Accounts for two thirds of pituitary adenomas presenting clinically
- Benign tumours > 1 cm in diameter
- Arise from the anterior lobe
- Majority are non-secreting; prolactin is the commonest hormone secreted, followed by GH
- Exert symptoms via mass effects:
  - Bitemporal hemianopia
  - Hydrocephalus
  - Cranial nerve palsies
  - Diabetes insipidus
- Apoplexy is a rare complication:
  - Massive haemorrhage into pituitary gland
  - Severe headache, visual loss, obtunded

Imaging features

Plain X-ray
- Enlarged sella turcica

- Erosion of sella floor ('double floor' if asymmetrical erosion)
- Erosion of anterior and posterior clinoids

CT
- Mass of soft-tissue density, which enhances homogeneously

MRI
- Solid, enhancing mass, which may contain cystic areas
- Lateral displacement of ICA flow void
- Macroadenomas typically do not occlude the ICA

Craniopharyngioma

- Benign tumour arising from cell remnants of Rathke's cleft
- Two thirds occur in children
- Majority are suprasellar with an intrasellar component
- Typically large lesions, which exert symptoms via mass effects:
  - Bitemporal hemianopia
  - Hydrocephalus
  - Cranial nerve palsies
  - Diabetes insipidus

Imaging features

Plain film
- Majority have enlarged sella turcica
- Erosion of sella floor and clinoids
- Visible calcifications within sella (in 90% of paediatric cases and 30% of adult cases)

CT
- Large cystic or solid mass with calcifications
- Avid enhancement of solid components

MRI
- Heterogeneous appearance
- Cystic areas are high signal on T2WI
- Calcifications are areas of signal void

Rule of threes for adult craniopharyngioma

- One third occur in adults
- 30% contain calcifications
- Third ventricle floor is an ectopic site

Suprasellar mass lesions

Common causes in adults

- Macroadenoma (superior extension)
- Meningioma
- ICA aneurysm

Common causes in children

- Craniopharyngioma
- Hypothalamic hamartoma
- Optic glioma of chiasma

Less common causes

- Lymphoma
- Germinoma
- Histiocytosis X
- Sarcoidosis
- Tuberculosis
- Metastases
- Dermoid or epidermoid
- Arachnoid cyst

Hypothalamic hamartoma

- Well-defined mass projecting down from the tuber cinereum
- Causes precocious puberty
- Isointense to grey matter on T1WI and T2WI
- Does not enhance (other non-enhancing suprasellar masses are dermoids, epidermoids and arachnoid cysts)

Lymphoma

- Non-Hodgkin's type
- Infiltration of hypothalamus, infundibulum and pituitary, which appear enlarged and of high attenuation on non-contrast CT
- Display avid enhancement

Suprasellar germinoma

- Malignant germ cell tumour
- 20% arise in the infundibulum
- Infiltrating mass
- Display avid enhancement

Pineal germinoma

- 80% arise in the pineal gland
- Commonest pineal gland tumour
- Occur in children and young adults
- Cause precocious puberty
- Parinaud's syndrome (upward gaze palsy)
- Infiltrating soft tissue mass
- Enhances avidly
- Hydrocephalus (aqueductal obstruction)
- CSF 'drop metastases'

Histiocytosis X

- Disseminated form (Hand–Christian–Schüller disease) can cause pituitary infiltration
- Typically a disease of childhood causing diabetes insipidus
- Loss of normal high signal from posterior lobe on T1WI
- Pituitary and infundibulum display avid enhancement

Pituitary metastases

- Breast is the commonest primary site
- Hypothalamic and infundibular metastases are much commoner than pituitary metastases

Suprasellar meningioma

- 10% of all meningiomas
- Most commonly arise from tuberculum sella or planum sphenoidale
- Can invade the cavernous sinus and occlude the ICA
- Can cause pneumosinus dilatans of the sphenoid sinus
- Blood supply is via posterior ethmoidal branches of ICA
- CT and MR features are the same as for meningiomas elsewhere

NICE head injury guidelines

Main indications for head CT within 1 hour of assessment:

- Glasgow coma scale < 13 at any time since the injury
- Any signs of skull base fracture
- Any bleeding tendency with loss of consciousness at time of injury
- Any convulsions following the injury
- Age > 65 years with loss of consciousness at time of injury
- Any problems with speaking, reading or writing
- Any problems with balance, walking or changes in eyesight

Skull vault fractures

Linear fracture

- Commonest type of skull fracture (> 70%)
- Commonest in squamous temporal bone
- Fine lucent line on plain film versus vascular groove (corticated margins, branching)
- Become less lucent as they heal, but may remain visible for years

Depressed fracture

- Second commonest fracture type
- Caused by a direct blow
- Commonest in frontoparietal region
- Usually comminuted
- Focal area of increased density on plain film
- CT is mandatory to assess for underlying brain damage
- High risk of brain injury if depressed > 5 mm

Growing fracture

- Fracture causing a tear in the underlying dura
- Herniation of CSF or brain parenchyma into fracture
- Fracture slowly widens, 'growing' over several months
- Associated with brain injury and seizures

Diastatic fracture

- Fracture extension into a suture
- Mainly occurs in children
- Lamboid suture is the most commonly involved
- Suture widened > 2 mm

Skull base fractures

Clinical features

- Associated with vascular injuries, cranial nerve damage and meningitis
- Battle sign (mastoid bruising)
- Raccoon eyes (periorbital bruising)
- Haemotympanum (blood behind an intact tympanic membrane)
- CSF rhinorrhoea or otorrhoea, usually apparent at time of injury

---

Skull base anatomy

Formed by several bones:
- Orbital plate of frontal bone
- Cribriform plate of ethmoid bone
- Sphenoid bone
- Temporal bone (squamous and petrous parts)
- Occipital bone
- Clivus

Imaging features

- Indirect radiological signs
  - Sphenoid sinus air–fluid level
  - Pneumocephalus

Orbital plate fracture

- Associated with frontal sinus fractures
- Fracture fragment can 'blow in' to the orbit
- Entrapment diplopia of superior rectus or superior oblique muscles

Temporal bone fractures

- Longitudinal (80% of cases)
  - Fracture line runs vertically through middle ear cavity
  - Ruptures tegmen tympani and tympanic membrane

- CSF otorrhoea and bleeding from external auditory canal
- Ossicular dislocation with conductive deafness
- Loss of malleus–incus articulation ('ice cream cone') on axial CT
- Sensorineural deafness, vertigo and seventh nerve palsy may occur but are uncommon
- Transverse (20% of cases)
  - Fracture line runs horizontally through middle ear cavity
  - Tympanic membrane intact
  - Haemotympanum and CSF rhinorrhoea
  - Commonly involves bony labyrinth
  - Sensorineural deafness, vertigo and seventh nerve palsy are common

Traumatic intracranial haemorrhage

Extradural haematoma

- Accumulation of blood between the dura and periosteum
- 90% caused by a temporal bone fracture with laceration of underlying middle meningeal artery
- 10% caused by tearing of a dural venous sinus
- High-pressure bleeding, which 'strips' dura away from the skull
- Haematoma confined by strong dural attachments at suture lines
- Initial loss of consciousness followed by a lucent interval
- Sudden rapid deterioration caused by rising intracranial pressure
- Majority present to hospital within 3 days of the injury
- Mortality is approximately 15% but higher if age > 65 years or if Glasgow coma scale < 8
- Requires urgent neurosurgical evacuation
- Outcome is usually good because there is minimal underlying brain injury

Imaging features

CT
- Biconvex, high-attenuation extra-axial collection
- Overlying fracture line

- Does not cross a suture line unless fracture runs through suture
- Can cross the midline (mainly seen in venous bleeds)
- Exerts considerable 'mass' effect because of rapid pressure rise

MRI
- Signal characteristics depend on age of the blood products
- Thin, low-signal line of dura separated from the inner skull table

Subdural haematoma

- Accumulation of blood between the leptomeninges and dura
- Tearing of bridging veins which cross through the subdural space (connecting cortical veins to dural venous sinuses)
- Elderly people and alcoholics are at risk, owing to cerebral atrophy and 'stretching' of bridging veins
- Caused by an acceleration–deceleration injury or minor trauma
- Initial event is often subclinical
- Clot slowly expands, with gradual development of pressure effects
- Rarely caused by rupture of a vascular malformation
- Around 15% are associated with a skull fracture
- Commonest location is over the cerebral convexities
- Posterior interhemispheric subdural is associated with non-accidental injury
- Bilateral in 20% of adult cases and 80% of paediatric cases
- Underlying brain damage is common, e.g. haemorrhagic contusion

Imaging features of acute subdural haematoma (0–7 days old)

CT
- Crescent-shaped, high-attenuation extra-axial collection
- Can appear isodense in anaemic patients
- Can spread over entire surface of cerebral hemisphere
- Can track along the tentorium or into interhemispheric fissure
- Does not cross the midline

Imaging features of subacute subdural haematoma (7–21 days)

CT
- Isodense extra-axial collection which exerts 'mass' effect
- Medial displacement of grey–white matter interface

MRI
- High signal on T1WI (methaemoglobin)

Imaging features of chronic subdural haematoma (>21 days)

CT
- Low-attenuation extra-axial collection, which exerts 'mass' effect
- High-attenuation areas within lesion (caused by acute-on-chronic bleeding)
- Layering of hyperdense material posteriorly; 2% calcify

Cerebral contusion

- Caused by direct trauma or acceleration–deceleration injuries in which the brain parenchyma strikes bony ridges of the inner skull
- Haemorrhagic focus primarily involves the superficial grey matter
- Often bilateral, occurring in a 'coup–contrecoup' pattern
- Commonest sites are the temporal and frontal lobes
- Seizures are common
- 20% expand, requiring neurosurgical intervention

Imaging features

CT
- Initial scan may be normal or show a focus of high attenuation
- Surrounding low-attenuation oedema develops overs days
- Oedema can cause significant mass effect and herniation
- Typically becomes isodense by 2 weeks

MRI
- Modality of choice, especially for posterior fossa contusions
- T2 gradient echo is most sensitive sequence for blood products
- 0–2 days: low T1 low T2, deoxyhaemoglobin

- 3–7 days: high T1 low T2, methaemoglobin (intracellular)
- 7–14 day: high T1 high T2, met deoxyhaemoglobin (extracellular)
- Chronic: low T1, low T2, haemosiderin

Traumatic subarachnoid haemorrhage

- Commonest cause of subarachnoid blood
- Associated with other injuries e.g. intracerebral contusion, fracture

Imaging features

CT
- Focal area of high-attenuation blood within the superficial sulci, which may extend into the rest of the subarachnoid space

Diffuse axonal injury

- Multiple small traumatic lesions at grey–white matter junction
- Caused by rotational acceleration–deceleration shearing forces
- Commonest type of injury in severe closed head trauma
- Usually associated with severe impairment of consciousness
- Poor long-term prognosis

Location (with increasing severity of injury)

- Frontal and temporal lobes
- Posterior aspect of corpus callosum
- Brainstem

Imaging features

CT
- Usually normal: 80% are non-haemorrhagic
- May see multiple petechial haemorrhages at grey–white interface

MRI
- Modality of choice
- Multiple small elliptical high-signal lesions on T2WI and FLAIR
- Haemorrhage seen as low-signal foci within these lesions

Brain herniations

- Caused by an expanding mass within the rigid cranial vault

Subfalcine herniation

- Commonest type of herniation
- Caused by laterally placed mass in a cerebral hemisphere
- Medial aspect of ipsilateral frontal lobe is displaced across the midline under the falx cerebri with compression of ipsilateral lower limb motor areas and ACA

Imaging features

Axial CT
- Midline shift (bowing of falx cerebri)
- Effacement of ipsilateral frontal horn
- Dilated contralateral frontal horn, with compression of the foramen of Munro
- Can cause ACA territory infarction

Transtentorial herniation

- Caused by a mass in the middle cranial fossa
- Uncus (medial aspect of temporal lobe) is displaced down through the transtentorial hiatus with compression of midbrain, ipsilateral third cranial nerve and PCA

Imaging features

Axial CT
- Effacement of ipsilateral lateral ventricle
- Dilatation of contralateral lateral ventricle and temporal horn
- Widened ipsilateral ambient cistern
- Can cause PCA territory infarction

Tonsillar herniation

- Caused by raised intracranial pressure or posterior fossa mass
- Downward displacement of cerebellar tonsils through the foramen magnum, with compression of the cardiorespiratory centres

Imaging features

Axial CT
- Tonsils visible at level of the dens

Sagittal CT and MRI
- Tonsils > 5 mm below the foramen magnum

Brachial plexus

Anatomy

- Brachial plexus is composed of the C5, C6, C7, C8 and T1 nerves
- Each nerve is formed from a dorsal and ventral nerve root
- Roots accompanied by a dural sleeve as far as the exit foramen

Traumatic injury

- Nerve root injuries are usually caused by closed traction
- Considerable force is required, e.g. high-speed road traffic accidents
- Associated with multiple life-threatening injuries
- Commonest injury pattern is avulsion of all C5–T1 nerve roots, producing a flaccid monoplegia

Imaging features

MRI
- Traumatic meningocele (tearing of dural sleeve with CSF leak)
- Avulsion of spinal nerve roots from the cord

Spinal cord injury

- Cord most commonly injured in cervical and thoracolumbar junction regions, usually caused by a fracture dislocation
- May also be caused by a burst fracture resulting from an axial loading injury with retropulsed vertebral body fragments

Cord oedema

- Long segment of high signal seen within cord on T2WI
- Greatest chance of neurological recovery

Cord haemorrhage

- Central low-signal areas are seen within the high-signal oedema
- Prognostically worse than oedema alone

Cord transaction

- No chance of neurological recovery

Cervical spine fractures

Normal intervals

- Atlantodens interval < 3 mm in an adult, < 5 mm in a child
- 2 mm subluxation allowed at C2–C3 and C3–C4 in a child < 8 years of age

Odontoid fractures

Type 1

- 4% of odontoid fractures
- Fracture through upper aspect of odontoid process

Type 2

- 66% of odontoid fractures
- Fracture through base of odontoid
- Best seen on open-mouth 'peg' view
- Unstable injury
- High risk of non-union, and requires surgical fixation

Type 3

- 30% of odontoid fractures
- Extension of fracture into body of C2
- Best seen on lateral view: disruption of Harris' ring

Mimics of an odontoid fracture

- Os odontoideum
- Ossiculum terminale
- Aplasia of dens
- Hypoplastic dens

Flexion tear-drop fracture

- Very unstable injury

- Associated with quadriplegia
- Most commonly occurs at C5

Imaging features

Plain X-ray

- Avulsion of anteroinferior vertebral body corner
- Posterior 'fanning' of spinous processes
- Widening of posterior disc space

Extension tear-drop fracture

- Stable injury
- Most commonly occurs at C2 or C3 level

Imaging features

Plain X-ray

- Widening of anterior disc space
- Fracture of articular pillar
- Narrowing of interspinous distance

Hangman's fracture

- Hyperextension injury
- Axial loading on posterior elements by occiput
- Oblique fracture through posterior arch of C2
- Unstable injury, but spinal cord usually not injured
- Fracture may extend into foramen transversarium

Jefferson fracture

- Axial loading injury
- Burst fracture of C1
- 'Peg' view shows widened lateral spaces

Clay shoveller's fracture

- C7 spinous process fracture
- Stable injury

Non-traumatic subarachnoid haemorrhage

Berry aneurysms

- 2% of the population have an intracranial aneurysm
- 90% of these are saccular 'Berry' aneurysms
- 20% are multiple
- Majority are asymptomatic
- Some cause local pressure effects, e.g. third nerve palsy with PCOM aneurysm
- 1% risk of rupture per year with aneurysms >5 mm

Associations of berry aneurysms

- Adult polycystic kidney disease
- Fibromuscular dysplasy
- Marfan's syndrome
- Ehlers–Danlos syndrome
- Coarctation of the aorta

Location

- 90% in the anterior circulation
  - ACOM (commonest)
  - PCOM
  - MCA bifurcation
  - Ophthalmic artery
- 10% in the posterior circulation
  - Basilar tip
  - PICA

Giant saccular aneurysm

- >2.5 cm
- Located at skull base, e.g. cavernous part of ICA
- Middle-aged women
- Peripheral calcifications
- Usually presents with symptoms of mass effect

Mycotic aneurysm

- Associated with bacterial endocarditis and intravenous drug use
- Typically small and peripherally located
- High risk of rupture

Aneurysm rupture: subarachnoid haemorrhage

- Presents with severe headache ('hit on the head with a hammer'), neck stiffness and photophobia
- 20% mortality
- 60% complete recovery
- 20% residual deficit

Imaging features in the first 48 hours

CT
- Modality of choice: non-contrast CT has > 95% sensitivity
- High-attenuation blood seen in CSF cisterns
- Blood may also be seen in the ventricles, as a result of reflux
- Location of blood is clue to location of aneurysm
  - ACOM: anterior interhemispheric
  - MCA: sylvian fissure
  - PICA: fourth ventricle

Imaging features beyond 48 hours

MRI (Modality of choice)
- Modality of choice
- FLAIR is best sequence
- Blood seen as areas of high signal

Imaging features beyond 7 days

- By day 7 only 50% of subarachnoid haemorrhages are visible with CT
- Any blood seen beyond 2 weeks on CT suggests a rebleed
- CSF xanthochromia is positive in all patients after 12 hours

- Xanthochromia persists for around 2 weeks
- Repeated subarachnoid haemorrhage causes meningeal signal voids from haemosiderin

Management pathway for subarachnoid haemorrhage

- CT or lumbar puncture demonstrates subarachnoid blood
- Angiography to identify and locate the aneurysm
- Treatment of aneurysm to prevent rebleeding with endovascular coiling or craniotomy and aneurysm clipping

Cerebral angiography in subarachnoid haemorrhage

Catheter angiography

- Injection of both carotids and vertebrals ('four-vessel' angiogram)
- Aneurysms are lobulated and arise from arterial bifurcations
- Best test for showing aneurysm morphology and vascular spasm
- Shows only intraluminal portion of aneurysm (not wall clot)
- Carries an approximately 1% risk of stroke

MR angiography

- Detects 90% of aneurysms of > 3 mm diameter

Time of flight

- Repeated excitations with a short TR saturate stationary tissue
- Fresh blood entering the slice is unsaturated and appears bright
- Slow flow and in-plane flow can mimic occlusion
- Technique of choice for cerebral angiography

Phase contrast

- Application of a positive gradient to moving blood followed by a negative gradient produces a detectable 'phase' shift, which is proportional to flow velocity and is not affected by slow flow and in-plane flow
- Long examination times and lower spatial resolution than TOF

CT angiography

- Detects 90% of aneurysms of > 5 mm diameter
- Aneurysms at the skull base may be obscured by bone artefacts

> **Angiogram-negative subarachnoid haemorrhage**
>
> - 10% of cases
> - CT or lumbar puncture shows subarachnoid blood
> - Angiogram demonstrates no aneurysm
> - Blood tends to be localised around the midbrain
> - Represents perimesencephalic venous bleeding
> - Typically has an excellent prognosis

Complications of subarachnoid haemorrhage

- Rebleeding
  - Acute clinical deterioration
  - Most commonly seen within first 48 hours
- Arterial vasospasm
  - Can cause cerebral infarction (2% of all strokes)
  - Mainly ACA territory (ACOM aneurysm)
- Non-communicating hydrocephalus
  - Can develop within first few hours
  - Blood products blocking the CSF pathways, e.g. aqueduct of Sylvius
- Communicating hydrocephalus
  - Occurs beyond first week
  - Blockage of arachnoid granulations due to meningeal fibrosis

Arteriovenous malformation

- Abnormal connection between arterial and venous systems
- No intervening capillary bed, just a nidus of thin-walled vessels
- Vascular stenoses and aneurysms are common within the nidus
- 0.1% of the population have an intracranial arteriovenous malformation

- Commonest symptomatic cerebral vascular malformation
- 80% are supratentorial, and the parietal lobe is the commonest location
- 2% are multiple (associated with Osler–Weber–Rendu syndrome)

Clinical manifestations

- Intracranial haemorrhage is the commonest clinical manifestation
  - 2% per year risk, 40% lifetime risk
  - Usually an intraparenchymal bleed
  - Rarely ruptures into the subarachnoid space
  - 5% risk of rebleed in the year following a first haemorrhage
- Seizures
  - The larger the aneurysm the greater the risk
- Progressive neurological deficit
  - Caused by stealing of blood from adjacent vascular territories

Increased risk of haemorrhage

- Size < 3 cm
- Exclusive central venous drainage
- Periventricular location

Imaging features

Plain X-ray
- Prominent vascular grooves and calcifications sometimes seen

CT
- Focal area of mixed attenuation
- 30% contain calcifications
- Adjacent brain atrophy from ischaemic steal
- 20% not visualised on non-contrast scans
- Dense enhancement of serpiginous vessels ('bag of worms')

- Enlarged supplying arteries and draining veins

MRI
- Modality of choice
- Central nidus vessels are of variable signal intensity
- Supplying arteries and draining veins identified in > 50% of cases
- Adjacent parenchymal volume loss and gliosis (high T2 signal)
- Variable appearance of associated haemorrhage
- Gadolinium is of limited value because of inconsistent enhancement

Catheter angiography
- Demonstrates vascular anatomy better than MR angiography or CT angiography
- Majority supplied by pial branches of ICA
- Characteristic early filling of draining veins caused by shunting

Cavernous angioma

- Well-defined collection of dilated intraparenchymal vascular channels, which are prone to recurrent intralesional haemorrhage
- Commonly multiple, especially in Osler–Weber–Rendu syndrome
- 50% are an incidental finding
- 50% present with seizures

Imaging features

CT
- Small, round, high-attenuation lesion (20% are calcified)
- Enhances post contrast
- Usually in a subcortical location

- *MRI*
- T2 is the most sensitive sequence
- Well-defined lesion of mixed signal intensity (blood products)
- Low-signal rim of haemosiderin

Multiple sclerosis

- Idiopathic inflammatory demyelinating disease of the CNS
- Commonest in young adults and the middle-aged and temperate climates; more common in women
- Diagnosis requires objective evidence of lesions disseminated in time (new lesions on follow-up scans) and space (multiple lesions)
- Starts as perivenous inflammation progressing to demyelination
- Mainly affects white matter but lesions in grey matter are also seen
- Relapsing–remitting clinical course, with optic neuritis, spastic paraparesis, ataxia, nystagmus and urinary incontinence
- Lumbar puncture shows CSF lymphocytosis and oligoclonal IgG bands
- Visual evoked potentials show delayed but well-preserved waveform

Imaging features

CT
- Low-attenuation periventricular lesions (low sensitivity)

MRI
- Most sensitive investigation
- Plaques are typically ovoid lesions 5–15 mm in diameter
- Plaques are low signal on T1
- Plaques are high signal on T2, proton-density weighted and FLAIR sequences
- Typical distribution of MS plaques
  - Perpendicular to ventricles (Dawson fingers)
  - Juxtacortical U-fibre
  - Corpus callosum
  - Temporal lobes
  - Brainstem
  - Cerebellum
  - Spinal cord
- Acute plaques
  - Display mild surrounding oedema and 'mass effect'
  - Enhance for up to 8 weeks (blood–brain barrier breakdown)
  - Variety of enhancement patterns, e.g. homogeneous, ring-like
  - Slowly decrease in size but do not disappear completely
- Chronic plaques
  - Number of plaques correlates with duration of disease
  - No surrounding oedema or 'mass effect'
  - No enhancement (blood-brain barrier intact)
  - Associated cerebral atrophy

MRI sequences in multiple sclerosis

FLAIR
- Best sequence for supratentorial lesions
- Poor for posterior fossa and spinal cord lesions

Proton-density weighted
- More sensitive than T2WI for brain lesions
- Best sequence for spinal cord lesions

McDonald MRI criteria for multiple sclerosis

- Dissemination in space, with at least three of the four following features:
  - One gadolinium-enhancing brain or cord lesion or nine T2-hyperintense brain or cord lesions
  - One or more brain, infratentorial or cord lesions
  - One or more juxtacortical U-fibre lesions
  - Three or more periventricular lesions
- Dissemination in time
  - A gadolinium-enhancing lesion detected more than 3 months after initial clinical event

Causes of periventricular high T2 signal lesions

- Small vessel ischaemia
- Virchow–Robin spaces (dark on FLAIR)
- Multiple sclerosis
- Migraine
- Vasculitis (systemic lupus erythematosis, Behçet's disease, Wegener's granulomatosis)
- Sarcoidosis
- Lyme disease
- Acute disseminated encephalomyelitis
- HIV infection, progressive multifocal leukoencephalopathy
- Radiotherapy

Acute disseminated encephalomyelitis

- Monophasic inflammatory demyelinating disease
- 10–14 days following infectious illness or vaccination
- Affects children more than adults
- Presents with change in mental state, seizures and focal neurological signs
- Increased risk of subsequently developing MS
- 10% mortality

Imaging features

CT
- Usually normal

MRI
- Multifocal high T2 signal lesions
- Predilection for white matter, basal ganglia and thalamus
- Most lesions shrink or disappear on follow-up scans

Features distinguishing acute disseminated encephalomyelitis from multiple sclerosis

- Younger age group
- Monophasic illness
- Larger more ill-defined lesions
- Majority of lesions enhance

Central pontine myelinolysis

- Caused by rapid correction of hyponatraemia (> 15 mm in 24 hours)
- Typically occurs in malnourished alcoholics
- Rapid demyelination with quadriparesis and bulbar palsy
- Commonly fatal

Imaging features

CT
- Low attenuation in pons

MRI
- High T2 signal in pons

Alcohol and the CNS

Wernicke's encephalopathy

- Caused by thiamine (vitamin B1) deficiency
- May progress to Korsakoff's dementia
- Clinical triad of ataxia, nystagmus and ophthalmoplegia

Imaging features

- Imaging triad
  - Symmetrical high T2 signal in medial thalamus
  - Mamillary body atrophy
  - Enlargement of third ventricle

Marchiafava–Bignami syndrome

- Alcohol-induced demyelination of corpus callosum

Cerebral and cerebellar atrophy

- Especially affects the vermis

Anatomy

The eyeball (globe)

- Positioned anteriorly in the orbit, closer to roof than floor, nearer to lateral than medial wall
- Around 24 mm in anteroposterior diameter
- Lens separates small anterior from large posterior segment
- Anterior eyeball contains aqueous humour
- Posterior eyeball contains vitreous humour

Layers of the eyeball

- Outer sclera is fused with dura and arachnoid sheaths of the optic nerve and is continuous anteriorly with the transparent cornea
- Uveal layer comprises, from back to front, the choroid, ciliary body and iris, which form a continuous, highly vascular structure
- Inner retinal layer extends from the optic nerve to a point just posterior to the ciliary body

Muscles of ocular motility

- Four rectus muscles arise posteriorly from the annulus of Zinn, a fibrous band continuous with periosteum and dura of optic canal
- From this common origin the muscles pass forward as a muscle cone to be inserted into the sclera of the eyeball
- The optic nerve sheath complex, which enters the orbit through the optic canal, runs within the muscle cone (intraconal)
- Superior oblique muscle arises above the annulus of Zinn and runs forward along the superomedial orbital wall to the trochlea, where it turns to insert on the posterosuperior aspect of eyeball
- Inferior oblique muscle arises anteriorly, below and lateral to lacrimal fossa and inserts on the posteroinferior aspect of eyeball

Orbital foramina and contents

Optic canal
- Lies in lesser wing of sphenoid, close to the orbital apex
- 5–6 mm in diameter and 8–12 mm long
- Connects the middle cranial fossa with the orbital cavity
- Transmits optic nerve sheath complex, ophthalmic artery and surrounding sympathetic plexus

Superior orbital fissure
- Thin cleft between the greater and lesser wings of sphenoid
- Separates the lateral wall and roof of the orbit posteriorly
- Connects the middle cranial fossa with the orbital cavity
- Transmits third, fourth and sixth cranial nerves and the ophthalmic division of the fifth cranial nerve as well as the superior and inferior ophthalmic veins
- The superior ophthalmic vein runs from medial to lateral over the superior aspect of the optic nerve

Causes of a wide superior orbital fissure

- ICA aneurysm
- Carotid–cavernous sinus fistula
- Neurofibroma
- Haemangioma

Inferior orbital fissure
- Lies between the greater wing of the sphenoid and the maxilla
- Separates the lateral wall and floor of the orbit posteriorly
- Connects the pterygopalatine fossa and the inferotemporal fossa to the orbital cavity
- Closed by the periorbita and the muscle of Müller
- Transmits maxillary division of fifth cranial nerve, the zygomatic nerve (a branch of

the maxillary nerve) and the emissary veins

Bony margins of the orbit
- Roof: orbital plate of frontal bone and lesser wing of sphenoid
- Medial wall: ethmoid bone, lacrimal bone, frontal process of maxilla and body of sphenoid
- Floor: orbital surface of zygomatic bone, orbital plate of maxillary bone and orbital process of palatine bone
- Lateral wall: zygomatic bone and greater wing of sphenoid

Nerve supply of the orbital muscles

- Lateral rectus: sixth cranial nerve
- Superior oblique: fourth cranial nerve
- All other muscles: third cranial nerve
- Mnemonic: LR6–SO4–3

Visual field defects: relationship between structure affected and clinical defect

Optic nerve: monocular blindness
Optic chiasma: bitemporal hemianopia
Optic tracts: incongruous homonymous hemianopia
Lateral geniculate bodies: incongruous homonymous hemianopia
Optic radiations: incongruous homonymous hemianopia
Occipital cortex: congruous homonymous hemianopia

Imaging of the eye

Ultrasound
- Performed using an 8 MHz or a 10 MHz probe
- Can be placed on closed lid or anaesthetised conjunctiva
- Aqueous and vitreous humour are normally echo-free
- Cornea, lens and retrobulbar fat are echo-bright
- Extraocular muscles and optic nerve are echo-poor with respect to the retrobulbar fat surrounding them
- Individual layers of the globe cannot be resolved separately
- Most sensitive modality for detecting retinal detachment

CT
- Modality of choice for assessing orbital trauma
- Lens is of high attenuation compared with adjacent structures

MRI
- Modality of choice for assessing orbital soft tissues, optic nerve sheath complex, chiasma, cavernous sinus and cranial nerves
- Fat saturation images help delineate the optic nerve and surrounding subarachnoid CSF from adjacent retrobulbar fat

Papilloedema
- Disc swelling from raised intracranial pressure
- Usually bilateral
- Causes include a space-occupying lesion, benign intracranial hypertension, hydrocephalus and cerebral oedema

Papillitis
- Refers to disc swelling from other causes (not papilloedema)
- Optic neuritis: viral infection, multiple sclerosis, systemic lupus erythematosus and other vasculitides
- Optic nerve infiltration: sarcoidosis, leukaemia, lymphoma
- Infection: syphilis, cytomegalovirus infection, lyme disease, toxoplasmosis
- Vascular: anterior ischaemic optic neuropathy, central retinal vein occlusion, diabetic papillopathy

Optic neuritis

- Sudden onset reduced vision
- Painful eye movements
- Swollen optic nerve, which enhances
- Usually resolves spontaneously

Horner's syndrome

- Ptosis, meiosis and pseudoenophthalmos with or without anhydrosis
- Caused by any interruption of sympathetic supply to the orbit
- Brainstem causes include multiple sclerosis, syringomyelia and lateral medullary syndrome
- Peripheral causes include Pancoast's tumour, cervical sympathectomy operation and carotid dissection (which is painful)

Causes of enophthalmos

- (Eye shrunken in orbit)
- Orbital rim fracture (blow-out)
- Parinaud's syndrome
- Dehydration

Third nerve palsy

- Ptosis, fixed dilated pupil, eye turned down and out
- Medical causes (which are painless) include any mononeuritis, e.g. diabetes
- Surgical causes (which are painful) include PICA aneurysm

Thyroid eye disease

- Lymphocytic infiltration of orbital contents that spares the globe
- Caused by long-acting thyroid stimulating antibodies
- Particularly affects the muscle cone and orbital fat; inferior rectus muscle followed by medial rectus muscle are the muscles most commonly involved
- There is no correlation with blood thyroxine level
- 10% of patients are euthyroid; it can be first presentation of Graves
- Classically occurs following treatment of hyperthyroidism
- Females affected four times more than males
- 80% of cases are bilateral
- Gradual onset of painless bilateral proptosis and ophthalmoplegia

- Commonest cause of unilateral and bilateral proptosis in adults
- Rarely can cause optic atrophy from raised intraorbital pressure
- Disease usually 'burns out' within 2–3 years

Imaging features

CT
- Proptosis: globe protrusion > 21 mm anterior to the lateral orbital wall
- Swollen muscle bellies with sparing of their tendinous insertions
- Hypertrophy and increased density of the retrobulbar fat
- Swollen optic nerve sheath complex

MRI
- Swollen muscle bellies have a smooth edge
- Muscles of low signal on T1WI and T2WI in chronic stage
- Thin 'stretched' optic nerve

Ultrasound
- Swollen muscle bellies are echo-bright
- In severe cases there may be flow reversal in ophthalmic vein

Causes of intraorbital muscle swelling

- Graves ophthalmopathy
- Pseudotumour
- Acromegaly
- Orbital cellulites
- Orbital myositis
- Leukaemia
- Lymphoma
- Metastases
- Sarcoidosis
- Vasculitides
- Carotid–cavernous sinus fistula
- Cavernous sinus thrombosis

Orbital pseudotumour

- Idiopathic lymphocytic infiltration of orbital contents
- Associated with vasculitis, sarcoidosis and retroperitoneal fibrosis

- Disease of middle-aged adults: equal incidence in men and women
- Commonest cause of an intraorbital mass in an adult
- Rapid onset of painful proptosis and ophthalmoplegia
- Majority of cases are unilateral
- Diagnosis of exclusion because it mimics infection, lymphoma and sarcoidosis
- Can affect any orbital structure but five main disease patterns exist:
  - Lacrimal (commonest)
  - Diffuse, mainly involving orbital fat and muscle cone
  - Periscleritis
  - Myositis
  - Perineuritis

Imaging features

- There is a wide spectrum of findings

CT
- Unilateral proptosis
- Swollen lacrimal gland
- Swollen muscle bellies and tendons
- Infiltrative mass lesion

MRI
- Swollen muscle bellies have a 'ragged' edge
- Muscles of low signal on T1WI and T2WI in chronic stage
- Thickened optic nerve sheath complex
- Characteristic avid enhancement of sclera, optic nerve and mass

Tolosa–Hunt syndrome

- Spread of inflammatory process into cavernous sinus via superior orbital fissure or orbital apex
- Retro-orbital pain and cranial nerve palsies

Orbital varix

- Intraorbital varicose veins that dilate with Valsalva manoeuvre or coughing and cause intermittent proptosis
- One third develop phleboliths within the varix

Imaging features

Ultrasound
- Echo-poor collection of vessels
- Intralesional venous flow increases with the Valsalva manoeuvre

CT
- Ideally performed with jugular vein pressure
- Serpigenous collection of vessels which enhance avidly

Orbital tumours

Intraconal tumours

- Optic glioma
- Optic meningioma
- Haemangiomas
- Melanoma
- Metastases
- Retinoblastoma

Extraconal tumours

- Dermoid
- Rhabdomyosarcoma
- Lymphoma
- Orbital extension of adjacent tumours

Optic glioma

- Commonest tumour of the optic nerve
- Presents with progressive reduction in visual acuity
- Majority occur in children and are of low histological grade
- Rare in adults, but typically high grade with a poor prognosis
- Associated with neurofibromatosis type 1 (not type 2)
- Commonly extends through optic canal into the chiasm

Imaging features

MRI (modality of choice)
- Modality of choice
- Lesion central, within optic nerve sheath complex
- Obliteration of surrounding subarachnoid space
- Isointense on T1WI, high signal on T2WI
- Avid contrast enhancement

Causes of enlarged optic canal (> 5 mm)

- Optic glioma
- Orbital pseudotumour
- Graves' ophthalmopathy
- Ophthalmic artery aneurysm
- Neurofibroma
- Sarcoidosis

Not caused by raised intracranial pressure, which narrows the canal

Optic meningioma

- Majority occur in adults, arising from arachnoid cap cells
- Associated with neurofibromatosis type 2 (not type 1)
- Progressive reduction in visual acuity
- Usually confined to the orbit

Imaging features

CT
- Modality of choice
- Enlarged optic nerve sheath complex
- 50% are calcified
- Display peripheral enhancement: 'tram track' sign in the axial plane and 'ring' sign in the coronal plane

Causes of enlarged optic nerve sheath complex

- Optic neuritis
- Orbital pseudotumour
- Graves ophthalmopathy
- Optic glioma
- Optic meningioma
- Leukaemia
- Lymphoma
- Subarachnoid haemorrhage
- Ophthalmic artery aneurysm
- Sarcoidosis

Haemangioma

Capillary haemangioma

- Proptosis in a newborn
- 90% have a cutaneous haemangioma
- Spontaneously involute in first year of life

Choroidal haemangioma

- Can cause retinal detachment in young adults
- Associated with Sturge–Weber syndrome
- Can involve any part of the choroid

Cavernous haemangioma

- Proptosis in an adult
- Large intraconal vascular channels
- Phleboliths may form within them
- Well-defined lesion appearing as high signal on T2WI

Melanoma

- Commonest ocular malignancy of adulthood
- Arises in choroidal layer of the globe
- Extends posteriorly, and the majority cause retinal detachment

Imaging features

Ultrasound
- Very sensitive test, with 95% accuracy
- Ill-defined echo-bright mass
- Detached retina, seen as an undulating bright line parallel to back of globe

MRI
- Modality of choice for assessing extrascleral extension
- Appears as a 'contrasting mass'
  - T1WI: vitreous humour is dark and melanoma is bright
  - T2WI: vitreous humour is bright and melanoma is dark

Metastases

- Majority occur in the highly vascular choroidal layer
- Common, but majority remain clinically silent
- In a child, commonest primary tumours are neuroblastoma are Ewing's sarcoma
- In an adult, commonest primary tumours are carcinoma of the breast and lung

Imaging features

Ultrasound
- Ill-defined echo-bright mass (cannot be distinguished from a melanoma)

MRI
- Key feature distinguishing it from a melanoma is isointensity of the metastatic lesion on T1WI)

Retinoblastoma

- Commonest ocular malignancy of childhood
- One third are hereditary and are usually bilateral
- Two thirds occur sporadically and are usually unilateral
- Clinically, patients have leukocoria (white pupil)
- Tumour mass arises from posterior aspect of the globe
- Propensity for extension along the optic nerve
- Meningeal metastases can occur via subarachnoid space

Causes of leukocoria (white pupil)

- Retinoblastoma (50% of cases)
- Retinopathy of prematurity
- Coats' disease
- Persistent hyperplastic vitreous
- Toxocariasis infection
- Congenital cataract

Imaging features

Ultrasound
- Echobright mass
- Foci of calcification (80%)
- Retinal detachment (100%)

MRI (modality of choice)
- Modality of choice
- Appears as a 'contrasting mass'
  - On T1WI, vitreous humour is dark and tumour is bright
  - On T2WI, vitreous humour is bright and tumour is dark
- Calcifications seen as areas of signal void

Poor prognostic signs (>50% mortality)

- Invasion of choroidal layer
- Lack of calcifications
- Extension along the optic nerve
- Contrast enhancement

Dermoid

- Common benign tumour that presents in childhood
- Contains tissue from all three germ cell layers
- Commonest location is superolateral aspect of the anterior orbit

Imaging features

CT
- Low attenuation
- May contain calcifications

MRI
- High signal on T1WI and T2WI
- May contain calcifications

Rhabdomyosarcoma

- Commonest childhood intraorbital malignancy (mean age 7 years)
- 60% arise in the genitourinary system, 40% in the head and neck
- Arises from the orbital soft tissues (not the muscles)
- Orbital disease presents with rapid onset of proptosis and visual loss
- 80% occur posterior to globe in the extraconal space
- 20% occur within the tissues of the eyelid
- Aggressive expansile soft tissue mass
- Metastasises to lungs and bone
- Responds well to radiotherapy
- Ill-defined enhancing soft tissue mass with bone destruction seen on CT

Lymphoma

- Majority are non-Hodgkin's B-cell type
- Presents with painless proptosis (mean age 60 years)
- Commonest locations are anterior extraconal space, lacrimal gland and extraocular muscles
- Expansile soft tissue mass with no characteristic imaging features
- Commonly calcifies following chemotherapy or radiotherapy

Orbital trauma

Orbital rim fractures

- Direct blow to the orbit causes an acute pressure rise
- Decompression via a 'blow-out' fracture
- Inferior wall is the commonest location followed by medial wall

Inferior wall

- Tear-drop sign of inferior rim fracture
- Air–fluid level in maxillary sinus
- Orbital emphysema

Medial wall

- Fracture of lamina papyracea
- Ethmoid sinus opacification
- Orbital emphysema

Complications

- Entrapment diplopia of inferior rectus, inferior oblique or medial rectus muscles
- Infraorbital nerve damage causing periorbital paraesthesia

Vitreous haemorrhage

- Ultrasound is modality of choice
- Echo-bright debris seen within the normally echo-free vitreous

Carotid–cavernous sinus fistula

- Base of skull fracture causing laceration of intracavernous ICA
- Rarely caused by rupture of an ICA aneurysm
- ICA communicates with cavernous sinus and arterial blood feeds the ophthalmic veins, causing pulsatile proptosis
- Palsy of all nerves passing through the cavernous sinus
- Orbital structures are markedly oedematous
- Pressure induced optic neuropathy if not treated promptly

Imaging features

MRI
- Dilated cavernous sinus and superior ophthalmic vein

Catheter angiography
- ICA contrast leak with early filling of superior ophthalmic vein

Lacrimal apparatus

Anatomy

- The oval-shaped lacrimal gland is lodged in the lacrimal fossa on the medial side of the zygomatic process of the frontal bone
- Divided into a small inferior part and a large superior part by the aponeurosis of levator palpebrae superioris
- Produces tears that drain by 12 or so small ducts into the lateral extent of the superior fornix
- Tears accumulate in the medial canthal area
- Drainage is via the superior and inferior lacrimal puncta, located on the medial aspect of the upper and lower eyelid margins
- Puncta are continuous with the superior and inferior canaliculi, which drain into the nasolacrimal sac, which is housed within a bony fossa, formed anteriorly by the frontal process of maxillary bone and posteriorly by the lacrimal bone
- The nasolacrimal sac narrows inferiorly to become the nasolacrimal duct (approximately 20 mm in length) which runs within the bony nasolacrimal canal
- The nasolacrimal canal is approximately 2 mm in diameter and has a slightly posterolateral course; it is formed laterally by medial wall of maxillary sinus and medially by the lacrimal bone
- It opens through the valve of Hasner into the inferior meatus, beneath the inferior turbinate

Enlarged lacrimal gland

Causes

- Infection (dacryocystitis)
- Orbital pseudotumour
- Sarcoidosis
- Sjögren's syndrome
- Lymphoma
- Pleomorphic adenoma (commonest benign tumour)
- Adenoid cystic carcinoma (commonest malignant tumour), which arises in the orbital part of the gland, extends posteriorly and is associated with adjacent bony sclerosis

Mikulicz's syndrome

- Enlarged lacrimal and salivary glands

Causes

- Sarcoidosis
- Sjögren's syndrome
- Lymphoma
- Leukaemia
- Tuberculosis

Nasolacrimal duct obstruction

- Presents with excessive eye watering (epiphora)

Causes

- Congenital: imperforate valve of Hasner
- Post-infectious
- Post-traumatic
- Iatrogenic, e.g. sinus drainage operations

6.11 Spine

Anatomy

- Spinal cord extends from the medulla oblongata to the conus medullaris
- Conus lies at L3 level at birth; it is normally above L2 in adulthood
- 31 pairs of spinal nerves originate from the cord, and each pair has an anterior and posterior nerve root
- C1–C7 spinal nerves exit above the corresponding pedicle
- C8 nerve exits above the T1 pedicle
- Thoracic and lumbosacral nerves exit below the corresponding pedicle
- Spinal nerves take a downward course from the cord to exit foramen; this is most pronounced in the lumbosacral region
- Nerves exiting below the level of the conus (the cauda equina) are contained within an expanded dural sac which ends at S2
- The cord expands in two regions:
  - Cervical (most pronounced), between C3 and T2
  - Thoracic, between T9 and T12

Filum terminale

- Thin (normally < 2 mm) fibrous filament that projects downwards from the apex of the conus and attaches to first coccygeal segment
- Continuous with the pia matter lining the cord
- Surrounded by descending nerves of the cauda equina

Central canal of spinal cord

- Continuous with the fourth ventricle
- Has a short fusiform dilatation within the conus (the terminal ventricle)
- Extends for a short distance into the filum terminale
- Position within the cord changes over its course
  - Anterior in cord in the cervical and thoracic spine
  - Central in cord in the lumbar spine
  - Posterior in cord in the conus medullaris

Cross sectional anatomy

- Central H-shaped region of grey matter
- Anterior horns contain cell bodies of the motor neurones
- Posterior horns contain cell bodies of the sensory neurones
- White matter tracts are located peripherally
  - Dorsal columns sense vibration and proprioception
  - Lateral columns sense pain and temperature

Blood supply

- Single anterior spinal artery
  - Formed from a branch of each vertebral artery
  - Descends anteriorly in the midline sulcus
  - Supplies anterior two thirds of the cord
- Paired posterolateral spinal arteries
  - Each arises from PICA (branch of the vertebral artery)
  - Descend along posterolateral aspect of the cord
  - Supply posterior third of cord
- Radiculomedullary arteries
  - Branches of the intercostal arteries
  - Enter spinal canal through the vertebral foramina
  - Anastomose with the spinal arteries around the cord
  - Play a major role in reinforcing cord blood supply
  - Largest radicular branch is the artery of Adamkiewicz, which arises from a left intercostal artery between T9 and T12

Arteriovenous malformations

Arteriovenous fistula

- Account for 80% of spinal arteriovenous malformations
- Acquired lesion, which usually presents in middle age

- Abnormal communication between a radiculomedullary artery and intradural veins, which leads to cord hypoperfusion
- Thoracic cord is the commonest location
- Patients present with slowly progressive back pain and leg weakness, which mimics spinal stenosis
- A recognised complication is thrombosis of the draining veins with rapid cord infarction (the Foix–Alajouanine syndrome)

Imaging features

MRI
- Flow voids from large dural veins in region of fistula
- Signs of associated cord infarction
  - High T2 signal in paired anterior grey matter horns: earliest sign
  - High T2 signal develops in paired posterior horns ('butterfly sign')
  - High T2 signal of entire cord cross-sectional area
  - Cord enhancement: late sign indicating infarction

Intramedullary arteriovenous malformation

- Accounts for 20% of spinal arteriovenous malformations
- Congenital lesion which usually presents in young adults
- Thin-walled vessels within the cord parenchyma connect the arterial and venous systems and are prone to haemorrhage
- Even distribution throughout the cord
- Patients present with sudden onset of upper or lower limb neurology

Imaging features

MRI
- Intramedullary blood breakdown products

Cord ischaemia

Causes
- Trauma
- Atherosclerosis
- Aortic dissection
- Hypotension, e.g. following repair of abdominal aortic aneurysm
- Vasculitis
- Arteriovenous fistula
- Hypercoagulable states

Evolution of MRI findings in cord ischaemia
1. High T2 signal in paired anterior grey matter horns: earliest sign
2. High T2 signal develops in paired posterior horns ('butterfly sign')
3. High T2 signal of entire cord cross-sectional area
4. Cord enhancement: late sign indicating infarction

Myelitis

Causes

- Multiple sclerosis (commonest cause)
- Vasculitis, e.g. systemic lupus erythematosus
- Acute disseminated encephalomyelitis
- Viral infection, e.g. AIDS-related human T lymphotropic virus-1 infection
- Sarcoidosis

Multiple sclerosis

- Involves spinal cord without brain lesions in 10% of cases
- Cervical spine is the most commonly affected region

Imaging features

MRI
- Proton density and T2 short T1 inversion recovery (STIR) are the most sensitive sequences

- FLAIR is a poor sequence for spinal cord multiple sclerosis
- Eccentric high-signal plaques that align parallel to long axis of corpus callosum
- Plaques typically occupy less than half the cross-sectional area of the cord
- Plaques typically extend over less than three vertebral body lengths
- Plaques show enhancement in the acute phase

Arachnoiditis

- Inflammation of the subarachnoid space
- Commonest cause is following spinal surgery
- Other causes include meningitis and subarachnoid haemorrhage myodil contrast agent (used in myelograms); some are idiopathic

Imaging features

MRI
- Most cases occur below the level of the conus
- Nerve roots are clumped centrally or adhere peripherally to dural sac (empty sac sign)

Subacute combined degeneration of the cord

- Caused by pernicious anaemia (atrophic gastritis) and low levels of vitamin B12 in macrocytic anaemia
- Dorsal columns of cord affected first

Imaging features

MRI
- Can be normal
- Cervical spine is the most commonly involved
- Continuous long segment of high T2 signal in dorsal columns

Epidural fibrosis

- Common cause of failed back surgery
- Fibrous tissue accumulates in the epidural space, causing localised pressure effects

Imaging features

MRI
- Gadolinium is used to distinguish between fibrous tissue and recurrent disc herniation
- Epidural fibrosis enhances avidly (because it is highly vascular)
- Disc herniation enhances little if at all

Epidural haematoma

- Epidural space contains fat and the epidural venous plexus
- Haemorrhage is venous, and the thoracic spine is the commonest location
- Most bleeds are posterior because the dura is fixed to vertebral bodies
- Patients present with sudden-onset back pain or lower limb paralysis
- Causes include lumbar puncture, trauma, anticoagulant medication, haemophilia and arteriovenous malformation

Imaging features

MRI
- Sagittal sequences best demonstrate the collection of blood
- Anterior focal displacement of the dural sac (curtain sign)
- Blood breakdown products have variable signal characteristics

Epidural abscess

- Spread of infection from adjacent discitis or osteomyelitis
- Rarely caused by haematogenous spread
- Staphylococcus aureus is the commonest pathogen
- Thoracic spine is the commonest site involved
- Most abscesses are located anterior to the dural sac
- Present with back pain, fever and raised white cell count or C-reactive protein
- Can cause cord compression with acute neurological features

Imaging features

MRI
- T2WI show high-signal, ovoid lesion that extends over several levels

- T1WI post-contrast shows linear enhancement along posteriorly displaced dura and around margins of abscess (pus does not enhance)

Vertebral body metastases

- Lung and breast and myeloma are the commonest primary tumours in adults

Imaging features

MRI
- Vertebral body collapse fracture
- T1WI shows low signal foci compared with normal high-signal marrow fat
- T2 STIR shows high-signal foci compared with saturated 'dark' fat
- Standard T2 sequences are unreliable for detecting metastases

Discitis
Pyogenic discitis

- Usually caused by blood bourne spread
- Risk factors include spinal surgery and intravenous drug use
- Staphylococcus aureus is the commonest pathogen
- Non-specific symptoms of low back pain and fever
- Usually confined to one disc space and adjacent vertebral bodies
- Complications are paravertebral and epidural abscess formation

Imaging features

Plain X-ray
- It is several weeks before changes can be detected
- Early features are narrowing of the disc space and irregularities of the endplate
- Late features are endplate sclerosis and bony fusion

Technetium-99m bone scan
- Detects changes much earlier than plain radiographs

MRI
- Modality of choice (sensitivity > 90%)
- Endplates have low T1 and high T2 signal
- High T2 signal within the affected disc
- Disc shows marked contrast enhancement

Tuberculous discitis

- Caused by spread of infection from the basivenous plexus
- Commonest site is the thoracolumbar junction region

Pathophysiology and imaging features

- Infection begins at the endplate (characteristic focal defect)
- The adjacent disc becomes involved but destruction here is slow and disc space height is typically preserved in the early stages
- Infection tracks beneath the anterior or posterior longitudinal ligaments to involve multiple vertebral bodies with collapse and kyphosis
- Complications are paravertebral and epidural abscess formation

Degenerative disc disease
Imaging features

MRI
- Loss of normal T2 signal of nucleus pulposus (caused by dehydration)
- Narrowed intervertebral disc space
- Endplate changes
  - Modic type I: low T1 and high T2 signal, caused by oedema
  - Modic type II: high T1 and high T2 signal, caused by fat (the commonest type)
  - Modic type III: low T1 and low T2 signal, caused by sclerosis
- Weakened annulus fibrosis and posterior longitudinal ligaments

Disc bulge

- Weakened annulus fibrosus

Disc protrusion

- < 3 mm beyond the vertebral margin
- Ruptured annulus fibrosus, intact nucleus pulposus

Disc herniation

- > 3 mm beyond the vertebral margin
- Ruptured annulus fibrosus and posterior longitudinal ligament

- Commonest at C5–C6, C6–C7 and L4–L5, L5–S1 levels
- Posterolateral herniation is commonest pattern

Atlantoaxial subluxation

- Atlantodens interval > 3 mm in an adult and > 5 mm in a child

Causes

- Trauma
- Pharyngitis or retropharyngeal abscess
- Congenital (trisomy 21, Marfan's syndrome, Morquio's syndrome)
- Rheumatoid arthritis
- Juvenile rheumatoid arthritis
- Ankylosing spondylitis
- Systemic lupus erythematosus
- Os odontoideum
- Aplasia of the dens
- Gout
- Calcium pyrophosphate dihydrate disease

Spinal fusion

Causes

- Diffuse idiopathic skeletal hyperostosis
- Ankylosing spondylitis
- Juvenile rheumatoid arthritis
- Reiter's syndrome
- Psoriasis
- Infections (pyogenic infection more commonly than tuberculosis)
- Klippel–Feil syndrome

Ankylosing spondylitis

- Seronegative spondyloarthropathy
- Typically occurs in young males
- HLA-B27 positive in 95% of cases
- Insidious onset of low back pain and stiffness

Imaging features

Plain X-ray
- Bilateral sacroiliitis
- Sclerosis and squaring of vertebral body corner (Romanus lesion)
- Calcification of the annulus fibrosis (syndesmophyte)

- Discovertebral erosions and disc calcification
- Calcification of supraspinous ligament (dagger sign)
- Ankylosis of apophyseal and costovertebral joints

Complications of ankylosing spondylitis

- Spinal fractures
- Apical fibrosis
- Aortic regurgitation
- Amyloidosis
- Atrioventricular conduction defects
- Atlantoaxial subluxation

Diffuse idiopathic skeletal hyperostosis

- Typically occurs in males >50 years age
- HLA-B27 positive in 30% of cases
- Associated with retinoids (vitamin A analogues)
- Commonest in thoracic spine
- Causes back stiffness and reduced range of movements

Imaging features

Plain X-ray
- Flowing right-sided paravertebral ossification over four or more vertebral levels
- Osteophytes are on anterolateral aspects of vertebral bodies
- Disc spaces well maintained and often calcified
- Ligamentous ossification and osteophytosis in pelvis or lower limbs

Diffuse idiopathic skeletal hyperostosis versus ankylosing spondylitis

- No corner erosions
- No sacroilitis
- No apophyseal joint ankylosis

Spondylolisthesis

Lytic spondylolisthesis

- Caused by repetitive minor trauma
- Occurs in young athletes, e.g. fast bowlers
- Bilateral stress fractures of pars interarticularis
- Widened spinal canal and foraminal stenosis

Imaging features

Plain X-ray
- 'Scottie dog' view: lateral spine with patient turned 45°
- Most commonly occurs at L5–S1 level
- Break in neck of 'Scottie dog'
- L5 vertebral body slips forward but posterior elements stay behind
- Posterior step is above level of slip

CT
- Continuous facet sign on axial sections

Degenerative spondylolisthesis

- Caused by severe apophyseal joint osteoarthritis
- Occurs in the elderly
- No pars interarticularis fractures
- Narrowed spinal canal and foraminal stenosis

Imaging features

Plain X-ray
- Most commonly occurs at L4–L5 level
- Apophyseal degenerative changes
- L4 vertebral body and posterior elements slip forward
- Posterior step is at the level of slip

Spinal stenosis

- Commonest sites are cervical and lumbar spine

Causes

- Congenital: achondroplasia, trisomy 21, Morquio's syndrome
- Degenerative: hypertrophy of facet joints or ligamentum flavum, disc herniation
- Fracture

- Paget's disease
- Giant vertebral body haemangioma with collapse
- Vertebral metastases with collapse
- Epidural lipomatosis

Plain X-ray signs

Widened interpedicular distance

Causes

- Trauma (burst fracture)
- Longstanding raised intraspinal pressure
  - Ependymoma
  - Communicating hydrocephalus
- Dural ectasia
  - Neurofibromatosis type 1
  - Marfan's syndrome
  - Ehlers–Danlos syndrome
- Myelomeningocele and associated conditions
  - Syringomyelia
  - Diastematomyelia

Posterior scalloping

Causes

- Longstanding raised intraspinal pressure
- Dural ectasia
- Acromegaly
- Achondroplasia
- Mucopolysaccharidoses, e.g. Morquio's syndrome

Achondroplasia

- Autosomal dominant
- Rhizomelic dwarfism (short humerus and femur)

Anteroposterior lumbar X-ray:
- Progressive narrowing of interpedicular distance
- Rounded iliac bones
- Horizontal acetabular roofs

Lateral lumbar X-ray:
- Posterior scalloping and inferior beaking
- Short pedicles (spinal stenosis)

Sclerotic pedicle

Causes
- Unilateral spondylolysis in chronic stage
- Lysis of contralateral pedicle
- Lymphoma
- Osteoid osteoma

Absent pedicle

Causes
- Lytic metastasis
- Multiple myeloma
- Giant cell tumour
- Aneurysmal bone cyst
- Congenital absence

Narrow intervertebral disc spaces

Causes
- Degenerative change
- Scheuermann's disease
- Discitis (pyogenic infection more common that tuberculosis)
- Ankylosing spondylitis
- Ochronosis

Hint
• Diffuse idiopathic skeletal hyperostosis: joint spaces are well maintained • Metastases: do not affect the joint space

Intervertebral disc calcification

Causes
- Any cause of chondrocalcinosis
- Degenerative changes
- Ankylosing spondylitis
- Diffuse idiopathic skeletal hyperostosis
- Discitis
- Trauma
- Spinal fusion

Causes of chondrocalcinosis
• Wilson's disease • Hyperparathyroidism • Haemochromatosis • Idiopathic • Pseudogout • Acromegaly • Diabetes • Onchronosis • Gout

Intramedullary spinal tumours

Ependymoma
- Commonest cord tumour in adults
- Associated with neurofibromatosis type 2
- Arise from ependymal cells lining the central canal
- Commonest location is in the conus medullaris
- Recognised ectopic sites: presacral, broad ligament of ovary
- Low-grade slow growing tumour: average 3 years to presentation

Imaging features

Plain X-ray
- Posterior scalloping
- Wide interpedicular distance
- Pedicle erosion

MRI
- Localised fusiform expansion of cord by spherical solid mass
- Mildly low signal on T1WI and T2WI
- Homogeneous enhancement
- Common findings at upper and lower poles of tumour are polar cysts, cord syrinx and the 'cap' sign (a haemosiderin rim from prior haemorrhage)

Astrocytoma

- Commonest cord tumour in children
- Commonest location is the thoracic spine
- Low grade slow growing tumour

Imaging features

Plain X-ray
- Posterior scalloping
- Wide interpedicular distance
- Pedicle erosion

MRI
- Localised fusiform expansion of the cord
- More cystic ill-defined lesion than ependymoma
- Eccentrically located
- Heterogeneous enhancement of solid components
- Common findings at upper and lower poles of tumour are polar cysts and cord syrinx
- Tumour haemorrhage is uncommon

Haemangioblastoma

- 20% of all haemangioblastomas occur in the spinal cord
- 20% associated with von Hippel–Lindau disease

Imaging features

MRI
- Large cystic mass with an enhancing mural nodule
- Prominent flow voids from vessels feeding the nodule
- Adjacent cord syrinx
- No calcification

Medullary metastases

- Primary tumours include carcinoma of the lung (commonest), carcinoma of the breast and melanoma
- Commonest location is cervical and thoracic cord

Imaging features

MRI
- Small foci of high T2 signal (best seen on T2 STIR)
- Extensive surrounding oedema and avid enhancement

Extramedullary intradural spinal tumours

Leptomeningeal carcinomatosis

- Tumour seeding along the pia and arachnoid layers
- Commonest causes in children are medulloblastoma, ependymoma, germinoma and pinealoblastoma
- Commonest causes in adults are metastases from breast, lung, melanoma or lymphoma

Imaging features

MRI
- Nodular leptomeningeal enhancement
- Serial lumbar punctures more sensitive than MRI

Meningioma

- 10% of all meningiomas are spinal
- Slowly growing dura-based lesion
- Extrinsic cord compression with radiculopathy or myelopathy
- Commonest location is the dorsal thoracic spine

Imaging features

MRI
- Signal characteristics as per other meningiomas

Nerve sheath tumours

- Benign, slow growing tumours arising from spinal nerve roots

- Dumbbell shaped lesions with an intra- and extradural component
- Grow out through neural foramina (widened on plain X-ray)
- Two main types: neurofibroma and schwannoma

Neurofibroma

- Associated with neurofibromatosis type 1
- Cervical spine is the commonest location
- No enhancement

Schwannoma
- Cervical spine is the commonest location
- Avid enhancement

Extradural tumours

Epidural metastases

- Commonest extradural spinal tumour
- Commonest location is the dorsal lumbar spine
- Commonest primary tumours are carcinoma of the breast, carcinoma of the lung, melanoma and lymphoma

Chordoma

- Locally invasive and destructive malignant tumour
- Arises from embryonic notochord remnants
- Mean age 60 years
- 20% have metastases at time of diagnosis from the liver or lung
- Location
  - Clivus (35%)
  - Vertebrae (15%)
  - Sacrum (50%)
  - Maxilla, mandible or scapula (rare)

Chordoma of the sacrum

- Commonest sacral tumour

- Presents with low back pain
- Large presacral mass (average 10 cm)
- Extends anteriorly, displacing the bladder and rectum

Causes of a presacral mass

- Chordoma
- Rectal carcinoma
- Anterior meningocoele
- Teratoma
- Metastases
- Ependymoma

Chordoma of the clivus

- Large expansile tumour
- Anteriorly invades the sphenoid sinus and nasopharynx
- Superiorly invades the sella turcica, cavernous sinuses or orbits
- Laterally invades the cerebellopontine angle
- Posteriorly invades the pons

Imaging features

CT
- Low-attenuation soft tissue mass with bone destruction
- Tumour matrix contains bone fragments and calcifications in 50% of cases

MRI
- Low-signal tumour contrasts with clivus marrow fat on T1WI
- Heterogeneous lesion containing cystic areas and foci of calcification on T2WI
- Heterogeneous enhancement

Nuclear imaging
- No uptake on Technetium-99m bone scan

Anatomy

- The temporal bone is composed of two parts
  - Squamous part, which forms the floor of the middle cranial fossa
  - Petrous part, which houses middle and inner ear cavities and mastoids

Middle ear cavity

Mesotympanum

- Central portion of middle ear cavity
- Lateral wall is formed by tympanic membrane, which attaches superiorly to the scutum and inferiorly to the limbus
- Medial wall has four components, from top to bottom:
  - Bulge of the lateral semicircular canal
  - Bulge of the facial nerve canal
  - Oval window (where the stapes footplate attaches)
  - Bulge of the cochlea promontory

Hypotympanum

- Inferior portion of middle ear cavity
- Connects to the Eustachian tube orifice
- A thin plate of bone separates it from the jugular bulb

Epitympanic recess

- Superior portion of middle ear cavity
- Contains head of the malleus and body of the incus
- Lateral wall is formed by the scutum
- Connects to mastoid air cells via a posterior opening, the aditus

Prussak's space

- Region between the scutum and the head of malleus

Tegmen tympani

- Thin plate of bone, which forms the roof of the middle ear cavity
- Separates the middle ear from the middle cranial fossa

Bony ossicles

- Lateral process of malleus attaches to the central portion of the tympanic membrane the pars tensa
- Round head of malleus articulates with the incus in the epitympanic recess: 'icecream cone' on axial section
- Incus articulates with the stapes, which attaches to the oval window via its footplate
- Tensor tympani muscle (mandibular nerve) attaches to malleus
- Stapedius muscle (supplied by the eighth cranial nerve) attaches to body of the stapes

Internal auditory canal

- Bony canal running from cerebellopontine angle to the inner ear
- Transmits seventh and eighth cranial nerves
- Seventh cranial nerve lies anterior to the eighth at the meatus
- The porus acousticus is the posterior bony lip of the meatus
- Internal auditory canal divided into superior and inferior sections by a bony septum
- Superior contains facial nerve and superior vestibular nerve
- Inferior section contains the cochlear and inferior vestibular nerve
- These nerves pierce a bony plate to reach the cochlea and vestibular apparatus
- The seventh nerve then runs anteriorly before bending around the cochlea to enter the facial canal in the medial wall of the middle ear cavity, where it runs posteriorly

CT in temporal bone imaging

- High-resolution images acquired by using 1–2 mm slice thickness
- Performed via a low-amperage, high-voltage technique
- Coronal imaging lowers the orbital dose

Pathology

Otitis media

- Middle ear infection
- Usually a clinical diagnosis

Imaging features

CT and MRI
- Middle ear opacification and fluid levels in the mastoids

Gradenigo's syndrome

- Apical petrositis secondary to otitis media
- Triad of features
  - Otitis media
  - Lateral rectus palsy (supplied by the sixth cranial nerve)
  - Retro-orbital pain (supplied by the fifth cranial nerve)
- May also get excessive lacrimation through involvement of the greater superficial petrosal nerve

Imaging features

CT and MRI
- Mastoid opacification
- Bone destruction
- Enhancing inflammatory tissue at petrous apex

Otitis externa

- Infection of the external ear canal
- Associated with diabetes
- Commonest pathogen is Pseudomonas
- Presents with otalgia and purulent discharge
- Left untreated can cause osteomyelitis and even meningitis
- CT or MRI are used to assess the extent of local invasion

Exostosis of the external auditory canal

- Common benign tumour
- Associated with swimming in cold water
- Bony overgrowth that can narrow or obliterate the canal
- A secondary cholesteatoma may form adjacent to the exostosis

Cholesteatoma

- Benign, slow growing accumulation of epithelial debris in the middle ear cavity

Congenital cholesteatoma

- Accounts for 2% of cholesteatomas

- Failure of normal involution of fetal epidermoid cell rests
- Usually arises centrally within middle ear cavity
- Presents in childhood with conductive deafness
- No history of otitis media
- Tympanic membrane is intact

Acquired cholesteatoma

- Accounts for 98% of cholesteatomas
- Accumulation of squamous epithelial cells in the middle ear cavity
- Arises in epitympanic recess (Prussak's space)
- Usually presents with conductive deafness
- Can cause meningitis, brain abscesses, sigmoid sinus thrombosis, facial nerve palsy and sensorineural deafness
- Associated with chronic otitis media
- Tympanic membrane is perforated (usually a pars flaccida perforation)

Imaging features

CT (early)
- Soft tissue mass between the scutum and the head of malleus
- Erosion of the scutum
- Medial displacement or erosion of the ossicles

CT (late)
- Non-enhancing soft tissue mass filling the middle ear cavity
- Extension through aditus to involve the mastoid air cells
- Superior erosion through tegmen tympani
- Erosion into the seventh cranial nerve canal and bony labyrinth

MRI
- Soft tissue mass is isointense to brain on T1WI
- Mass is mildly high signal on T2WI

Cerebellopontine angle lesions

- Three main types of lesions
  - Acoustic schwannoma (80%)
  - Meningioma (10%)
  - Epidermoid (5%)

- Other causes of lesions
  - Arachnoid cyst
  - Trigeminal schwannoma
  - Cholesterol granuloma
  - Dermoid
  - Metastases
  - Endolymphatic sac tumour

Acoustic schwannoma

- Benign, slow growing tumour of the eighth cranial nerve
- Associated with neurofibromatosis type 2 (bilateral schwannoma is pathognomonic of this condition)
- Majority arise from the superior vestibular portion within the internal auditory canal
- Tumour expands within IAC and exits proximally into the cistern of the cerebellopontine angle, where it usually grows posteriorly (anterior growth is limited by the facial nerve)
- Tumour encases adjacent neurovascular structures
- Unusual cause of progressive unilateral sensorineural deafness
- Rarely presents with facial nerve palsy

Imaging features

CT
- Widening of the internal auditory meatus
- Erosion of the porus acousticus
- Dumbbell shaped soft tissue mass which enhances avidly
- No calcifications

MRI
- Tumour is high signal on T2WI, and large tumours contain cystic areas
- Tumour enhances avidly on post-gadolinium T1WI; this is the best modality for detection of very small lesions

---

Anterior inferior cerebellar artery

- First branch of the basilar artery
- Runs through the cistern of the cerebellopontine angle
- Normally enhances post-contrast
- Can mimic a small acoustic neuroma

Meningioma

- Displays typical features on CT and MRI

Meningioma versus acoustic schwannoma: distinguishing features

- No widening of the internal auditory meatus
- No erosion of the porus acousticus
- Dural tail enhancement in 70% of cases
- Adjacent temporal bone hyperostosis
- Calcified in 20% of cases
- High attenuation with non-contrast CT

Epidermoid

- Benign congenital lesion
- Slow build-up of squamous epithelial cells (like a cholesteatoma)
- Encases the adjacent neurovascular structures
- Presents in middle age with seventh and eighth cranial nerve palsies
- More than 50% occur at the cerebellopontine angle
- Can also occur in the suprasellar region

Imaging features

CT
- Low-attenuation (fat-density), lobulated lesion
- 20% are calcified
- No enhancement

MRI
- Variable signal depending on fat and water content
- Commonly high signal on T2WI

Epidermoid versus acoustic schwannoma: distinguishing features

- No widening of the internal auditory meatus
- No erosion of the porus acousticus
- Calcified in 20% of cases

> **Epidermoid versus arachnoid cyst: distinguishing features**
>
> MRI FLAIR
> - Epidermoids retain some signal
> - Arachnoid cysts that are filled with CSF appear dark
>
> MRI (DWI)
> - Epidermoids appear bright (because of restricted diffusion)
> - Arachnoid cysts appear dark

Childhood deafness

Causes

- 50% are acquired, particular through infection in utero (notably the TORCH infections: Toxoplasmosis; Other infections, e.g. HIV, syphilis; Rubella; Cytomegalovirus; Herpes)
- 50% are hereditary
  - Mondini malformation
  - Enlarged vestibular aqueduct syndrome
  - Otosclerosis

Mondini malformation

- Incomplete formation of the cochlea, which has 1.5 turns instead of the normal 2.5
- Causes congenital sensorineural deafness
- Associated with Pendred's syndrome

Imaging features

CT and MRI
- Cystic dilatation of the cochlea and vestibular apparatus

Enlarged vestibular aqueduct syndrome

- Aqueduct is a narrow bony canal in the petrous temporal bone
- It contains the endolymphatic duct, which drains endolymph from the inner ear to the endolymphatic sac in the posterior cranial fossa
- In this condition the aqueduct is abnormally dilated

- Associated with Pendred's syndrome
- Causes a progressive sensorineural deafness in childhood
- Onset of deafness is associated with minor head trauma

Imaging features

CT
- Enlarged vestibular aqueduct (> 1.5 mm)

> **Pendred's syndrome**
>
> Autosomal-recessive condition with:
> - Sensorineural deafness
> - Mondini malformation
> - Enlarged vestibular aqueduct
> - Goitre

Otosclerosis

- Idiopathic deafness caused by bony sclerosis
- Usually bilateral, with onset around puberty
- Identical imaging appearances to those seen in osteogenesis imperfect; stapes–oval window articulation seen in 90% of cases

Imaging features

CT
- In conductive deafness, thickened stapes and excess soft tissue at the oval window; 10% involves cochlea
- In sensorineural deafness, cochlea appears thickened and sclerotic

> **Temporal bone sclerosis and deafness**
>
> Occurs in:
> - Paget's disease
> - Fibrous dysplasia
> - Osteopetrosis
> - Meningioma
> - Otosclerosis
> - Osteogenesis imperfecta
> - Syphilis

Anatomy

The nose

- Upper one third of the external nose is bony; the lower two thirds is cartilaginous
- The septum is composed of the ethmoid bone, vomer and quadrilateral cartilage
- Each lateral nasal wall has three medial projections: the upper, middle and lower turbinates (conchae)
- The cavities are lined by ciliated respiratory epithelium
- Communicates posteriorly with the nasopharynx via the choana
- Blood supply is from the anterior and posterior ethmoidal arteries (branches of the ophthalmic artery) and the sphenopalatine artery (the terminal branch of the maxillary artery)

Paranasal sinuses

- Frontal sinus drains into the frontal recess
- Maxillary sinus drains via the infundibulum and hiatus semilunaris
- Anterior ethmoid air cells drain into the ethmoid infundibulum
- These drainage pathways unite as the osteomeatal complex, which opens into the middle meatus (between the middle and inferior turbinates)
- Sphenoid sinus and posterior ethmoid air cells together drain via the sphenoethmoidal complex, which opens into the superior meatus (between the middle and superior turbinates)

Functional endoscopic sinus surgery (FESS)

- Minimally invasive technique using a fibreoptic endoscope
- Used to restore mucociliary drainage in patients with chronic sinus disease unresponsive to medical therapy
- Preoperative CT is mandatory
- Useful for defining sinus anatomy and extent of sinus disease

Structures vulnerable to injury

- Several important structures are vulnerable to injury at FESS and CT provides vital information to the surgeon regarding these

Anterior ethmoidal artery

- Originates from the ophthalmic artery and runs medially between the superior oblique and medial rectus muscles
- Enters the anterior ethmoid sinus via the cribroethmoid foramen and courses medially along its superior aspect before piercing the cribriform plate to enter the anterior cranial fossa
- Marks the superolateral boundary for FESS.

Optic nerve

- Related to the posterior ethmoid air cells (especially the Odoni cell anatomical variant) and the superolateral aspect of the sphenoid sinus

ICA

- Intimately related to the sphenoid sinus
- A deviated intersphenoid septum may attach to the carotid canal
- Rarely the thin bone separating the ICA and the sphenoid sinus is absent.

Ethmoid roof

- Thin piece of bone composed of the cribriform plate and fovea ethmoidalis
- Easily damaged, causing a CSF leak
- Such leaks may not present clinically for several weeks, in contrast to those caused by skull base fractures, which are usually evident immediately

Anatomical variants

- Concha bullosa: a large pneumatised middle turbinate, which can obstruct the

ethmoid infundibulum or osteomeatal complex
- Haller cells: ethmoid air cells extending beneath the floor of the orbit; they are intimately related to the maxillary infundibulum and, if large, can obstruct it
- Odoni cell: a posterior ethmoid air cell that extends superiorly and laterally to abut the optic nerve.

Nasal septal perforation

Causes

- Cocaine
- Septal surgery
- Nasal intubation
- Wegener's granulomatosis and other vasculitides
- Sarcoidosis
- Lymphoma
- Tuberculosis
- Syphilis

Bacterial sinusitis

- Inflammation of the paranasal sinus mucosa
- Begins as a viral infection with secondary bacterial invasion
- Risk factors
  - Cystic fibrosis
  - Kartagener's syndrome (situs inversus, bronchiectasis)
  - Nasal septal deviation
  - Horizontal uncinate process
- Commonest site is isolated maxillary sinusitis, followed by frontal sinusitis
- Least common site is sphenoethmoidal sinusitis
- If acute sinusitis does not resolve adequately with medical therapy (decongestants, antibiotics), chronic sinusitis may develop.
- FESS is used in these cases to improve sinus drainage

Imaging features

CT and plain X-ray
- Acute sinusitis: air–fluid level in sinus (secretions of water attenuation)

- Chronic sinusitis: mucosal thickening (secretions of soft-tissue attenuation)

Complications

- Orbital cellulitis
- Intracranial extension (meningitis, abscesses, subdural empyema)
- Mucocele

Mucormycosis

- Fungal sinusitis affecting immunocompromised patients and patients with diabetics
- Aggressive infection, which can spread to the orbits, cavernous sinus and brain

Imaging features

CT and plain X-ray
- Sinus opacification without air–fluid level
- Adjacent bony destruction
- High attenuation on CT (contains manganese)

Mucocele

- End stage of a chronically obstructed paranasal sinus ostium
- Causes include chronic sinusitis, nasal polyps and osteomas
- Sinus fills with secretions
- Commonest expansile lesion of the paranasal sinuses
- Commonest site is frontal sinus
- Can cause proptosis, diplopia, visual loss and CSF rhinorrhoea
- An important complication is secondary infection (mucopyocele), which behaves like a large abscess and is a surgical emergency

Imaging features

CT
- Expanded sinus opacified by low-attenuation material
- Pressure erosion or sclerosis of sinus wall
- May contain peripheral calcifications
- Rim enhancement post-contrast (tumours enhance centrally)

MRI
- Variable signal depending on duration:
- Acute: high signal on T2WI (because of high water content), low T1
- Chronic: low signal on T2WI (because water has been resorbed), low T1

> **Causes of sinus opacification and bone destruction**
>
> - Inverting papilloma
> - Lymphoma
> - Fungal sinusitis
> - Squamous cell carcinoma
> - Wegener's granulomatosis
> - Juvenile angiofibroma
> - Tuberculosis

Nasal polyps

- Inflammatory swellings of the sinonasal mucosa
- Associated with allergic and infective rhinitis
- Common in adults
- Rare in children unless associated with cystic fibrosis
- Usually bilateral within maxillary or ethmoid sinuses
- Well-defined soft tissue masses
- Frequent cause of sinus obstruction

Antrochoanal polyp

- Large unilateral polyp arising from the maxillary antrum
- Typically occurs in young adults
- Widens the sinus ostium and extends back into the middle meatus
- A large polyp can pass through the posterior choana into the nasopharynx

Fibrous dysplasia

- Developmental disease of bone
- Normal marrow is replaced by fibrous tissue

- Well-defined, expansile, lucent lesion with a ground-glass texture
- 80% are monostotic (localised to a single bone)
- Commonest sites are the ribs, the femoral neck and the craniofacial area

Craniofacial fibrous dysplasia

- Frontal bone is the commonest site, and it can obliterate the frontal sinus
- Lesion widens the diploic space but spares the inner table
- Skull base lesions are usually sclerotic
- Can mimic a variety of other lesions, e.g. meningioma
- Symptoms include headaches and facial deformity (proptosis)
- 0.5% risk of transformation into osteosarcoma or fibrosarcoma

Imaging features

Plain X-ray
- Wide range of appearances; can be lucent, sclerotic or mixed

CT
- Expansile lesion with a ground-glass texture

MRI
- Low T1, low T2, with intense enhancement

Technetium-99m bone scan
- Increased uptake

Wegener's granulomatosis

- Necrotizing vasculitis of small and medium-sized arteries
- Positive for classical antineutrophil cytoplasmic antibodies (cANCA), specifically proteinase-3 (PR3)
- 80% have nose and paranasal sinus involvement
- Causes bloody sinus discharge, epistaxis and collapse of the nasal septum
- Other findings
  - Otitis media
  - Subglottic stenosis
  - Arthritis
  - Neuropathy (mononeuritis multiplex)

- Multiple lung cavitatory lesions (in 90% of cases)
- Glomerulonephritis (in 90% of cases, and the commonest cause of death)

Benign tumours

Inverting papilloma

- Commonest benign tumour of the paranasal sinuses
- Peak incidence in the sixth decade
- Possible viral aetiology (human papilloma virus)
- Commonest location is lateral nasal wall
- Polypoid growth with mass effect, causing proptosis and facial deformity
- Requires complete surgical excision because approximately 10% transform into squamous cell carcinoma

Imaging features

CT
- Polypoid soft tissue mass
- Adjacent bony deformity or destruction

MRI
- Intermediate signal on T2WI and high signal in adjacent inflamed tissues

Osteoma

- Slow growing, bone-forming tumour
- Majority occur in the frontal sinuses
- Usually an incidental plain film finding
- Can obstruct the frontoethmoidal complex, causing a mucocele
- If large can cause facial deformity and proptosis
- Multiple osteomas are associated with Gardner's syndrome

Imaging features

Plain X-ray
- Solid, homogeneous, well-defined radiodensity

CT
- Modality of choice to assess local pressure effects

Gardner's syndrome

Autosomal-dominant inheritance

TRIAD:
- Multiple osteomas
- Colonic polyposis
- Soft tissue tumours, e.g. desmoids, and increased risk of duodenal and other carcinomas

---

Malignant tumours

Squamous cell carcinoma

- Commonest paranasal malignant tumour, accounting for 80% of cases
- Can arise from inverting papilloma
- Majority arise in the maxillary sinus
- Soft tissue mass with bone destruction
- 20% of patients have cervical lymphadenopathy at time of diagnosis

Lymphoma

- Account for 5% of malignant tumours of the sinuses
- Majority are non-Hodgkin's B-cell lymphomas
- Peak incidence in the seventh decade
- Presents with nasal obstruction
- Commonest location is the maxillary sinus, followed by the nasal cavity
- Bulky soft tissue mass with bone destruction
- No specific imaging features to distinguish it from squamous cell carcinoma

Metastases

- Rare
- Commonest primary is renal cell carcinoma
- Commonest sinus involved is maxillary sinus
- Typically presents with epistaxis (because they are hypervascular)

Esthesioneuroblastoma

- Rare
- Neurogenic tumour arising from the olfactory sensory epithelium in the roof of the nasal cavity (undersurface of the cribriform plate)
- Bimodal age distribution, with peak incidences among teenagers and in the sixth decade
- Presents with nasal obstruction, epistaxis and anosmia
- Locally aggressive with submucosal spread in all directions: through the cribriform plate into the frontal lobes, into the orbits and into the ethmoid sinuses
- 20% of patients have cervical lymphadenopathy at time of diagnosis
- Treatment is surgical resection and radiotherapy
- High rate of recurrence

Imaging features

CT and MRI

- Enhancing mass in the upper nasal cavity with local bone destruction

Causes of anosmia
• Old age
• Frontal lobe tumours
• Olfactory groove meningioma
• Esthesioneuroblastoma

Anatomy

Parotid gland

- Composed of superficial and deep lobes
- Larger superficial lobe lies anterior to the mastoid process, ramus of mandible and masseter muscle
- Smaller deep lobe passes between ramus of mandible anteriorly and styloid process posteriorly (stylomandibular tunnel)
- Parotid 'tail' is a small inferior extension, which wraps around the angle of the mandible
- Facial nerve exits from the stylomastoid foramen and runs through the gland in a plane between superficial and deep lobes
- Parotid gland normally contains around 20 intraparotid lymph nodes
- The retromandibular vein and ECA pass upwards through the parotic gland and deep to the nerve (with the artery deep to the vein)
- Parotid duct (Stensen's duct) runs along the surface of masseter muscle before turning medially to pierce buccinator muscle
- Parotid duct opens into the mouth above the second upper molar tooth

Submandibular gland

- Lies medial to the body of mandible in the submandibular fossa
- Wedged between the mylohyoid and digastric muscles
- Separated from parotid by deep cervical fascia and Kuttner's node
- Continuous with a smaller, deep part, which passes around the posterior border of mylohyoid to lie deep to this muscle
- Submandibular duct (Wharton's duct) opens into the floor of the mouth beside the frenulum of the tongue
- Similar ultrasound appearance to the parotid gland

Sublingual gland

- Lies in the floor of the mouth beneath the mucus membrane and above the mylohyoid muscle
- Drained by several small ducts into the floor of the mouth, posterior to the submandibular duct orifice.

Minor salivary glands

- The greatest concentration of these small submucosal glands is in the hard and soft palates
- They are also found in the side walls of the oral cavity and on the oropharynx, lips and tongue

Infections

- Can be viral, e.g. mumps, or bacterial
- Stones predispose to bacterial infections

Imaging features

Ultrasound
- Swollen glands are echo-poor with a heterogeneous texture

Sjögren's syndrome

- Clinical triad
  - Xerostomia (dry mouth), with enlarged salivary glands
  - Keratoconjunctivitis sicca (dry eyes), with enlarged lacrimal glands
  - Autoimmune disease, e.g. rheumatoid arthritis, systemic lupus erythematosus, scleroderma
- Progressive non-obstructive salivary gland duct dilatation
- Associated with an increased risk of salivary gland lymphoma

Imaging features

Ultrasound
- Enlarged salivary glands
- Containing multiple small round echo-poor areas
- Increased vascularity seen on colour Doppler scans

Sialogram
- Multiple small cavities of contrast accumulation

MRI
- Enlarged glands containing multiple cysts of varying sizes
- Speckled 'honeycomb' appearance on T2WI

Sarcoidosis

- Salivary glands involved in 30% of cases
- Painless enlargement

Imaging features

Ultrasound
- Enlarged glands, echo-poor

CT
- Enlarged glands with multiple small foci of high attenuation

---

Uveoparotid fever (Heerfordt's syndrome)

TRIAD
- Bilateral uveitis
- Bilateral parotitis
- Facial nerve palsies

Salivary gland stones

- 80% of stones occur in the submandibular gland
- 20% of stones occur in the parotid
- Majority of stones are radiopaque

Imaging features

Ultrasound
- Echo-bright foci with post-acoustic shadowing
- Commonest location of submandibular stones is within the duct

Sialogram
- Filling defects, associated strictures and proximal duct dilatation

Ranula

- Mucus-retention cyst causing a swelling on the floor of the mouth
- Most commonly involves the sublingual glands

- Occasionally extends below the mylohyoid muscle and presents as a neck swelling ('plunging ranula')
- If large may cause dysphagia and airway compromise
- CT and MRI are used to assess the extent of these large lesions

---

Benign salivary gland tumours

- 80% of benign tumours occur in the parotid gland
- The smaller the gland involved, the more likely the tumour is to be malignant

Pleomorphic adenoma

- Commonest benign salivary gland tumour, accounting for 80%
- Majority found in superficial lobe of parotid
- Tend to recur following removal
- Malignant transformation is recognised

Imaging features

Ultrasound
- Well-defined, echo-poor, oval mass with post-acoustic enhancement
- May contain areas of dystrophic calcification
- Perilesional blood flow with small branches running centrally

MRI
- Very high signal on T2WI

Adenolymphoma (Warthin's tumour)

- Accounts for 10% of benign salivary gland tumours
- Commonest location is in tail of parotid gland (the superficial lobe)
- Commoner in men than women
- 10% are bilateral
- Well-defined mass lesion
- More complex appearance than pleomorphic adenoma

Imaging features

Ultrasound
- Well-defined, echo-poor lesion with internal echoes

CT
- Heterogeneous cystic or solid lesion

Parotid haemangioma

- Commonest parotid mass in young children
- Develops in first few months of life
- Progressively enlarges over subsequent months
- Most spontaneously regress by teenage years

Imaging features

Ultrasound
- Echo-poor mass (because it contains vascular spaces)
- Displays internal blood flow

MRI
- Soft tissue mass containing prominent flow voids

Malignant salivary gland tumours

Mucoepidermoid tumour

- Commonest malignant salivary gland tumour
- Majority occur in the parotid gland
- Commonest malignant parotid tumour

- Present as a hard 'craggy' mass and facial nerve palsy

Cylindroma (adenoid cystic carcinoma)

- Commonest in females, with an average age of 60 years
- Commonest malignant tumour of the minor salivary glands
- Uncommon in the parotid gland
- Aggressive tumour with a propensity for early perineural spread

Imaging features

Ultrasound
- Ill-defined lesion of mixed echotexture
- Infiltration around adjacent vessels
- Cervical lymphadenopathy

CT and MRI
- More accurate than ultrasound at assessing the degree of local invasion and perineural involvement

Metastases

- Commonest primary tumours are melanoma and squamous cell carcinoma
- Imaging features are non-specific
- On ultrasound, typically appear as small echo-poor lesions

Anatomy

- Vertical fibromuscular tube extending from skull base to cricoid cartilage, where it merges with the oesophagus
- Lies in front of the cervical prevertebral fascia and behind the nasal cavity, oral cavity and larynx
- There are three layers
  - Mucosa, the innermost layer
  - Submucosa (also known as the pharyngobasilar fascia)
  - Muscular layer, the outer coat composed of superior, middle and inferior pharyngeal constrictors
- Constrictor muscles diverge anteriorly but form a continuous overlapping posterior layer
- The pharynx is described in three parts
  - Nasopharynx: skull base to level of soft palate
  - Oropharynx: soft palate to hyoid bone
  - Laryngopharynx: hyoid bone to cricoid cartilage (C6)

Nasopharynx

- Continuous anteriorly with the nasal cavity through the choana
- Lined by respiratory epithelium
- Roof is applied to the skull base and slopes beneath sphenoid bone and clivus
- Lateral walls supported by superior pharyngeal constrictor muscle
- Eustachian tube pierces its lateral walls on either side
- Torus tubarius is a ridge posterior to each tubal orifice, formed by the levator veli palatine muscle and the cartilaginous portion of the eustachian tube
- Behind these ridges are the paired lateral pharyngeal recesses of Rosenmüller
- The submucosal layer contains numerous minor salivary glands and lymphoid tissue
- The adenoids are aggregations of lymphoid tissue in the midline roof; they are prominent in children and regress from puberty onwards

Oropharynx

- Lies posterior to the oral cavity: circumvallate papillae of the tongue mark the transition point
- Includes posterior one third of the tongue and the lingual tonsils
- Contains two muscular folds in its lateral walls, the palatoglossal arch (anteriorly) and the palatopharyngeus arch (posteriorly)
- Between these arches lie the palatine tonsils

Waldeyer's ring

- Ring of lymphoid tissue that lies around the oropharynx and the nasopharynx
- Includes the adenoids and the lingual and palatine tonsils

Laryngopharynx

- Lies posterior to the larynx
- Continuous inferiorly with the oesophagus
- Contains two deep lateral recesses (the piriform fossae)
- Lateral walls are supported by the inferior pharyngeal constrictor muscle
- An anatomical weak point where its lower fibres diverge is called Killian's dehiscence; this is the site of a Zenker diverticulum

Thornwald cyst

- Developmental thin-walled cyst (notochordal remnant)
- Occurs in 2% of the population
- Located in midline on the posterior wall of nasopharynx
- Contains proteinaceous fluid
- Can become infected and rupture

Imaging features

CT
- Low-attenuation and non-enhancing lesion

MRI
- High signal on T1WI and T2WI

Benign tumours of the pharynx

Juvenile angiofibroma
- Commonest benign tumour of the nasopharynx
- Very locally aggressive and highly vascular
- Supplied by maxillary or ascending pharyngeal artery
- Mean age 15 years
- Occurs almost exclusively in males
- Commonest clinical features are nasal speech (caused by nasal obstruction), severe recurrent epistaxis and facial deformity
- Arises in region of the sphenopalatine foramen at the junction of the nose and nasopharynx
- Biopsy is contraindicated

Pathways of tumour invasion
- Lateral invasion
  - Into the pterygopalatine fossa, which is widened in 90% of cases
  - Through the pterygomaxillary fissure, which is widened in 90% of cases
  - Into the infratemporal fossa
  - Erosion of the medial pterygoid plate
- Superior invasion
  - Into the sphenoid sinus (in 70% of cases) and the middle cranial fossa
- Inferior invasion
  - Into the soft palate and the oropharynx
- Posterior invasion
  - Filling the nasopharyngeal airway
- Anterior invasion
  - Into the nasal cavity

Imaging features
CT
- Soft tissue mass that enhances early and avidly
- Modality of choice to assess extent of local invasion and bony destruction

MRI
- Prominent flow voids are seen within the lesion (which contains large vessels)

Malignant tumours of the pharynx

Nasopharyngeal carcinoma (70%)
- Accounts for 70% of malignant tumours of the pharynx
- Squamous cell carcinoma
- High incidence in Chinese and other Asian men
- Associated with Ebstein–Barr virus
- Aggressive tumour that infiltrates into adjacent tissue spaces
- Late presentation is typical
- Most tumours arise in the lateral fossa of Rosenmüller
- 90% of patients have lymphadenopathy at time of diagnosis
- Lateral retropharyngeal nodes of Rouvière and the cervical chain lymph nodes (most commonly levels II and V) are commonly involved

Pathways of tumour invasion
- Lateral invasion (earliest)
  - First sign is obliteration of fat strip between tensor palatine and levator palatine muscles
  - Grows into parapharyngeal space, obliterating the fat there
  - Further lateral extension is into the masticator space
- Anterior invasion
  - Blocks the Eustachian tube orifice, causing otitis media and mastoiditis
  - Into the pterygopalatine fossa
  - Into the posterior aspect of the nasal cavity
- Posterior invasion
  - Into the retrostyloid space, which contains the carotid sheath and the ninth, tenth and eleventh cranial nerves
  - Into the prevertebral muscles
- Superior invasion
  - Into the skull base and sphenoid sinus
  - Through the foramen lacerum (which contains the ICA) and into cavernous sinus
  - Through the foramen ovale into the middle cranial fossa

Masticator space

- Lateral to the parapharyngeal space
- Contains muscles of mastication (the medial and lateral pterygoids, masseter and temporalis)
- Ramus of mandible
- Mandibular nerve

Imaging features

CT
- Soft-tissue attenuation mass

MRI
- Modality of choice
- Isointense to muscle on T1WI, which is the best sequence to assess for obliteration of the fat plane
- Intermediate signal on T2WI
- Solid tumour elements enhance avidly

Non-Hodgkin's lymphoma

- Accounts for 20% of malignant tumours of the pharynx
- Arises in lymphoid tissue of Waldeyer's ring
- Disease of the elderly, presenting with nasal obstruction
- Bulky soft tissue mass, which grows in a circumferential pattern
- Late invasion of parapharyngeal spaces
- Presence of large non-necrotic cervical lymph nodes
- Systemic signs, e.g. splenomegaly
- Imaging features suggestive of lymphoma

Cystic adenoid carcinoma

- Accounts for 10% of malignant tumours of the pharynx
- Commonest malignant tumour of the minor salivary glands
- Soft palate is the commonest site
- Aggressive lesion that invades the adjacent parapharyngeal spaces
- Early perineural spread into the skull base and cavernous sinuses

Pathology of related spaces

Retropharyngeal space
- Between pharyngeal constrictor muscles anteriorly and prevertebral muscles posteriorly
- Contains fat and lymph nodes
- A mass here displaces the prevertebral muscles posteriorly

Retropharyngeal abscess
- Spread of infection from tonsils

Nodal metastases
- Common in head and neck squamous cell cancers
- Lateral nodes in the retropharyngeal space are the nodes of Rouvière, which are involved early in nasopharyngeal carcinoma

Prevertebral space
- Deep to the retropharyngeal space
- Extends from the skull base to the superior mediastinum
- Pathology here displaces the prevertebral muscles anteriorly

Contents of the prevertebral space

- Prevertebral muscles (longus coli and capitis)
- Vertebral artery and veins
- Phrenic nerve
- Scalene muscles
- Brachial plexus

Pre-vertebral abscess
- Anterior spread from vertebral body osteomyelitis

Metastatic invasion
- Anterior extension of vertebral body metastases

Parapharyngeal space

- Slit-like space located lateral to the nasopharynx, between the pharyngeal constrictor muscles and the masticator space
- The styloid process, ICA and jugular vein lie posteriorly
- Bounded superiorly by the skull base
- Contains fat, mandibular nerve branches and the ascending pharyngeal artery
- Important anatomically in that it can be invaded by several tumours
  - Posterolateral invasion by tumours in the deep lobe of the parotid gland
  - Medial invasion by nasopharyngeal carcinoma
  - Posterior invasion by vagus nerve paraganglioma
  - Inferior invasion by carotid bulb paraganglioma

Paraganglioma

- Rare, slow growing tumour that arises from paraganglia cells
- Amine precursor uptake decarboxylase (APUD)-type tumours
- Commonest site is the adrenal (phaeochromocytoma)
- Head and neck paragangliomas occur at four main sites
  - Carotid bulb
  - Vagus nerve
  - Jugular bulb
  - Cochlear promontory

Carotid bulb paraganglioma

- Arises from paraganglia cells within the adventitia of the carotid bulb
- Commonest paraganglioma of the head and neck (accounting for 60%)
- Slow growing, pulsatile neck mass at the anterior border of sternocleidomastoid, just lateral to the hyoid bone.
- 2% secrete catecholamines
- 5% undergo malignant transformation

Imaging features

Ultrasound
- Oval, well-defined, echo-poor mass in the lateral neck
- Splays the (CCA bifurcation
- Encases the CCA but does not narrow it

CT
- Well-defined soft tissue mass that has homogeneous intense enhancement

MRI
- Solid areas of high signal with flow voids on T2WI
- 'Salt-and-pepper' appearance

Angiogram
- Intense blush (because it is a highly vascular tumour)
- Head and neck paragangliomas are supplied by the ascending pharyngeal artery and its branches

Nuclear scan
- Indium-111 octreotide is highly sensitive for these tumours

Vagus nerve paraganglioma

- Arises from paraganglia cells of the vagus nerve perineurium
- Commonest at the nodose ganglion
- Slow growing, painless neck mass behind the angle of the mandible
- Characteristically displaces the ICA anteromedially and internal jugular vein posterolaterally
- Large tumours can invade into the parapharyngeal space
- 25% invade the sympathetic ganglia, causing a Horner's syndrome

Jugular bulb paraganglioma (glomus jugulare)

- Arises from paraganglia cells in the adventitia of the jugular bulb
- Causes pulsatile tinnitus
- Expands to erode the jugular foramen
- Can invade superiorly into the middle ear cavity

- Can invade posterosuperiorly along the jugular vein into the posterior cranial fossa
- Can cause jugular vein thrombosis
- Involvement of adjacent cranial nerves (ninth, tenth and eleventh) is Vernet's syndrome

Jugular foramen

- Between petrous temporal and occipital bones
- Posteromedial to the styloid process
- Separated from hypotympanum above by a thin plate of bone
- Asymmetrical (right is larger than left)
- Contains the jugular vein, inferior petrosal sinus, and the ninth, tenth and eleventh cranial nerves (the twelfth cranial nerve exits the skull via the hypoglossal canal)

Cochlear promontory paraganglioma

- Arises from paraganglia cells of the tympanic plexus (ninth and tenth cranial nerves) on the cochlear promontory
- Commonest tumour of the middle ear
- Presents with pulsatile tinnitus and conductive deafness
- Red tumour mass seen behind the eardrum
- Tumour remains confined to the middle ear cavity

Causes of pulsatile tinnitus

- Glomus jugulare (commonest)
- Glomus tympanicum
- No cause identified
- Meningioma
- Carotid dissection
- Carotid fibromuscular hyperplasia
- Aberrant ICA

Anatomy

Divisions of the larynx

- Supraglottic region: the epiglottis to the upper border of the true cords
- Glottic region: the true cords
- Subglottic region: below the true cords to the trachea
- False cords are situated just above the true cords
- A thin cleft between them is called the ventricle
- A small pouch projects laterally from each ventricle (the saccule)
- The arytenoid cartilages lie posteriorly on the upper surface of the cricoid cartilage and span the level of the ventricle
- Each arytenoid cartilage has a vocal process where the true cords attach
- Thyroarytenoid muscle makes up the bulk of the true cords

Paraglottic space

- Lateral space between inner lining of larynx and thyroid cartilage
- Contains fat and lymphatics
- Inferiorly it contains the thyroarytenoid muscle
- An important site of supraglottic tumour extension

Pre-epiglottic space

- Anterior space between thyroid cartilage or the thyrohyoid membrane and the epiglottis
- Continuous inferiorly with the paraglottic space
- Contains fat and lymphatics
- Another important site of supraglottic tumour extension
- A key area radiologically in that extension into the pre-epiglottic space cannot be assessed endoscopically

Piriform fossae

- Paired lateral recesses of the laryngopharynx, which make up the posterior wall of the paraglottic space on each side
- Help to channel food towards the oesophagus during swallowing
- Tumours here can invade into the paraglottic space and reach the vocal cords

Benign tumours of the larynx

Squamous papilloma

- Commonest benign tumour of the larynx
- Caused by human papilloma virus
- Commonly occur on the vocal cords
- Presents with hoarseness, stridor, haemoptysis and recurrent chest infections
- In children, usually multiple (laryngeal papillomatosis)
- In adults, usually solitary
- Complications include airway compromise
- Can spread to involve the trachea, bronchi or lungs
- Transformation into squamous cell carcinoma can occur but is rare

Malignant tumours of the larynx

Laryngeal carcinoma

- Vast majority are squamous cell carcinomas
- Risk factors are smoking and alcohol

Supraglottic tumours

- Account for 35% of laryngeal carcinomas
- Present late
- Metastases common at time of diagnosis
- Spread into the paraepiglottic space and the paraglottic space and to the jugular lymph nodes
- Optimal surgery is partial laryngectomy, preserving the true cords

Contraindications to partial laryngectomy, i.e. requires total laryngectomy

- Thyroid cartilage invasion
- Cricoid cartilage invasion
- Extension into the true cords
- Extension into the piriform fossae

- CT and MRI are complementary to endoscopic evaluation of these tumours
- Imaging provides information regarding endoscopic 'blind spots', e.g. nodal disease
- Signs of cartilage invasion (CT is modality of choice) are cartilaginous erosions and soft tissue beyond the outer margins of cartilage (seen on axial image)

Glottic tumours

- Account for 50% of laryngeal carcinomas
- Present early with hoarseness
- Typically arise from anterior half of the cord
- Metastases uncommon at time of diagnosis (the true cords have no lymphatics)
- Optimal surgery is laser resection if very localised; if more advanced, surgery is a vertical hemilaryngectomy (removing the true and false cord on one side)

Contraindications to hemilaryngectomy, i.e. requires total laryngectomy

- Tumour extending across anterior commissure to involve more than one third of the opposite cord
- Thyroid cartilage invasion
- Cricoid cartilage invasion
- Extension superiorly into the false cord
- Inferior extension > 1 cm

Subglottic tumours

- Rare
- Present late

- Usually represent inferior extension of a glottic tumour
- Metastases common at time of diagnosis
- Paraoesophageal and mediastinal lymph nodes may be involved
- Requires total laryngectomy because the cricoid cartilage is invariably involved
- Majority are non-operable, owing to extensive invasion into surrounding structures, e.g. the trachea

Other pathology

Laryngocele

- Dilatation of either saccule of the laryngeal ventricle
- Caused by raised intraglottic pressure
- 80% unilateral
- Filled with air or fluid
- Increases in size with Valsalva manoeuvre
- 50% caused by a laryngeal tumour obstructing the saccule
- Also associated with glass blowing and excessive coughing
- A large tumour can extend through the thyrohyoid membrane to present as an anterior neck mass

Subglottic stenosis

- Worse on inspiration (unlike tracheomalacia, which is worse on expiration)
- May be congenital
- Other causes include post-tracheostomy, prolonged endotracheal tube placement, Wegener's granulomatosis and relapsing polychondritis

Extramedullary plasmacytoma

- Rare
- Discrete mass of monoclonal plasma cells within the soft tissues
- 90% occur in the head and neck
- Commonest sites are the upper airways and conjunctiva
- Lobulated soft tissue mass with local bone and cartilage destruction
- CT or MRI is used to assess extent of local invasion prior to resection

Rheumatoid arthritis

- Can affect the cricoarytenoid joint, but there are no specific radiological findings

Trauma

Cricoid and thyroid fractures

- Vertical fractures are easily identified by axial CT

- Horizontal fractures are best assessed by coronal reformats

Cricoarytenoid joint dislocation

- Normally the arytenoid cartilages are seen symmetrically, perched on the cricoids
- Asymmetry of cartilage in axial plane images

Anatomy

- Each half of the mandible is composed of
  - Horizontal body
  - Angle
  - Vertical ramus
  - Coronoid process anteriorly
  - Condylar process posteriorly
- The mandible houses the mandibular canal, which runs from the inner aspect of the ramus to open on the external aspect of the body (mental foramen)
- The inferior alveolar nerve (a branch of the mandibular nerve) and the inferior alveolar artery are contained within the mandibular canal

Temporomandibular joint (TMJ)

- Synovial joint between condyle and temporal bone
- Contains a biconcave fibrocartilagenous disc
- Disc lies slightly anteriorly when the mouth is closed
- Disc moves posteriorly to a neutral position when the mouth is open

TMJ subluxation

- The disc lies very anterior in both the closed and open positions
- T1 MRI is the best sequence to assess subluxation

TMJ arthritis

- Rheumatoid arthritis is the commonest cause
- Erosions mainly occur on the condylar head
- T2 MRI is the best sequence to assess arthritis

Mandibular pathology

Mandibular hypoplasia (micrognathia)

- Can be part of a congenital syndrome, e.g. Pierre Robin syndrome, Turner's syndrome, Treacher–Collins syndrome, progeria
- Acquired causes include juvenile rheumatoid (Still's disease) and fetal alcohol syndrome

Mandibular fractures

- Commonest site is the condylar neck, followed by the ramus, the angle and the body
- Fractures are commonly bilateral (the mandible acts like a bony ring)
- Occlusal films can help detect subtle fractures

Cystic lesions of the mandible

Radicular cyst (apical cyst)

- Commonest jaw cyst (accounting for 60%)
- Inflammatory cyst at root of a carious tooth (tooth decay)
- Caused by proliferation of cells of Malassez in the periodontal ligament
- Well-defined, unilocular cyst

Residual cyst

- Occurs following tooth extraction

Odontogenic keratocyst

- Developmental cyst arising from dental lamina cell rests
- Most occur in the ramus of the mandible (rarely in the maxilla)
- Well-defined, unilocular cyst with corticated margins
- 50% recur following removal
- Multiple cysts are associated with Gorlin's syndrome

Gorlin's syndrome

- Multiple basal cell carcinomas
- Multiple mandibular keratocysts
- Skeletal anomalies
- Extensive soft tissue calcification (of the falx cerebri and tentorium)

Dentigerous cyst

- Arises from the crown of an impacted or unerupted tooth
- Third mandibular molar is the commonest site
- Well-defined, corticated, cystic lesion containing the impacted tooth
- Rarely develops into an ameloblastoma

Ameloblastoma

- Benign but locally aggressive tumour, which expands into adjacent soft tissues
- Peak age is sixth decade
- Two thirds arise from enamel cells around a tooth
- One third arise from enamel cells in dentigerous cyst wall
- 75% occur in the mandible, 25% in the maxilla
- Expansile multilocular cystic lesion containing daughter cysts
- Commonly recurs following removal
- CT and MRI are used to assess extent of local invasion
- Rare unicystic variant, which has a better prognosis and is more common in the maxilla
- Plain X-rays cannot reliable distinguish between ameloblastoma, dentigerous cyst and odontogenic keratocyst

Other cystic jaw lesions

- Brown tumour
  - Seen in hyperparathyroidism (primary > secondary)
  - Commonest sites are the jaw, pelvis and ribs
  - Bone is resorbed by osteoclasts and replaced by fibrous tissue
  - Expansile lytic lesion
- Myeloma (common)
- Metastases (uncommon), typically from the breast or lung
- Haemangioma
- Eosinophilic granuloma ('floating teeth')
- Fibrous dysplasia
- Simple bone cyst
- Aneurysmal bone cyst
- Ossifying fibroma

  - Encapsulated expansile benign neoplasm
  - Composed of fibrous tissue and osteoid
  - Slow growing, but cause facial asymmetry
  - Lucent cyst with varying degrees of calcification
  - Intense uptake on bone scan
- Cementoma
- Odontoma
  - Hamartoma
  - Well-defined, cystic lucency
  - Contains calcifications and tooth-like structures
- Stafne bone cyst
  - Incidental finding
  - Aberrant lobe of submandibular gland causing a well-defined depression in the body of mandible

Lamina dura

- Cortical bone that lines the tooth socket
- Seen as a thin white line around the root
- Separated from the tooth by the radiolucent periodontal ligament

Causes of erosion of the lamina dura

- Re-modelling disorders
  - Hyperparathyroidism, e.g. renal osteodystrophy
  - Fibrous dysplasia
  - Paget's disease
  - Anaemia
  - Osteoporosis
  - Cushing's syndrome (steroids cause demineralisation)
- Tumours, cysts and other lesions
  - Ameloblastoma
  - Metastases
  - Radicular cyst
  - Dentigerous cyst
  - Odontogenic keratocyst
  - Ossifying fibroma
  - Osteomyelitis
  - Periodontitis
  - Eosinophilic granuloma
  - Cretinism (not adult-onset hypothyroidism)
  - Burkitt's lymphoma

Burkitt's lymphoma
• Highly malignant non-Hodgkin's lymphoma
• Endemic in west African children
• Malaria acts as a co-factor with Ebstein–Barr virus
• Grossly destructive lesion of mandible with a large soft tissue component
• Abdominal and ovarian involvement is common
• Responds well to chemotherapy

Teeth

Normal development

- Total of 20 deciduous teeth
- Eruption starts at 6 months of age
- Continues until 2–3 years of age
- These are replaced by permanent teeth between 6 and 12 years of age
- No deciduous teeth remain > 12 years of age
- Total of 32 permanent teeth
  - four maxillary and four mandibular molars
  - two maxillary and two mandibular canines
  - four maxillary and four mandibular incisors
- Usually all permanent teeth are present by 18 years of age (but this is variable)

Supernumerary teeth

- Extra teeth nearly always occur in the maxilla
- Associated with Gardner's syndrome and idiopathic hypoparathyroidism

Anatomy

- Divided into two triangles by the sternocleidomastoid muscle (SCM)

Anterior triangle

- Borders
  - SCM posteriorly
  - Mandible superiorly
  - The midline
- Further subdivided by the hyoid bone into the suprahyoid triangle and the infrahyoid triangle

Contents of the suprahyoid triangle

- Submandibular and submental nodes – level I
- Submandibular gland

Note: The floor is the mylohyoid muscle; structures deep to this are in the sublingual space, e.g. the sublingual gland

Contents of the infrahyoid triangle

- Carotid arteries and internal jugular veins
- Strap muscles of the neck
- Level VI lymph nodes
- Larynx, trachea and thyroid gland

Posterior triangle

- Borders
  - Trapezius posteriorly
  - SCM anteriorly
  - Clavicle inferiorly
- The floor is formed by four muscles: the splenius capitis, levator scapulae, scalenus medius and scalenus anterior

Contents of the posterior triangle

- Fat
- Level V lymph nodes
- Accessory (eleventh) cranial nerve
- Dorsal scapular nerve
- Brachial plexus
- Subclavian artery and vein

Head and neck lymph nodes

Cervical lymph nodes

- Left-sided neck nodes drain into the thoracic duct
- Right-sided neck nodes drain into the junction of the internal jugular vein and the subclavian vein
- Nodal level predicts survival in squamous cell carcinoma of the head and neck
  - Level I nodes have a 40% 5-year survival rate
  - Level V nodes a 4% 5-year survival rate
- Standard treatment of head and neck cancer with positive nodes is neck dissection with removal of all level I–V nodes, because metastases do not occur in any set order

Cervical lymph node classification

- Level I: submandibular and submental nodes
- Level II: cervical chain nodes deep to upper third of SCM (above level of hyoid bone on axial images)
- Level III: cervical chain nodes deep to middle third of SCM (below hyoid and above cricoid cartilage on axial images)
- Level IV: cervical chain nodes deep to lower third of SCM (below level of cricoid cartilage on axial images)
- Level V: posterior triangle nodes
- Level VI: nodes around thyroid gland
- Level VII: superior mediastinal nodes

Features of malignant head and neck nodes

- Enlargement
  - Level I and II nodes are normally slightly larger than level III–VII nodes
  - Normal nodes are larger and more conspicuous in children and young adults than in the elderly
  - Short axis measurements are used

Size criteria for head and neck nodes

- Levels I and II: > 10 mm by ultrasound, > 12 mm by CT or MRI
- Levels III–VII: > 8 mm by ultrasound, > 10 mm by CT or MRI

- Rounded shape: ration of maximum short axis to maximum long axis ratio > 0.6
- Loss of fatty hilum
  - Ultrasound shows loss of normal echo-bright centre
  - MRI shows low signal on T1WI and T2WI

MRI of lymph nodes

- T1WI and STIR are best sequences
- Intravenous contrast not required to tell nodes from vessels
- Intravenous contrast improves detection of necrotic nodes

- Central necrosis
  - CT shows low-attenuation centre and peripheral enhancement
  - MRI: T1WI post-contrast is the best sequence and shows peripheral enhancement
  - Ultrasound shows an echo-poor central cystic area
  - Tuberculous adenitis can mimic squamous cell carcinoma metastases
- Microcalcifications
  - Highly suggestive of papillary thyroid carcinoma
  - Coarse nodal calcification is seen in treated lymphoma and tuberculosis

- Peripheral blood flow pattern with colour Doppler ultrasound
  - Normal nodes have a central hilar flow pattern
- Extracapsular spread
  - Non-sharp, 'spiculated' margins
  - Absence of a clean fat plane around node

Ultrasound and fine-needle aspiration cytology

When used together, ultrasound and fine-needle aspiration cytology have > 90% accuracy in the detection of malignant lymph nodes

PET–CT in head and neck cancer

- PET–CT is developing an increasing role
- Can detect lesions as small as a few millimetres in diameter
- More sensitive than CT and MRI for nodal metastases
- Nodal uptake is size-dependent and is poor for nodes < 6 mm in diameter

Indications

- Staging of primary head and neck cancer
- Detection of locally recurrent disease after treatment
- Detection of unknown primary with positive neck nodes

Normal FDG-18 uptake in the head and neck

- Extraocular muscles
- Brain grey matter
- Fossae of Rosenmüller
- Pterygoid muscles
- Prevertebral muscles
- Tonsils
- Salivary glands
- Uvula
- Tongue and oral mucosa
- Mylohyoid
- Vocal cords if talking
- Strap muscles
- Brown fat

Anterior triangle pathology

Suprahyoid pathology

- Lymphadenopathy (level I and II nodes)
- Submandibular gland lesions
- Vagus nerve paraganglioma
- Plunging ranula

Infrahyoid pathology

- Lymphadenopathy (level VI nodes)
- Thyroglossal duct cyst
- Laryngocele
- Carotid bulb paraganglioma
- Neurofibroma
- Jugular vein thrombosis
- Branchial cleft cyst

Neurofibroma

- Nerve sheath tumour
- Commonest in cervical region
- Arises from spinal nerve roots, sympathetic chain and brachial plexus
- Multiple or plexiform neurofibromas are associated with neurofibromatosis type 1
- Only 10% of people with a solitary neurofibroma have neurofibromatosis type 1
- Well-defined, lobulated soft tissue mass

Imaging features

MRI
- Isointense on T1 to the adjacent strap muscles
- High signal on T2WI with a low signal centre
- Does not enhance

Jugular vein thrombosis

- Associated with central venous catheters and intravenous drug use
- Presents with a swollen neck with a firm palpable mass in the anterior triangle

Imaging features

Ultrasound
- Early: echo-poor clot expands the vein
- Late: echo-bright clot in a contracted vein

CT
- Wall enhancement of expanded vein

Branchial cleft cyst

- Developmental anomaly
- Caused by incomplete obliteration of the branchial apparatus
- Fluid filled cyst with or without a fistulous tract
- Lined by stratified squamous epithelium
- Typically present later in life (unlike a cystic hygroma)
- Prone to secondary infection: internal debris seen
- There are four types: first, second, third and fourth brachial cleft cysts

First branchial cleft cyst

- Accounts for 5% of cases
- Fistulous tract from parotid region to external auditory canal
- Classically presents in middle age with recurrent parotid abscesses and otorrhoea
- Can exert pressure on the seventh cranial nerve

Second branchial cleft cyst

- Accounts for 95% of cases
- Usually a cyst
- Anteromedial to SCM (anywhere in anterior triangle)
- Lateral to carotid arteries, and may extend medially between them
- Ultrasound shows echo-free lesion (internal echoes seen if infected)
- CT shows low-attenuation lesion with mild rim enhancement
- MRI shows lesion low on T1WI, high on T2WI

Third and fourth branchial cleft cysts (very rare)

- Very rare
- Fistulous tracts running from the piriform fossae to the border of SCM at the base of neck
- Third brachial cleft cyst lies adjacent to the laryngeal ventricle
- Fourth brachial cleft cyst lies adjacent to the recurrent laryngeal nerve

Posterior triangle pathology

- Lymphadenopathy (level V nodes)
- Cystic hygroma
- Tuberculous adenitis
- Lipoma
- Haemangioma of the trapezius

Cystic hygroma

- Developmental anomaly
- Failure of lymphatic sacs to connect with draining veins, which results in large cystic lymphatic spaces
- 80% occur in the neck, 20% in the axilla
- 80% are present at birth and associated with Turner's syndrome; trisomies 13, 18 or 21, Noonan's syndrome, or fetal alcohol syndrome
- Painless compressible and transilluminable mass in the posterior triangle
- Extends around muscles and blood vessels, with no displacement
- 10% extend down into the mediastinum
- Important complications are haemorrhage and infection causing enlargement and mass effect with tracheal or vascular compression

Imaging features

Ultrasound
- Multiple, thin-walled, cystic spaces
- Fluid–fluid levels seen if there is associated haemorrhage

CT
- Low-attenuation cystic lesion

MRI
- Typically low on T1WI, high on T2WI
- Variable appearance if there is intralesional haemorrhage

Tuberculous adenitis

- In adults mainly caused by *Mycobacterium tuberculosis*

- In children mainly caused by other mycobacteria, e.g. *Mycobacterium avium-intracellulare* complex
- Presents as a slow growing, painless neck mass
- Left untreated, the caseating nodes can weaken the overlying skin leading to sinus formation ('collar stud abscess')
- Posterior triangle is the commonest site
- Unilateral neck involvement is typical

Imaging features

Plain X-ray
- Chest X-ray is abnormal in only 25% of cases

CT
- Enlarged nodes with fluid attenuation centres
- Displays rim enhancement
- Can mimic metastases from a squamous cell carcinoma
- Coarse nodal calcifications may be seen after treatment

Lipoma

- Posterior triangle is a common location
- Well-defined, elliptical subcutaneous mass

Imaging features

Ultrasound
- Echo-bright with echogenic lines

CT and MRI
- Fat-containing lesion (high on T1WI and T2WI)

Anatomy

- Thyroid gland is composed of two lateral lobes and a midline isthmus; each lobe has an upper and lower pole
- Isthmus is positioned approximately level with the cricoid cartilage
- Each lobe lies between the trachea medially and the CCA and internal jugular vein laterally
- Normal craniocaudal length of each lobe is < 5 cm
- Normal anteroposterior diameter is < 2 cm
- Posterior to each lobe is the longus coli muscle
- 50% of people have an additional pyramidal lobe, which extends superiorly from the isthmus
- Arterial supply
  - Inferior thyroid artery: branch of the thyrocervical trunk
  - Superior thyroid artery: first branch of ECA
  - 5% of people also have a thyroid ima artery, a branch of the aorta or the brachiocephalic trunk
- Venous drainage
  - Via paired superior and middle thyroid veins to the internal jugular
  - Via multiple inferior thyroid veins to the brachiocephalic veins

Physiology

- Iodine in food is converted to iodide in the intestine and enters the circulation
- One quarter of the iodine is 'trapped' by the follicular cells of the thyroid and organified into thyroglobulin, from which tri-iodothyronine (T3) and thyroxine (T4) are produced
- Three quarters of the iodine is excreted by the kidneys
- The release of T3 and T4 is controlled via TSH as part of a negative feedback mechanism with the hypothalamus and pituitary gland

Normal imaging features

- Ultrasound shows homogeneous echotexture, brighter than the adjacent strap muscles
- CT shows high attenuation (because of the iodine content) and uniform enhancement
- MRI shows a slightly higher signal than the adjacent strap muscles on both T1WI and T2WI with uniform enhancement

Thyroid scintigraphy

Agents

- Iodine-123: slightly superior to technetium-99m-pertechnetate in all aspects of thyroid imaging, but more expensive and requires longer imaging times
- Iodine-131: principally used for assessment and treatment of thyroid cancer metastases; it delivers a much higher radiation dose than I-123
- Technetium-99m-pertechnetate: most widely used thyroid imaging agent in the UK. Can be performed without the patient having to stop thyroxine or carbimazole, but poor assessment of retrosternal thyroid tissue (owing to sternal attenuation)

Technetium-99m-pertechnetate

- Method
  - Given by intravenous injection
  - Imaged at 20 minutes
  - Pin-hole gamma camera is ideal
- Pertechnetate is trapped by thyroid gland but not organified into thyroglobulin and rapidly excreted by kidneys
- Normally there is uniform uptake of pertechnetate throughout both lobes of the thyroid
- Uptake also occurs in the salivary glands (patient is given a drink prior to imaging), the gastric mucosa and the choroid plexus

Causes of diffuse high uptake

- Graves' disease
- Early Hashimoto's thyroiditis
- Iodine deficiency
- Stopping antithyroid drugs (rebound phenomenon)
- TSHoma
- Lithium treatment
- Hydatidiform mole or choriocarcinoma

Causes of diffuse low uptake

- Subacute thyroiditis (de Quervain's thyroiditis)
- Established Hashimoto's thyroiditis
- Recent intravenous iodinated contrast, e.g. for an intravenous urogram
- Amiodarone treatment
- Thyroxine replacement therapy
- Anti-thyroid drugs, e.g. carbimazole
- Riedel's thyroiditis
- Congenital hypothyroidism
- Strumi ovari
- Thyroidectomy

- Hot nodule: a focal area of increased uptake, which indicates that a lesion is hyperfunctioning. The majority are caused by a secreting adenoma, and are almost never malignant (< 1% of cases)
- Cold nodule: a focal area of decreased uptake, which indicates that a lesion is hypofunctioning
  - 15% will be malignant if solitary
  - 5% will be malignant if multiple

Causes of a cold nodule

- Colloid cyst
- Non-secreting adenoma
- Focal area of thyroiditis
- Granuloma
- Abscess
- Parathyroid adenoma
- Thyroid carcinoma
- Thyroid metastases

Pathology
Thyroglossal duct cyst

Embryology of thyroid gland

- Arises from the tongue base (foramen cecum)
- Descends in the midline with thyroglossal duct
- Passes anterior to the hyoid bone
- Reaches its final position by seventh week of gestation

- Commonest congenital midline neck mass
- Arises from remnants of thyroglossal duct
- 80% are located in the midline, 20% are paramedian
- Present in young adults as a painless neck swelling
- May become secondarily infected
- Cyst moves upwards with swallowing and tongue protrusion
- 1% risk of developing thyroid carcinoma (majority are papillary)
- Even smaller risk of developing squamous cell carcinoma
- < 5% contain functioning ectopic thyroid tissue
- Mainly a clinical diagnosis; imaging is used to confirm diagnosis and assess extent of lesion prior to surgical removal
- Surgical procedure is the Sistrunk operation, whereby the cyst is resected along with the entire thyroglossal duct (including central portion of hyoid bone)
- Removal of the cyst alone is associated with a high rate of recurrence
- Preoperative technetium-99m-pertechnetate or iodine-123 scans are sometimes performed to confirm the presence of a normal thyroid gland before resection, i.e. to check that ectopic thyroid tissue in the cyst wall is not the patient's only thyroid tissue

Imaging features
Ultrasound
- Well-defined, cystic lesion embedded within the strap muscles

- Majority contain internal echoes as a result of proteinaceous debris

CT
- Fluid-attenuation lesion with a thin enhancing rim

MRI
- Typically low T1 high T2, but variable appearance depending on protein content

Graves' disease

- Autoimmune disorder caused by long-acting thyroid-stimulating (LATS) antibodies
- Predominantly affects young females
- Presents with smooth, painless goitre
- Raised T4 and low TSH

Imaging features

Ultrasound
- Diffusely enlarged and echo-poor
- Diffusely hypervascular 'thyroid inferno'
- Vessels have high flow velocities (> 50 cm/second) with colour Doppler scans
- Velocities return to normal (< 30 cm/second) after treatment

Scintigraphy
- Diffusely increased uptake throughout both lobes and the isthmus
- Hypertrophied pyramidal lobe

Complications

- Thyroid acropachy
  - Usually occurs in first year following treatment
  - Painless swelling of wrists or hands with finger clubbing
  - Asymmetrical, thick periosteal reaction along metacarpals and phalanges
- Graves' ophthalmopathy

Hashimoto's thyroiditis

- Commonest cause of hypothyroidism in developed countries
- Autoimmune disease caused by anti-thyroid antibodies
- Predominantly affects middle-aged females
- Diffuse lymphocytic infiltration of thyroid
- Gland is enlarged and non-tender and feels 'rubbery' to palpation

- 5% get an initial transient thyrotoxic state ('hashitoxicosis')
- Up to one third of patients will develop non-Hodgkin's lymphoma

Imaging features

Ultrasound
- Diffusely enlarged with a coarse echotexture
- Echo-poor micronodules

Scintigraphy
- Non-specific appearances
- Increased uptake in early stage
- Reduced uptake in established disease

Subacute thyroiditis (de Quervain's thyroiditis)

- Typically occurs 2 weeks after a viral respiratory tract infection
- Inflamed gland releases thyroxine with transient hyperthyroidism
- Causes fever and painful goitre
- Majority return to a euthyroid state over several months

Imaging features

Ultrasound
- Mildly enlarged and echo-poor thyroid
- Absent colour flow

Scintigraphy
- Diffusely decreased uptake

Amiodarone-induced thyroiditis

- Amiodarone is an iodine-containing anti-arrhythmic drug with a long half-life of 90 days
- 10% of patients taking it develop problems with thyroid function
- Causes a destructive thyroiditis or a Graves'-like condition

Multinodular goitre

- Benign nodular (adenomatous) hyperplasia
- Typically occurs in middle-aged females
- Causes a swollen neck with palpable nodules
- Retrosternal extension can cause tracheal compression

- Thyroid function is usually normal
- Occasionally a nodules is hypersecreting (Plummer's disease)

Imaging features

Ultrasound
- Asymmetrically enlarged gland (anteroposterior diameter of lobe > 2 cm)
- Contains multiple nodules of varying sizes
- Nodules can be purely solid, purely cystic or mixed

Scintigraphy
- Heterogeneous uptake by an enlarged gland
- May see discrete hot nodules on a background cold parenchyma
- A solitary cold nodule has a 5% risk of being malignant

Congenital hypothyroidism

- Diagnosed at birth via heel prick test
- Diagnosis confirmed via scintigraphy, which shows absent uptake

Riedel's thyroiditis

- Rare idiopathic chronic inflammatory disorder
- Dense fibrous tissue replaces normal thyroid parenchyma
- Associated with retroperitoneal and mediastinal fibrosis
- Fibrosis extends beyond thyroid capsule into adjacent structures
- Can cause stridor or dysphagia from compressive effects
- Hard, fixed and painless goiter
- One third of patients are hypothyroid
- Fine-needle aspiration biopsy cannot distinguish Riedel's thyroiditis from anaplastic carcinoma

Imaging features

Ultrasound
- Enlarged, echo-poor gland with ill-defined margins

CT
- Extensive areas of low attenuation throughout gland

MRI
- Low signal on T1WI and T2WI

Scintigraphy
- Diffuse low uptake

Lingual thyroid

- Accounts for 90% of ectopic thyroid tissue (the mediastinum is another recognised ectopic site)
- Caused by arrest of normal descent from the foramen cecum
- More common in females
- 2% risk of developing thyroid carcinoma

Imaging features

CT
- High-attenuation, enhancing lesion at the base of the tongue

Thyroid nodule

- Assessed by a combination of ultrasound, scintigraphy and fine-needle aspiration cytology

Imaging features

Ultrasound
- Features suggestive of a benign nodule:
  - Purely cystic lesion
  - Cystic lesion with 'comet tail' artefacts
  - Thin uniform echo-poor halo
  - Peripheral coarse calcifications
  - Perilesional blood flow
- Features suggestive of a malignant nodule:
  - Microcalcifications
  - Irregular margins
  - Irregular halo around lesion
  - Invasion of local structures
  - Intralesional blood flow
  - Lymphadenopathy

Scintigraphy
- 15% risk of malignancy if a solitary cold nodule
- 5% risk of malignancy if multiple cold nodules

Fine-needle aspiration cytology
- Ultrasound and scintigraphy cannot reliably distinguish benign from malignant nodules
- When combined with fine-needle aspiration cytology the overall accuracy is around 90%
- However, cytology cannot distinguish follicular adenoma from carcinoma

Thyroid malignancy

- Head and neck irradiation is the major risk factor (latency > 5 years)

Papillary carcinoma

- Accounts for 70% of thyroid malignancies
- Low-grade malignancy usually affecting young adults
- Spreads early via lymphatics to adjacent neck nodes
- Irregular echo-poor mass containing microcalcifications
- Nodes contain punctuate microcalcifications
- Lymph node metastases have no bearing on overall prognosis
- Prognosis is generally excellent

Follicular carcinoma

- Accounts for 20% of thyroid malignancies
- Affects middle-aged females
- Intermediate-grade malignancy
- Spreads via bloodstream to lungs and bone
- Fine-needle aspiration biopsy cannot distinguish follicular adenoma from follicular carcinoma

Medullary carcinoma

- Accounts for 5% of thyroid malignancies
- Associated with multiple endocrine neoplasia type 2a (MEN-2a) and occurs in the teenage years
- Arises from C cells in the upper two thirds of the gland
- Secretes calcitonin but blood calcium levels are not affected
- Early spread to lymph nodes, lung and bone
- Echo-poor lesion containing calcifications
- Nodes are hypoechoic with dense calcifications
- Poor prognosis if there are metastases at time of diagnosis

---

Multiple endocrine neoplasia type 1 (MEN-1)

- Pituitary adenoma
- Pancreatic islet cell carcinoma
- Parathyroid adenoma or hyperplasia

Multiple endocrine neoplasia type 2a (MEN-2a)

- Medullary carcinoma thyroid (in 100%)
- Phaeochromocytoma (in < 50%)
- Parathyroid adenoma or hyperplasia (in < 50%)

Anaplastic carcinoma

- Accounts for 3% of thyroid malignancies
- Very aggressive infiltrative tumour affecting elderly patients
- Invades into adjacent muscles and vessels
- Necrotic tumour often containing foci of calcification
- Usually inoperable at time of diagnosis
- Treatment is with radiotherapy
- Mean survival is 6 months

Lymphoma

- Accounts for 2% of thyroid malignancies
- Non-Hodgkin's B-cell type tumour
- Affects middle-aged females with coexistent Hashimoto's thyroiditis
- Up to one third of patients with Hashimoto's thyroiditis develop it
- Usually a solitary echo-poor lesion

Metastases to thyroid

- Rare
- Usually occurs in the context of disseminated malignancy
- Commonest primary lesion is melanoma
- Usually a solitary echo-poor lesion

Treatment and follow-up

- Primary treatment is thyroidectomy with or without neck dissection
- T3 (short-acting) is taken for 4 weeks
- T3 is stopped for 2 weeks (to elevate TSH level)
- Whole body iodine-131 scan is performed to assess for metastases
- False-negative scans are seen in 20% (caused by non-functioning metastases)
- If serum thyroglobulin is raised and iodine-131 scan is negative, an F-18-DG PET scan is indicated
- PET is very sensitive for these non-functioning metastases

- High doses of iodine-131 are used to treat metastases
- Technetium-99m-pertechnetate is not suitable for whole-body scans because it is masked by background activity
- Iodine-131 is contraindicated in pregnancy and breast-feeding because it crosses the placenta and is excreted in breast milk
- Iodine-131 is more accurate for assessing thyroid bone metastases than conventional bone scans

Medullary carcinoma

Does not accumulate I-131, amd the following can be used:
- Technetium-99m(V) DMSA scan
- Iodine-131-MIBI scan
- Thallium-201 scan
- F-18-DG PET scan

Parathyroid glands

Anatomy and physiology

- Typically there are four parathyroid glands
- Situated posterior to the thyroid and anterior to longus coli muscle
- The two superior glands are deep to the midpart of each lobe
- The two inferior glands are deep to the lower pole of each lobe
- Up to 25% of people have more than four parathyroid glands
- Normal glands are not visible by ultrasound
- Parathyroid hormone (PTH) is secreted by the chief cells of these glands in response to low serum calcium levels
- PTH acts to elevate calcium levels by increasing osteoclastic bone resorption

Primary hyperparathyroidism

- 85% of cases caused by a parathyroid adenoma
- Rarer causes include parathyroid hyperplasia, ectopic PTH secretion (e.g. from squamous cell lung cancer), parathyroid carcinoma

- Increased PTH and increased serum calcium
- Complications include renal calculi, pancreatitis, nephrocalcinosis, chondrocalcinosis and subperiosteal resorptions
- Treatment is surgical removal of the adenoma

Preoperative adenoma localization investigations

Ultrasound
- Adenomas most commonly arise from the inferior glands
- Well-defined, oblong-shaped, echo-poor lesion
- Usually > 1 cm in diameter, and hypervascular
- Parathyroid carcinoma can have identical imaging features
- 20% are ectopic and not visible with ultrasound
- Ectopic sites include thymus, mediastinum and carotid sheath
- False positives may be caused by the longus coli muscle or a lymph node

Scintigraphy
- Technetium-99m-sestamibi (MIBI) scan
- Dual-phase study: intravenous injection with imaging at 20 minutes and re-imaging at 2 hours
- Scan covers cervical and thoracic regions (ectopic adenomas)
- MIBI washes quickly out off thyroid but is retained in abnormal parathyroids

Old method: subtraction study

- Technetium-99m-pertechnetate given first
- Taken up only by thyroid and washes out quickly
- Thallium-201 given second
- Taken up by thyroid and parathyroid glands
- Images are 'subtracted' to view the parathyroid glands
- Major limitation was that a thyroid nodule could mimic a parathyroid adenoma

Secondary hyperparathyroidism

- Increased PTH and increased serum calcium
- Usually due to chronic renal failure (lack of vitamin D activation)
- Compensatory hyperplasia of all four parathyroid glands

Tertiary hyperparathyroidism

- Increased PTH and increased serum calcium
- Long-standing hyperplasia develops into autonomous secretion

Hypoparathyroidism

- Increased PTH and increased serum calcium
- Tetany and convulsions
- Most commonly due to surgical removal of all four glands
- Rarely autoimmune

Pseudohypoparathyroidism

- Increased PTH and increased serum calcium
- Caused by end organ resistance to PTH
- Clinical features include short stature, short fourth metacarpals, moon face and intellectual impairment

Pseudopseudohypoparathyroidism

- Normal biochemistry
- Phenotypically the same as pseudohypoparathyroidism

Reversible posterior leukoencephalopathy

- Brain capillary leak syndrome with widespread cerebral oedema
- Failure of autoregulation following acute blood pressure elevation
- Misnomer as anterior changes are well recognised
- Causes headaches and cortical visual loss
- Progresses to infarction if blood pressure not promptly controlled

Imaging features

MRI
- Bilateral confluent areas of white matter high T2 signal
- Commonly affects centrum semiovale of occipital lobes
- Changes typically resolve with treatment over 1–2 weeks
- Appears dark on DWI (increased diffusion)

Basal ganglia

Anatomy

- Basal ganglia comprise:
  - Caudate nucleus
  - Lentiform nucleus (globus pallidus, putamen)
  - Claustra
  - Amygdaloid body

Low-attenuation lesions in the basal ganglia

- Hypoxia
- Hypoglycaemia
- Wilson's disease
- Toxins – carbon monoxide, methanol, cyanide, barbiturates

Basal ganglia calcifications

- Idiopathic (50%)
- Hyperparathyroidism
- Hypoparathyroidism, pseudohypoparathyroidism, pseudopseudohypoparathyroidism

- TORCH infections
- Cockayne syndrome (demyelinating disease of childhood)
- Down's syndrome
- Tuberous sclerosis
- Mitochondrial diseases
- Toxins (carbon monoxide, lead)

Neurocysticercosis

- Caused by ingestion of pork tapeworm larvae
- Faecal–oral spread
- Endemic in developing countries
- Commonly involves the CNS causing meningoencephalitis
- Parenchymal calcified cystic lesions with homogeneous or rim enhancement
- Intraventricular cysts with hydrocephalus

High T2 signal thalamic lesions

- Wernicke's encephalopathy
- New-variant Creutzfeldt-Jakob disease
- Wilson's disease
- Acute disseminated encephalomyelitis (40% have thalamic involvement)
- Lacunar infarcts
- Lead poisoning
- Hallervorden–Spatz disease
- Reye's syndrome
- Leigh's disease
- Biliary encephalopathy

Wilson's disease

- Autosomal-recessive disorder
- Low levels of caeruloplasmin
- Copper deposition in tissues
- Eyes show Kayser–Fleisher ring
- Cirrhosis
- Basal ganglia show low T1, high T2 signal
- Copper has only weak paramagnetic effects and therefore appears as low signal on T1WI

Normally enhancing structures

Enhancing structures on both CT and MRI

- Pituitary gland (anterior and posterior lobes)
- Infundibulum
- Nasal turbinates
- Sinonasal mucosa
- Choroid plexus
- Pineal gland
- Cavernous sinuses
- Extraconal eye muscles

Enhancing structures on CT

- Arterial structures, e.g. circle of Willis
- Dural venous sinuses and deep veins

Enhancing structures on MRI

- Thin short linear segments of dural enhancement

Normally calcified structures

- Choroids plexus
- Basal ganglia
- Pineal gland
- Dura
- Habenula
- Falx cerebri and cerebellum
- Tentorium
- Clinoid ligaments

Skull vault thickening

Generalised thickening

- Severe anaemias
- Acromegaly
- Hyperparathyroidism
- Osteopetrosis
- Shunted hydrocephalus

Focal thickening

- Paget's disease
- Meningioma
- Fibrous dysplasia
- Hyperostosis frontalis

Hair-on-end skull

- Hereditary anaemias
  - Thalassaemia
  - Glucose-6-phosphate dehydrogenase deficiency
  - Spherocytosis
  - Sickle cell disease
- Neuroblastoma metastases

Epilepsy

- Idiopathic, or caused by a structural brain lesion acting as a focus
- Identification of focus via electroencepholography, MRI or PET scanning
- Commonest structural lesion is hippocampal sclerosis

Hippocampal sclerosis

- Highly epileptogenic abnormality
- Associated with temporal lobe epilepsy
- 80% can be cured with an anterior temporal lobectomy

Imaging features

MRI
- Hippocampal atrophy and enlarged temporal horn on T1WI
- High signal in atrophic hippocampus on T2WI

F-18-DG PET
- Decreased uptake in epileptogenic temporal lobe

Other structural lesions that can cause epilepsy

- Stroke: commonest cause in those aged > 50 years
- Cavernous angioma
- Primary or secondary brain tumours
- Arteriovenous malformation
- Post infectious, e.g. neurocysticerosis
- Phakomatoses
- Neuronal migration anomalies, e.g. heterotopias (grey matter in abnormal location), pachygyria (paucity of gyri), agyria (absent gyri), schizencephaly (CSF-filled transcerebral cleft)

Dementia

Causes

- Alzheimer's disease (60% of cases)
- Multi-infarct dementia (20% of cases)
- Other causes (20% of cases): Lewy bodies, Pick's disease, Parkinson's disease, Korsakoff's psychosis, Creutzfeldt-Jakob disease, depressive dementia

Reversible causes of dementia

- Normal pressure hydrocephalus
- Meningioma
- Hypothyroidism

Alzheimer's disease

- Slowly progressive loss of memory and cognition

Imaging features

CT and MRI
- Normal in early stages of disease
- Later prominent sulci and atrophy of medial temporal lobe

PET and HMPAO-SPECT
- Symmetric perfusion defects in posterior temporal and parietal lobes

Pick's disease

- Pre-senile onset (< 65 years)
- Enlarged frontal horns
- Frontotemporal atrophy and hypoperfusion

New-variant Creutzfeldt-Jakob disease

- Rapidly progressive dementia and myoclonus
- Occurs in young adults
- Caused by a prion protein

Imaging features

MRI
- Symmetrical high T2 signal in posterior thalami (pulvinar nuclei)

Normal MRI findings in the ageing brain

- Multiple patchy T2 white-matter hyperintensities
- Enlargement of sulci and ventricles
- Triangle-shaped frontal horn 'caps', best seen on T2WI
- Thin, smooth periventricular 'rims', best seen on T2WI
- Iron deposition in globus pallidus or putamen: low signal on T2WI

Trigeminal nerve (fifth cranial nerve)

- Supplies sensation to the face, the corneal reflex and the muscles of mastication
- Arises from ventral aspect of the pons
- Passes into the middle cranial fossa through Meckel's cave
- Forms its ganglion and divides into three branches, the ophthalmic nerve, the maxillary nerve and the mandibular nerve.

Ophthalmic nerve

- Runs in the lateral wall of the cavernous sinus (below the trochlear and oculomotor nerves and above the maxillary nerve) before exiting through the superior orbital fissure into the orbit
- Here it divides into lacrimal, frontal and nasociliary branches

Maxillary nerve

- Runs in the lateral wall of the cavernous sinus (being the most inferior nerve here) before exiting through the foramen rotundum into the pterygopalatine fossa
- Its main branch is the infraorbital nerve, which enters the orbit through the inferior orbital fissure and exits through the infraorbital foramen

Mandibular nerve

- Exits the skull before the cavernous sinus through the foramen ovale to reach the masticator space

Cerebral sulci

- Deep grooves that separate the cerebral lobes
- Pia mater dips into all the sulci
- Only the lateral sulcus has an arachnoid mater lining

Lateral sulcus (Sylvian fissure)

- Separates the frontal and temporal lobes
- Contains branches of the middle cerebral artery

Central sulcus of Rolando

- Runs upwards from the lateral sulcus
- Separates the frontal and parietal lobes
- Separates the precentral motor gyrus from postcentral sensory gyrus

Parieto-occipital sulcus

- Separates the parietal and occipital lobes

Calcarine sulcus

- Separates the temporal and occipital lobes

Germinoma

- 80% occur in the pineal gland
- Commonest pineal tumour)
- 20% occur in the suprasellar region
- Malignant germ-cell tumour
- Causes precocious puberty and Parinaud's syndrome (upward gaze palsy)
- Causes hydrocephalus as a result of aqueductal obstruction

Imaging features

CT
- Infiltrating calcified soft tissue mass
- CSF seeding ('drop' metastases)

Causes of vertebral ossifications

- Paravertebral ossification
  - Diffuse idiopathic skeletal hyperostosis
  - Reiter's syndrome
  - Psoriasis
- Syndesmophytes
  - Ankylosing spondylitis
  - Ochronosis (alkaptonuria)

Bibliography

Books

Adam A, Dixon A, Grainger RG, Allison DJ (eds). Grainger & Allison's Diagnostic Radiology, 5th edn. Edinburgh: Churchill Livingstone, 2009.

Sutton D, Reznek R, Murfit J. Textbook of Radiology and Imaging, 7th edn. Edinburgh: Churchill Livingstone, 2002.

Haaga JR, Lanzieri CF. CT and MR Imaging of the Whole Body, 4th edn. St Louis: Mosby.

Hansell DM, Armstrong P, Lynch DA, Page McAdams H. Imaging of the Diseases of the Chest, 4th edn. Philadelphia: Mosby, 2004.

Webb R, Muller NL, Naidich DP. High Resolution CT of the Lung, 4th edn. Philadelphia: Lippincott Williams & Wilkins, 2008.

Dahnert W. Radiology Review Manual, 6th revised edn. Baltimore: Lippincott Williams & Wilkins, 2007.

Helms CA. Fundamentals of Skeletal Radiology, 3rd edn. London: Elsevier, 2005.

Weissleder R, Wittenberg J, Harisinghani MMGH, Chen JW, Jones SE, Patti JW. Primer of Diagnostic Imaging, 4th edn. Philadelphia: Mosby, 2007.

Rogers LF. Radiology of Skeletal Trauma. New York: Churchill Livingstone, 2001.

Manaster BJ, May DA, Disler DG. Musculoskeletal Imaging: The Requisites, 3rd edn. Philadephia: Mosby, 2006

Blickman G, Parker BR, Barnes PD Paediatric Radiology: The Requisites, 3rd edn. Philadelphia: Mosby, 2009.

Zagoria RJ. Genitourinary Radiology: The Requisites, 3rd edn. Philadelphia: Mosby, 2004 .

Kopans DB. Breast Imaging, 3rd edn. Baltimore: Lippincott Williams & Wilkins Ltd, 2007.

Davies SG (ed.). Chapman & Nakielny: Aids To Radiological Differential Diagnosis, 5th edn. Edinburgh: Saunders, 2009.

Journals

American Journal of Neuroradiology: www.ajnr.org

American Journal of Roentgenology: www.ajronline.org

Radiographics: http://radiographics.rsna.org

Clinical Radiology: www.rcr.ac.uk, www.sciencedirect.com

On-line resources

e-medicine http://emedicine.medscape.com

Wheeless' Textbook of Orthopaedics. www.wheelessonline.com

www.radiologyassistant.nl

Index